A Minyan of Women

This book explores the diverse manner in which family dynamics shaped Jewish identities in ways that were unique and directly connected to their experiences within their families of origin. Highlighted is the diversity of experience of ethnic identity within members of a group of women who are similar in many respects and who belong to an ethnic group that is often invisible. Jewish people, like members of other ethnic groups are often treated as if their identities were homogeneous. However, gender, social class, sexual orientation, factors surrounding immigration status, proximity of family members to the holocaust or pogroms, the number of generations one's family has been in the US and other salient aspects of experience and identities transform and inform the meaning and experience by group members.

The book explores these diversities of experience and goes on to highlight the way in which the intermingling of family dynamics and subsequent Jewish identity in these women is manifested in the practice of psychotherapy.

This book was published as a special issue of *Women and Therapy*.

Beverly A. Greene, PhD, ABPP is a Professor of Psychology at St. John's University and a practicing clinical psychologist in New York City. She is the author of nearly 100 publications, and recipient of nearly 30 national awards including the 2009 American Psychological Association's senior career award for Distinguished Contributions to Psychology in the Public Interest. She is recognized as an exemplary model and mentor in the practice, teaching, and training of mental health professionals who seek to better understand and improve the delivery of psychological services to socially marginalized people.

Dorith Brodbar, MA, MS. Ed, PhD is a counselor at the Borough of Manhattan Community College of the City University of New York and a clinical psychologist in an independent practice at Lindenhurst, N.Y. Dr. Brodbar has worked with deaf individuals and their families in academic and clinical environments including six years with deaf mothers and their hearing children in the Parent-Infant Therapeutic Nursery Program at the Lexington Center for Mental Health Services.

I loved this book, and so will you, if you are a psychotherapist, a woman, a Jew, as I am, or any one of the above. The insights which the contributors share will resonate with you as they did with me, even though each of us brings our unique perspective to our roles. Treat yourself to *A Minyan of Women*. It will be a rare experience.

Dorothy W. Cantor, Psy.D.
Former President, American Psychological Association

A Minyan of Women

Family Dynamics, Jewish Identity and Psychotherapy Practice

Edited by
Beverly A. Greene and Dorith Brodbar

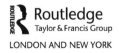

Routledge
Taylor & Francis Group

LONDON AND NEW YORK

First published 2011
by Routledge
2 Park Square, Milton Park, Abingdon, Oxfordshire OX14 4RN

Simultaneously published in the USA and Canada
by Routledge
711 Third Avenue, New York, NY 10017

Routledge is an imprint of the Taylor & Francis Group, an informa business

This book is a reproduction of *Women and Therapy*, vol. 33, issue 3/4. The Publisher requests to those authors who may be citing this book to state, also, the bibliographical details of the special issue on which the book was based.

Typeset in Times New Roman by Taylor & Francis

British Library Cataloguing in Publication Data
A catalogue record for this book is available from the British Library

ISBN13: 978-0-415-60882-4 (h/b)
ISBN13: 978-0-415-61065-0 (p/b)

Disclaimer
The publisher accepts responsibility for any inconsistencies that may have arisen in the course of preparing this volume for print.

For the gift that is my mother and her survival, past and present
For my 'othermothers', Lucy Turk and Florence Brown
For Christopher, Stephanie, Gabrielle and Quentin. . . .
With my hopes for their futures.
—Beverly Greene, New York, July 2010

In memory of my dear and good friend, Bonnie Sirvint Weber,
Taken too soon, you are always here in spirit.
—Dorith Brodbar, New York, July 2010

Contents

CONTENTS

CONTENTS

Notes on Contributors

Judith L. Alpert, PhD, is a professor of applied psychology at New York University and co-director of the Trauma and Violence Transdisciplinary Studies Program at NYU. In addition, she is a clinical professor and supervisor at the NYU Post-doctoral Program in Psychotherapy and Psychoanalysis. Her private practice is in New York City. She has received numerous national awards for scholarship and for service. A prolific author, she has edited four books and over 200 book chapters and articles, mostly in the areas of trauma, psychoanalysis, and women's issues. Dr. Alpert is the founder and past president of the Division of Trauma Psychology of the American Psychological Association.

Julie R. Ancis, PhD, is a professor in the Department of Counselling and Psychological Services at Georgia State University. She has published and presented in the area of multicultural competence, race and gender, university climate, and women's legal experiences. She is the author of several books, including *The Complete Women's Psychotherapy Treatment Planner*, published by Wiley, and *Culturally Responsive Interventions: Innovative Approaches to Working with Diverse Populations*, published by Taylor and Francis. Dr. Ancis's professional activities include serving on the editorial boards of the *Journal of Counseling and Development* and other counselling and psychology journals, as Colegal and legislative representative of the Georgia Psychological Association's Division F, and on the committee for the development of the American Psychological Association's Guidelines for Psychological Practice with Girls and Women. She is currently writing a book on women's legal experiences in the area of divorce and custody disputes.

Andrea J. Bergman, PhD, is a professor of psychology at St. John's University in New York and a clinical psychologist in independent practice. Dr. Bergman's research interests are focused on developmental psychopathology and the application of empirically validated treatments for underserved populations, such as emerging adults who have dropped out of high school and are experiencing multiple problems. Currently, she is involved in the development of a treatment program for emerging adults who have experienced problems such as academic failure, exposure to trauma, and substance abuse. Dr. Bergman is also interested in comorbidity of attention deficit/hyperactivity disorder and substance use disorders in older adolescents and phenomenology and comorbidity in psychopathology.

Dorith Brodbar, MA, MSEd, PhD, is a counsellor at the Borough of Manhattan Community College of the City University of New York and a clinical psychologist in independent practice in Lindenhurst, New York. Dr. Brodbar received her PhD in clinical psychology from the New School for Social Research in New York and her MSEd in school psychology from Long Island University in Brooklyn. Dr. Brodbar is a licensed psychologist and certified school psychologist. Her career has focused on working with deaf individuals and their families in academic and clinical settings. She spent six years working with deaf mothers and their hearing children in the Parent-Infant Therapeutic Nursery Program at Lexington Center for Mental Health Services. She has presented lectures in the areas of deafness, including such issues as diversity within deaf culture, deaf cultural identity and family dynamics, multiple marginalizations of deaf mothers within their hearing families, and the importance of facilitating communication between deaf/hearing and hearing/deaf parent–child dyads. Her work has also included working with individuals who have a broad range of disabilities, and she is currently involved in facilitating a peer mentoring program for and by college students with disabilities.

Laura S. Brown, PhD, ABPP, received her PhD in 1977 from Southern Illinois University at Carbondale. She has lived and practiced in Seattle since 1977 and is known as a leading theoretician and scholar of feminist therapy. A prolific author of groundbreaking scholarship in feminist psychology, she has received numerous national awards for distinguished contributions to psychology practice, education and training. Her passions include reading, aikido, and the pursuit of social justice. In 2006 she founded the Fremont Community Therapy Project, a low-fee feminist therapy training clinic.

Paula J. Caplan, PhD, is a clinical and research psychologist. She received her AB with honours from Radcliffe College of Harvard University and received her MA and PhD in psychology from Duke University. She is currently a research associate and project director of Voices of Diversity at the DuBois Institute at Harvard. She has been a lecturer at Harvard, teaching myths of motherhood, girls' and women's psychological development over the life span, and psychology of sex and gender. She is former full professor of applied psychology and head of the Centre for Women's Studies in Education at the Ontario Institute for Studies in Education, where she also headed the School Psychology and Community Psychology programs, and she is a former lecturer in women's studies and an assistant professor of psychiatry at the University of Toronto. She is the author of 10 books, co-editor of one book, and author of dozens of book chapters and articles in scholarly journals as well as of numerous articles and essays in popular publications. She has given nearly 400 invited addresses and invited workshops and done more than 1,000 media interviews.

Ellen Cole, PhD, is a professor of psychology and director of the Master of Science in Counselling Psychology program (MSCP) at Alaska Pacific University in Anchorage. She is past president of the Alaska Psychological Association and president-elect of the Society for the Psychology of Women, Division 35 of the American Psychological Association. She is certified as a Sex Therapist Diplomate by AASECT and a Fellow of APA. For 12 years Ellen co-edited the *Journal of Women & Therapy* and the Haworth Press book program "Innovations in Feminist Studies." She is the recipient of a variety of professional awards, including a Distinguished Publication Award and two awards for Jewish scholarship from the Association for

Women in Psychology, two Faculty Merit Awards for research from Alaska Pacific University, a Woman of Achievement award from Anchorage's YWCA, and a distinguished service award from the Alaska Psychological Association. Her most recent book, co-edited with Jessica Henderson-Daniel, is *Featuring Females: Feminist Analyses of Media*, published by the American Psychological Association in 2005. New projects include books on feminist retirement and the impact of global climate change on human welfare. Ellen plays tennis and has fast-walked four marathons in the past four years. She and her husband, Doug North, have four grown children and ten grandchildren.

Lillian Comas-Díaz, PhD, Lillian Comas-Díaz is the executive director of the Transcultural Mental Health Institute, a clinical professor at the George Washington University Department of Psychiatry and Behavioural Sciences and a private practitioner in Washington, DC. The former director of the American Psychological Association's Office of Ethnic Minority Affairs, Lillian was a faculty member at the Yale University Department of Psychiatry, where she also directed its Hispanic Clinic. As a clinician, scholar, and activist, Lillian is interested in reconciling liberation psychology, feminism, and multiculturalism. She has been a member of fact-finding delegations investigating human right abuses in Chile, the former Soviet Union, and South Africa. Lillian has written extensively on the interaction between culture, gender, ethnicity, race, social class, and mental health. She is the founding editor in chief of the American Psychological Association Division 45 official journal, *Cultural Diversity and Ethnic Minority Psychology*. Additionally, Lillian is an associate editor of the *American Psychologist* and serves on the editorial boards of several journals.

Sari Dworkin, PhD, is a professor of counsellor education at California State University, Fresno, and licensed as a psychologist and marriage and family therapist. She does pro-bono, part time private practice as a marriage and family therapist at a community counselling centre. Her specialty areas are lesbian, gay, bisexual and transgender client issues, and Jewish-American issues. In addition, she is a past president of Division 44, Society for the Psychological Study of Gay, Lesbian, Bisexual and Transgender Issues of the American Psychological Association (APA), and past chair of APA's Committee on Women in Psychology and the Committee on Lesbian, Gay, Bisexual, and Transgender concerns.

Elena J. Eisman, EdD, ABPP, is a licensed psychologist in Massachusetts. She is the executive director and director of professional affairs for the Massachusetts Psychological Association, is a faculty member at the Massachusetts School of Professional Psychology and has a small private practice in Newton Massachusetts. She has written and spoken widely in the areas of professional practice, assessment, and advocacy. She holds diplomas in clinical psychology and in family psychology from the American Board of Professional Psychology. She is currently serving her eighth term as chair of the Massachusetts Mental Health Coalition and is the current chair of the Policy and Planning Board of the American Psychological Association. She is the recipient of the Karl Heiser Award for State Level Advocacy and of the 2000 State Leadership Award.

Ruth E. Fassinger, PhD, is dean of the College of Education at California State University, Stanislaus, and professor emeritus at the University of Maryland, College

Park. She received her PhD in psychology from the Ohio State University in 1987 and joined the University of Maryland faculty after holding staff psychologist positions at the University of California/Santa Barbara and Arizona State University. Her primary research interests are in the psychology of women and gender, the psychology of work and career development, sexuality and sexual orientation, diversity and advocacy in the mental health arena, and the history of psychology. She is a fellow of the American Psychological Association (APA) in Divisions 17 (Society of Counselling Psychology), 35 (Society for the Psychology of Women), and 44 (Society for the Psychological Study of Lesbian, Gay, Bisexual, and Transgender Issues). She serves on APA's Board of Professional Affairs and the Committee on Professional Practice Standards, serves on the editorial board of *The Counselling Psychologist*, and has held offices in several APA divisions. She has received numerous awards for her scholarship, teaching, and professional contributions, including the Outstanding Achievement Award (APA Committee on Lesbian, Gay, and Bisexual Concerns), Early Career Scientist-Practitioner Award (Division 17), Distinguished Contributions to Education and Training Award (Division 44), and Outstanding Scientific Contributions to Psychology Award (Maryland Psychological Association). She maintains a psychotherapy and consultation practice specializing in issues related to gender, work, and sexuality.

Beth A. Firestein, PhD, is a psychologist in private practice in Loveland, Colorado. She specializes in working with bisexual, lesbian, gay and transgender individuals, couples and families. She is the editor of two books on bisexuality, *Bisexuality: The Psychology and Politics of an Invisible Minority* (Sage, 1996) and *Becoming Visible: Counseling Bisexuals across the Lifespan* (Columbia University Press, 2007). Iris Goldstein Fodor, PhD, is a professor in the Department of Applied Psychology at New York University and a psychotherapist in New York City. Her presentations and writings have focused women's issues and feminist therapy. Her papers have highlighted phobic anxiety disorders in women, women's body image, assertiveness training, and feminist therapy. She was a founding member of the Women's Studies Commission at New York University and taught Women and Mental Health. Iris Fodor is also a photographer whose work has focused on digital storytelling and narrative process in working with indigenous and immigrant children from diverse cultures.

Leah M. Fygetakis, PhD, GCEC, is a licensed psychologist and holds the additional credential of a graduate certificate in executive coaching. In the first two decades of her career, she worked primarily within university counselling services. She practiced at the University of Rochester as the coordinator of internship training and taught courses in psychology and women's studies. Later she directed the Boston University Counseling and Wellness Centre from 1990–2004. Dr. Fygetakis has been recognized by American Psychological Association's Society for the Psychological Study of Lesbian, Gay, Bisexual and Transgender Issues (Division 44) of the American Psychological Association with their Distinguished Contribution to Education and Training Award. She has also received honours from the Association for Women in Psychology for Best Unpublished Manuscript in Lesbian Psychologies for her groundbreaking work in understanding the interplay of the multiple identities of being Greek, female, and lesbian. That work spawned several presentations and a publication (as referenced in her commentary). Since leaving university work, she has been raising her children, serving as a board director for SpeakOUT Boston, and volunteering her time as an executive coach for the Social Innovation Forum. Recently, Dr. Fygetakis began her own business, Directed Success, focusing on executive coaching, women's leadership, and career development.

Judith M. Glassgold, PsyD, is a licensed psychologist and a visiting faculty member at the Graduate School of Professional Psychology at Rutgers University. She served the chair of the APA Task Force on Appropriate Therapeutic Responses to Sexual Orientation (2007–2009), past president of the New Jersey Psychological Association (2008), and president of the Society for the Psychological Study of Lesbian, Gay and Bisexual Issues (Division 44 of APA) (2004). She has written extensively on issues of psychotherapy and sexual orientation.

Beverly Greene, PhD, ABPP, is a professor of psychology at St. John's University and a practicing clinical psychologist in New York City. She is a fellow of seven divisions of the American Psychological Association (9, 12, 29, 35, 42, 44, and 45), of the Academy of Clinical Psychology, of the American Orthopsychiatric Association, and is a member of the Association for Women in Psychology. She has served in many leadership positions in the American Psychological Association (APA) and currently serves on the Division 35 executive board, the association's policy and planning board, and is a representative of Division 44 to the APA Council of Representatives. Dr. Greene holds a Diplomate in clinical psychology from the American Board of Professional Psychology, has served on the editorial boards of numerous scholarly journals, and is the author of nearly 100 publications in the psychological literature. Nine of those publications have received national awards as significant contributions to the psychological literature on women, women of colour, sexual minorities, African American women, and families. She is the founding co-editor of the APA Division 44 book series Psychological Perspectives on Lesbian, Gay & Bisexual Issues. She is also the recipient of numerous national awards that include the 1996 Outstanding Leadership Award from the APA Committee on Lesbian, Gay and Bisexual Concerns, 2000 APA Society for the Psychology of Women Heritage Award, APA Division 35 Psychotherapy with Women Research Award (1995, 1996, 2000), Association of Women in Psychology's (AWP) Distinguished Publication Award (1994, 2000), AWP's Women of Color Psychologies Publication Award (1991, 1995, 2000), 2003 APA Committee on Women in Psychology Distinguished Leadership Award, 2004 Award for Distinguished Senior Career Contributions to Ethnic Minority Research (APA Division 45), 2005 Stanley Sue Award for Distinguished Professional Contributions to Diversity in Clinical Psychology (APA Division 12), 2006 Helms Award for Scholarship and Mentoring (Teachers College, Columbia University Cross Cultural Roundtable), 2006 Florence Halpern Award for Distinguished Professional Contributions to Clinical Psychology (APA Division 12), 2007 Distinguished Scientific Contributions to LGB Psychology Award (APA Division 44), 2007 Distinguished Career Award (AWP), 2008 Carolyn Wood Sherif Award (APA Division 35), and 2009 APA Distinguished Contributions to Psychology in the Public Interest Senior Career Award. She is recognized as an exemplary model and mentor in the practice, teaching, and training of clinical psychologists and other mental health professionals who seek to better understand and improve the delivery of psychological services to socially marginalized people.

Marny Hall, PhD, LCSW, is a psychotherapist and author who lives and works in the San Francisco Bay Area. Her books include *The Lavender Couch, Sexualities, The Lesbian Love Companion*, and with Kimeron Hardin, *Queer Blues*. At her recent combo bris and bar mitvzah, she got her foreskin removed and her Yiddische Kop screwed on tight.

Kornelia Harari, PhD, received her doctorate in clinical psychology from St. John's University in 2006. She is a practicing clinical psychologist working at the Westchester Centre for Cognitive Therapy on the Upper East Side of Manhattan and Scarsdale. In addition to the identities discussed in this chapter, she is also a wife and mother to two wonderful little boys.

Carol R. Heffer, MA, is a licensed mental health counsellor in Independent Practice in South Burlington, Vermont. Ms. Heffer has advanced training in the treatment of dissociative disorders and trauma as well as three years of Gestalt training and advanced training in EMDR. Her practice focuses on high risk clients, many of whom have dissociative disorders. Her career has combined her interests in arts and counselling, which she considers one of the healing arts. She has served as a parole officer in New York City, a counselling supervisor for Planned Parenthood, and a counsellor and construction instructor for Youth Build Burlington. Youth Build is a program for at-risk youth that included education, job skills, leadership development, and counselling. Her skills include work for 14 years as a carpenter, general contractor, and construction educator as well as a graphic designer, artist, and printer. Carol brings all of these skills and experiences with diverse populations to her work with psychotherapy clients.

Clare G. Holzman, PhD, was born in 1942. She and the women's movement discovered each other as she was completing her training as a clinical psychologist in the early 1970s. After graduating she was a therapist at a residential treatment centre for adolescent boys for three years before starting a private practice as a feminist therapist in 1976. She was a member of the Women's Psychotherapy Referral Service and the Feminist Therapy Institute for many years and served on the board of directors of the former and the steering committee of the latter. She has volunteered as a helpline staffer at a community-based women's centre, a counsellor and supervisor at New York Women against Rape, and a counsellor and supervisor at the NYC Victim Services Agency. She has served on the editorial board of *Violence Against Women* and is currently on the editorial board of *Women and Therapy*. She joined the Be Present Inc. network in 1997 and served as the secretary of the board of directors from 2004 through 2009. Clare recently retired from private practice and is still trying to figure out where all that time went. She and her husband of 48 years live in New York City. She has two children and one astonishing grandchild.

Ellyn Kaschak, PhD, is professor emerita of psychology at San Jose State University. She was professor of psychology from 1974 to 2008, where she has also been the chairperson of the graduate program in marriage, family, and child counselling and director of the university's family counselling service. She is one of the founders of the field of feminist psychology, which she has practiced since its inception some 35 years ago and has published numerous articles and chapters on the topic as well as the award-winning *Engendered Lives: A New Psychology of Women's Experience.*

Additionally, Dr. Kaschak conducts research and clinical training, she speaks to related groups, nationally and internationally, and she has served as a consultant on gender and psychological issues to the vice president of Costa Rica. Dr. Kaschak is also the editor of the *Journal of Women and Therapy* and has published eight edited anthologies including *Minding the Body, A New View of Women's Sexual Problems, Intimate Betrayal: Domestic Violence in Lesbian Relationships and Assault on the Soul: Women in the former Yugoslavia*, co-edited with Dr. Sara Sharratt. Dr. Kaschak is the past chair of the Feminist Therapy Institute and a Fellow of Division 35 (the Psychology of Women), Division 12 (Clinical Psychology), Division 44 (Lesbian, Gay, and Bisexual Issues), Division 45 (Ethnic Minority Issues), and Division 52 (International Psychology of the American Psychological Association). She has received the Heritage Award of Division 35, the Distinguished Leader Award of the APA Committee on Women in Psychology, and the Feminist Therapy Institute Award for Outstanding Contribution to Feminist Psychology.

Hannah Lerman, PhD, is a feminist psychologist practicing in Las Vegas, Nevada, after many years of practice, primarily in Los Angeles. She is the author of two books, *A Mote in Freud's Eye: From Psychoanalysis to the Psychology of Women* and *Pigeonholing Women's Misery: A History and Critical Analysis of the Psychodiagnosis of Women in the Twentieth Century*. She also edited *The Handbook of Feminist Therapy*, the first publication of the Feminist Therapy Institute. She has also written about psychological and feminist ethics and twice compiled bibliographies of literature about sexual abuse of clients by professionals and clergy.

Marsha Pravder Mirkin, PhD, is an associate professor of psychology at Lasell College and a resident scholar (on leave) at the Brandeis Women's Studies Research Centre. Her work involves exploring the multiple and interwoven contexts and identities that inform our lives, our clients' lives, and our work together in psychotherapy. She also teaches and provides workshops about progressive psychological interpretations of biblical stories and the meaning they have in our lives today. Her latest books are *The Women who Danced by the Sea: Finding Ourselves in the Stories of our* Biblical Foremothers and an edited work with Karen Suyemoto and Barbara Okun titled *Psychotherapy with Women: Exploring Diverse Contexts and Identities*.

Elaine Pinderhughes, DSW, is professor emerita and former chair of the Clinical Sequence at Boston College Graduate School of Social Work. She received her AB degree summa cum laude from Howard University and her master's degree from Columbia University. Her practice experience has included clinical social work, supervision, and administration in child guidance settings and in mental health centres. She has extensive experience in private practice, has lectured on clinical practice, and has conducted diversity training in social agencies, mental health centres, public and private educational institutions, residency training programs in psychiatry and internal medicine, and in corporations both nationally and internationally. She is past president of the American Orthopsychiatric Association and has received numerous awards that include Massachusetts Psychological Association's Allied Professional Award, Greater Massachusetts Chapter of the National Association of Social Workers' Greatest Contribution to Social Work Education, Jesuit Book Award honourable mention, and the Award for Lifetime Achievement from American Family Therapy Academy. She has served as Lydia Rapoport

Professor at Smith College School of Social Work, Lucille Austin Fellow at Columbia University, and held the Moses Chair at Hunter College School of Social Work. Smith College has requested and is receiving her papers into its Sophia Smith Collection. In 2007 Boston College established the annual Elaine Pinderhughes Diversity Lecture in her honour. The author of numerous journal articles and book chapters, she has written three books published by Free Press: *Understanding Race, Ethnicity and Power: Key to Efficacy in Clinical Practice, The Power to Care: Clinical Practice Effectiveness with Overwhelmed Clients (co-author), and Group Work with Overwhelmed Clients* (co-author).

Sophia Richman, PhD, ABPP, is a psychologist licensed in New York and in New Jersey. She holds a diplomate in psychoanalysis from the American Board of Professional Psychology. In addition to her full time private practice, Dr. Richman is a supervisor at the New York University Postdoctoral Program in Psychotherapy and Psychoanalysis, a training analyst and supervisor at the Contemporary Center for Advanced Psychoanalytic Studies in New Jersey, and a faculty member of the Stephen A. Mitchell Centre for Relational Studies. Dr. Richman is a child survivor of the Holocaust and has written and lectured extensively about its long term psychological impact. She is the author of *A Wolf in the Attic: The Legacy of a Hidden Child of the Holocaust* (Routledge, 2002). The memoir, currently in its third printing, received the 2003 Award for Scholarship from the Jewish Women's Caucus of the Association for Women in Psychology. It is recommended reading by the New Jersey Commission on Holocaust Education.

Barbara Levine Rodriguez, PhD, ABPP (pseudonym), is a licensed psychologist with a diplomate in clinical psychology. She is a professor at a local university and has a private clinical and forensic practice. Her specialization has been in the area of child abuse and trauma.

Janis Sanchez-Hucles, MSEd, PhD, is a professor of psychology at Old Dominion University in Norfolk, Virginia, and a clinical psychologist in part time private practice in Virginia Beach, Virginia. She is a fellow of the American Psychological Association's Society for the Psychology of Women (Division 35) and serves on their executive board. Dr. Sanchez has been involved in developing and teaching courses in the psychology of women, the psychology of African Americans, and diversity issues in psychodynamic therapy. Her research has focused on clinical training, diversity, feminism, and leadership and her research grants have involved training women and minorities for careers in the sciences. She has become a national speaker and trainer in her areas of expertise and most recently has been actively training professionals in the health and mental health applications of cultural competency. Dr. Sanchez is the author of numerous book chapters and journal articles, including "Racism as a Form of Emotional Abuse," "Trauma: Racial and Cultural Factors in Domestic Violence for Families of Color," and "Women and Women of Color in Leadership: Complexity, Identity and Intersectionality." She has also written *The First Session with African* Americans: A Step by Step Guide and is a co-editor of Women and Leadership: Transforming Visions and Diverse Voices.

Barbara E. Sang, PhD, is a licensed clinical psychologist in independent practice in New York City, and has been for over 30 years. A lesbian activist since 1967, Sang has been associated with groundbreaking innovations in lesbian psychology. Dr.

Sang cofounded the Homosexual Community Counseling Centre in 1971 and was a leader in the development of its journal from 1974 to 1978. In 1977 she published a trailblazing scholarly paper on psychotherapy with lesbians. Her work spearheaded affirmative approaches to psychotherapies with lesbians when pathology models were dominant in organized mental health. Among her publications and research she is one of the editors of *Lesbians at Midlife: The Creative Transition*. She has received numerous awards for her work. In addition to her practice she is an artist with a particular focus on nature photography.

Rachel Josefowitz Siegel, MSW, is no longer the wandering Jew of her childhood. Now settled in a retirement community and enjoying old age, she is still a feminist change agent in her family, her Conservative congregation, her town, and her new home. She was the first recipient of the Association for Women in Psychology's Jewish Caucus Award for Distinguished Scholarship in the field of the psychology of Jewish women. She is also co-editor with Ellen Cole of *Celebrating the Lives of Jewish Women: Patterns in a Feminist Sampler*, and *Jewish Mothers Tell Their Stories: Acts of Love & Courage* (with Steinberg-Oren & Cole).

Louise Bordeaux Silverstein, PhD, is a professor of psychology at the Ferkauf Graduate School of Psychology at Yeshiva University, in the Bronx, New York. A fellow of the American Psychological Association, she is a past president of APA's Division of Family Psychology and a former Chair of the APA Committee on Women in Psychology. She is cofounder with Dr. Carl Auerbach of the Yeshiva University Fatherhood Project and co-author of *Qualitative Data: An Introduction to Coding and Analysis* (2003). Dr. Silverstein is the recipient of numerous awards that include the 2000 Association for Women in Psychology Distinguished Publication Award for *Deconstructing the Essential Father*, the 2006 Carolyn Attneave Award for Distinguished Contribution to Enhancing Diversity in Family Psychology from the Division of Family Psychology in the American Psychological Association. Dr. Silverstein is also an associate Eeditor of the American Psychological Association's journal *Men and Masculinity* and is a consulting editor for *Journal of GLBT Family Studies*.

Shanee Stepakoff, PhD, is a clinical psychologist and registered poetry therapist in New York City. A graduate of St. John's University, she began working with survivors of human rights violations in 1986 during a six-month stay at an ecumenical, anti-apartheid centre in South Africa. She was the psychologist for the United Nations war crimes tribunal (Special Court) in Sierra Leone and prior to that spent a year as psychologist/trainer for the Center for Victims of Torture's treatment and training program for Liberians living in the refugee camps of Guinea. She and six colleagues from this program won the American Psychological Association's 2006 International Humanitarian Award. Since February 2009, she provides psychotherapy and supervision in a clinic for Iraqi refugees in the Middle East. She has also provided training and consultation for organizations serving survivors of human rights abuses in Liberia, Zimbabwe, Cambodia, and several other countries. She has completed postdoctoral fellowships in trauma studies, child development, comparative psychoanalysis, and ethnopolitical conflict. An adjunct instructor of expressive therapies at Lesley University, her clinical and research interests focus on verbal truth-telling and the literary, visual, and performing arts as tools for individual and community healing in the aftermath of mass atrocities.

Frances K. Trotman, PhD, is a professor of psychology and psychological counselling at Monmouth University and has been a practicing psychologist in New Jersey for over 30 years. Dr. Trotman is a fellow of the American Psychological Association and has written books, articles, and other publications in the areas of individual and group psychotherapy with African-American women. In 2009, she was awarded the Association of Women in Psychology's Feminist Pioneer in the Psychology of Women's Award for her over 100 publications and presentations on the psychology of women since the 1970s.

Pratyusha Tummala-Narra, PhD, is a clinical psychologist and assistant professor in the Department of Counseling, Developmental and Educational Psychology at Boston College. She is a teaching associate at the Cambridge Health Alliance/Harvard Medical School. Dr. Tummala-Narra received her doctoral degree from Michigan State University and completed her postdoctoral training in the Victims of Violence Program at the Cambridge Hospital in Cambridge, Massachusetts. She founded and directed (1997– 2003) the Asian Mental Health Clinic at the Cambridge Health Alliance and was an assistant professor in psychiatry at Georgetown University School of Medicine. She was also the director of integrative research at the Michigan School of Professional Psychology, and she has been in clinical practice for over 12 years. She is the recipient of the Scholars in Medicine Fellowship from the Harvard Medical School. She has presented nationally and published peer-reviewed journal articles and book chapters on the topics of immigration, ethnic minority issues, trauma, and psychodynamic psychotherapy. Her research concerns the areas of racial and ethnic discrimination and health care disparities among ethnic minority communities. Dr. Tummala-Narra is currently the chair of the Multicultural Concerns Committee for Division 39 (Psychoanalysis) and a member of the Committee on Ethnic Minority Affairs (CEMA) in the American Psychological Association.

Karen Fraser Wyche, MSW, PhD, is a professor in the Department of Psychiatry and Behavioral Sciences and a co-investigator of the Terrorism and Disaster Center (National Child Traumatic Stress Network) at the University of Oklahoma Health Sciences Center. She is licensed as a psychologist and as a social worker in New York and Rhode Island, where she had part-time private practices. She is a fellow of the American Psychological Association in the Society for the Psychology of Women where she was awarded the Sue Rosenberg Zalk Award. She is also a fellow in the Society for Clinical Psychology and the Society for the Psychological Study of Social Issues, where she served from 1999–2002 as one of the nongovernmental association representatives from that division to the United Nations. She is past chair of APA's Committee on Women and Psychology and serves as a member of the Board for the Advancement of Psychology in the Public Interest. Her research and writings focus on understanding the role of gender, sociocultural, and socioeconomic factors in a variety of outcomes including mental and physical health, ethnic identity, and community based interventions. She has extensive experience in working with low income and minority communities in program evaluation, training of service providers, and community focused interventions. She is senior advisor to the HIV Center of Clinical and Behavioral Studies, New York State Psychiatric Institute, and Columbia University. Dr. Wyche has been a faculty member at a variety of public and private universities including Hunter College, Brown University, New York University, and University of Miami.

Sara E. Zarem, PhD, is a psychologist and psychoanalyst in private practice in New York City. A former supervising psychologist at the Lexington Center for Mental Health, she is an assistant adjunct professor of psychology at LaGuardia Community College in New York City and has served as a clinical supervisor in the doctoral clinical psychology program at St. John's University.

Foreword

As the editor of *Women and Therapy* I am proud to present this special issue, "A Minyan of Women: Family Dynamics, Jewish Identities, and Psychotherapy Practice." The stories of these women, their experiences, and the effects of those experiences on the shaping of their identities have certain commonalities and many differences. Many of the contributors practice a psychotherapy formed and informed, to varying degrees, by feminism. The writers have everything and nothing in common at the same time. In any seemingly homogeneous group, closer scrutiny begins to reveal the differences as well as the similarities, begins to highlight the texture and complexity. In the main it is to that project that this collection contributes. We wish to complicate the dominant narrative.

One might well ask why this topic is important. There are many women therapists who are Jews. Isn't this topic, in fact, quite ordinary? To this question, I answer a resounding *no*. It is often precisely when an issue appears to be ordinary or already fully mined that it can fade from view, becoming more ground rather than figure. We feminists know this all too well.

Both benefits and liabilities simultaneously accrue as a consequence of the contemporary American assumption that Jews are ordinary White people. In this country, that idea did not develop until long after the time of the massive wave of Jewish immigration at the turn of the twentieth century. As the children of these Jews began to be born as Americans, they were slowly but surely declared to be officially White. Gradually the signs posted in many parts of the American South that announced "No dogs or Jews" were taken down. Gradually the lynching ceased. A bit more gradually, the government compelled the large American corporations to remove their ubiquitous bans on hiring Jews. Eventually the quotas on acceptance of Jewish students to the major universities in the country were also declared illegal. After World War II, when the American government began to build miles of identical suburban housing for the families of returning soldiers, the officially sanctioned redlining of these instant communities excluded African Americans and other people of color but declared Jews to be White. Many of us who grew up in those suburbs did not know why our neighborhoods were all White and wrongly assumed that it was financial rather than racial (Brodkin, 1998).

Many do not know this shameful American history of former generations. If not kept alive by our memory, it begins to fade. We must not forget because in this erasure we risk losing our own identities and consequently being lost to ourselves, as well as to others. I consider this issue part of that remembering, just as feminism has been for women in general. As we have learned as feminists, the more that is remembered, the more there is to remember and to perceive in the complex texture of the present.

Ashkenazi Jews are now considered by the official decider to be White-skinned. Many other Jews are Sephardic or Mizrachi people of color, but this detail largely escapes notice in the American mind. I would suggest that even white-skinned Jews continue to occupy a certain liminal position between White people and people of color. They belong fully to neither group and retain centuries old marginal status in both. Yet we betray ourselves even as we speak the word "both." Such grouping is another false dichotomy, an oversimplification.

In the generation of the 1960s and 1970s, the American metaphor of a melting pot failed as it required those who melted to emerge from the mix as White. African Americans could not accomplish the trompe l'oeil in which Jews, Italians, and Irish immigrants had successfully participated. Instead, an interest in particulars of American identities began to emerge more fully through a homogeneous recollecting of specific groups and then emerged as standpoint theory and practice. Individuals identified and spoke as group members. This is perhaps the first stage in the development of collective identity and eventually must lead to greater complexity and texture within and between group members.

This issue is an important step in that developmental process, as the compilation, editing, and commentary on these collected stories is done by an accomplished senior African American feminist scholar, Beverly Greene, PhD, ABPP, along with her Jewish coeditor Dorith Brodbar, PhD. This combination produces dialogue and, at best, more complex and nuanced perspectives raising more questions than can be easily answered. It marks an important step in the complex feminist understandings of gender, ethnicity, and race, class and other important cultural influences on individual psychology, which is ultimately the purview of the psychotherapist. It is time on the cultural clock to open these dialogues between and not just within groups and individual group members. This issue takes a giant step in that direction.

Ellyn Kaschak, PhD
Editor, *Women and Therapy*

REFERENCE

Brodkin, K. (1998). *How Jews became white folk: And what that says about race in America*. Piscatoway, NJ: Rutgers University Press.

Introduction

A Minyan of Women: Family Dynamics, Jewish Identity and Psychotherapy Practice

> First of all I'm Jewish,
> The Rest is Commentary
> –Adrienne Smith, 1991[1]

In conservative and orthodox Judaism the quorum needed to recite important prayers is called a Minyan and traditionally consists of 10 men. This issue represents a collection of narratives, essays, and articles aimed at explicating the connections between family dynamics, the development and consolidation of an identity as a Jew, and the effects of Jewish identity on psychotherapy practice in a group of Jewish women who are psychotherapists. The narratives are followed by a series of commentaries by a diverse "minyan" of women who are also psychotherapists. While a traditional minyan is restricted in composition to 10 men, we have expanded that concept to include the multiple voices of the contributors to this volume and to those who discuss their work. Their numbers have illuminated a wider spectrum of ways of experiencing oneself as a Jew than non-Jews and perhaps many Jews might presume exist.

The contributors are psychotherapists with varying years of professional experience, from a range of backgrounds, socioeconomic class origins, sexual orientations, ages, and theoretical orientations. They range from those who come from Orthodox Jewish backgrounds to one author who grew up thinking her family was White, Anglo-Saxon Protestant only to find at the age of 30 that her parents, grandparents, and great-grandparents were Jewish. Each discusses, with the power that narratives beautifully capture, their own personal journey to the present understanding of who they are as Jewish women and what kinds of experiences were most salient in shaping those understandings. They explore their relationships with family members and how those relationships affected their sense of what it meant to be Jewish, whether or not their families accurately fit those definitions (by both the family definition as well as by how other Jews defined them), how they felt about the varying degree to which they "belonged" as Jews or did not, and their own conflicts about their Jewish identities.

1 Sang, B., Warshow, J. & Smith, A.J. (Eds.). (1991). Lesbians at Midlife: The Creative Transition. New York: Spinsters Ink.

While most of the contributors are or have been in independent practice, almost all have experience conducting psychotherapy in a range of settings and geographic locations, with a diverse range of clients. The editors
maintain that our personal identities, regardless of our formal training or
theoretical orientations, contribute greatly to who we are and how we use
ourselves as therapeutic instruments in the consulting room as therapists.
We also maintain that those personal identities of the people who trained
us and supervised our clinical work—not merely the didactic instruction
we receive—also affects the development of our professional therapeutic
"style" in both our attraction and aversion to a range of ways of approaching
and understanding the nature of the work we do as therapists. We believe
that those variables we have mentioned helped to shape the personal identities of the contributors and that their personal identities in turn shape their
desire to become psychotherapists. Those variables also shape the kinds of
therapists they become and the theoretical orientations they are drawn to
or value in their professional work and their relationships with their clients.

All of the narrative contributors are Jewish and live in a predominately
Christian society. Being Jewish can mean that one has a particular cultural
identity that differs from the dominant cultural narrative as well as from
the narratives of members of other socially marginalized or persecuted
groups. However, the narratives of our contributors highlight the reality that
the experience of being Jewish is as diverse as the women who tell their stories. We are provided with powerful examples of the range of differences in
the experience of a cultural identity, even in people who belong to the same
cultural or religious group. Some group members may feel as different from
one another as they do from members of the dominant culture. While they
share a great deal and there is clear overlap in many of their experiences,
their narratives are powerfully distinctive and speak to the uniqueness of
human experience.

A distinguished and diverse group of authors provide us with their commentary on these essays. Each contributor attempts to explicate what the
narrative elicited in them about their own struggles around identity and their
practice, what it tells us (through the non-Jewish lens of many of them) about
what it means to be Jewish, what it tells us about identity and its complexity
more broadly, and what it contributes to our understanding of people as psychotherapists. The eclectic group of commentators was designed to provide
us with a range of prisms through which to view these complex narratives
and to discuss their meaning from those diverse perspectives. We are pleased
to present them all to you in the hopes that they will help us better understand the complexity and intersectional nature of identity, the need to grasp
any individual's subjective sense of identification/disidentification with a
salient social group or groups they belong to and their relative importance,
and how to identify some of the variables that are a part of the development
of identities or lack thereof.

We would like to thank some of the individuals and institutions that made this volume possible. Beverly Greene would like to thank St. John's University for its generous granting of research reductions and research assistants, specifically Juliana Blitzer and Lisa Martin, without whom this undertaking would have been extremely difficult. Both editors would like to thank Dr. Sara Zarem for timely editorial assistance in the review of manuscripts submitted for the volume and Dr. Ellyn Kaschak for her invaluable assistance as midwife to the "birth" of this issue. We've had many important conversations with colleagues and friends that were relevant to shaping the ideas that contributed to the finished product. They are too numerous to mention, and we thank them all for their efforts.

Beverly Greene, PhD, ABPP
Dorith Brodbar, PhD
Guest Editors

Narratives

Sara, Without the "H"

SARA E. ZAREM

I was puzzled about why I was asked to participate on a panel of Jewish women discussing the different ways in which their Jewish identity affected their clinical work. I couldn't imagine that I had anything to contribute. I thought my being Jewish came up in my clinical work only reactively, when a client would bring it up through a comment or a query. I never imagined that my Jewish identity was so central to both my personal and professional life.[1]

In taking up the challenge I wondered, what does it mean to *me* to be a Jew? What do I mean by my Jewish identity? I am a Jew by ethnic and cultural identification, not religious. Although I have a Jewish name, Sara, it is spelled in the non-Jewish way, without an "h." On hearing my name, you wouldn't know this, because Sara spelled with or without the "h" sounds the same. When I speak to religious Jews, I feel very much Other. I cannot connect with their faith, their observance of the many rituals, their immersion in Jewish scripture, or their veneration of the Hebrew language. I sometimes wish I could believe; I can imagine the sense of community, continuity, and transcendence being a religious Jew might bring, but I cannot connect in this way. When I go to synagogue, I remain an outsider, neither comprehending the Hebrew that is being spoken or sung nor feeling a spiritual connection to God. If I feel anything, it is through the music, and the feeling is one of sadness and loss. I remember attending a recent bar mitzvah for a son of a close friend of mine. Listening to the music and incantations I suddenly felt profoundly sad. I realized that I was both yearning and mourning: yearning for a more spiritual connection to my Jewishness and mourning the dual loss of my mother and belongingness in a Jewish community.

So let me begin with my mother. I didn't know my mother well. She died of breast cancer when I was 19 and she was a private, secretive person.

---

[1] I would like to express my deep appreciation and gratitude to Dr. Beverly Greene for her inspiration in creating this project and inviting me to participate.

When I would be curious about her life, of her own growing up and life before her marriage to my father, and would ask her questions about her girlhood, she would stiffen, becoming visibly anxious and pained. I soon learned that these questions were not welcome and I stopped asking. I disconnected from my curiosity. My mother never, unbelievable as this sounds, mentioned her parents—not their names, snippets of memories about them, or made a passing comment about a mannerism, trait, or characteristic that either parent had. Her own background had, in a very real sense, vanished. It was an absence, a void. While I think her own past must have been much alive to her as she often drifted off, absorbed in her own thoughts, as though she were remembering another world. But for me, my grandparents, their lives, and my mother's own feelings about them were a void.

Yiddish was my mother's native language. She was, according to an aunt, born here, but her parents were immigrants from "the old country," somewhere in Russia or Poland. Family rumor had it that my mother's parents were quite orthodox and that when they arrived here, they decided to become Americanized. This was much before the current interest in multiculturalism, when the goal was assimilation. I imagine that when my mother was growing up, to be an immigrant, a poor, non-English speaking Jew, was shameful. By the time I came along, in the 1950s, whatever pains my mother had suffered as a first generation American could not be spoken of, and she was determined that neither my sister nor I would suffer any taint of immigrant (read: different) status. She named me after my grandmother, Sarah, but left off the last "h," which marked the name as Jewish.

I never learned Yiddish. My father didn't speak Yiddish. He grew up in a very nonreligious family where they were Jews in name only. Although he did have a bar mitzvah, he describes his family as very nonreligious, and there is a good deal of Jewish/Christian intermarriage among his siblings. My parents never went to temple and never celebrated the Jewish holidays in any serious way. We might have latkes on Chanukah and light a menorah, but there was no ceremony over lighting the candles, songs sung, or stories told. Rather, Chanukah was an excuse to get eight gifts. On the High Holy Days we visited with my mother's extended family, but nothing religious was ever mentioned or practiced. Rather, it was an excuse for a get-together and pot roast. My parents once sent me to religious school to learn Hebrew, but I felt uncomfortable being the sole emissary from the family to set foot inside a synagogue. Try as I might, I couldn't wrest meaning from the oddly shaped letters and sounds that were Hebrew. My attempts to learn Hebrew didn't last long. With hindsight I imagine that learning Hebrew was associated with unraveling secrets that I wasn't supposed to know, whether they were the secrets of the ancient language or secrets about my mother's family. Knowledge of Hebrew signified the forbidden. Despite the absence of religious ritual in our household, my mother strongly identified culturally and ethnically as Jewish. She joined and was active in Hadassah, a woman's organization that raised money for Israel. She spent hours on the phone doing the 1950s equivalent of telemarketing, and Hadassah meetings provided a social outlet as well as cultural connection for her. My mother never denied her Jewishness; she simply did not advertise or celebrate it. Jewishness was connected with survival and loss (Israel as post-Holocaust refugee), secular study, and learning and a love of the arts. My mother made us aware of the persecution the Jews had suffered over the years, although she never spoke of losing any of her own family in the Holocaust. Wary of non-Jews, she preferred for us to socialize with other Jewish children but did not insist on it since she was adamantly committed to liberal, humanistic values. Her goal for me was clear: a college education. And this, more than anything, is the sense of Jewishness I retain: a reverence for learning and education. Perhaps in my mother's family of origin, particularly if the rumor that they were orthodox was true, education was something reserved for boys, not girls. By the time my mother was of college age she had been orphaned and was living with her eldest sister and brother-in-law. As an outsider in that family, there was no money or support for a college education, and she went to work immediately after high school. My being a college graduate was the female version of the Jewish stereotype "my son, the doctor." I did become a doctor, just not an MD.

I have always thought that there was a split in my mother about her Jewishness, part of her proud and part of her ashamed. This split was/is played out between my sister and me. I, like my mother, continued in the secular version of Jewishness, however my sister has rejected her Jewishness completely. Married to a Catholic man, raising her children as Catholic, she has dissociated herself from her Jewish roots. She did not convert to Catholicism yet she considers herself "not Jewish" and is offended when/if I wish her a Happy Jewish New Year. Her attitude toward being Jewish parallels my mother's discomfort in being from an immigrant family. It feels shameful and low class. My sister will easily tell you that she was raised by a Jewish family, that her birth certificate says she is Jewish, and she will proudly cook Jewish food that my mother made (mondel bread), but she'll say that she is not Jewish. She rejects any Jewish identity. It is a part of her to be buried, not spoken about.

For both my sister and I, Jewishness is connected to our mother. Since I knew so factually little about my about my mother, I cannot relinquish the importance of the Jewishness I perceived in her and feel connected to. To lose this is to lose an inextricable part of her. I was the studious child who would achieve my mother's dream of college and an education. I was symbolically the boy. My sister, who had more academic difficulty and was socially shy and inhibited, was the problematic daughter, the girl who would remind my mother of second class citizenship and outsiderness. My sister, in rejecting her Jewishness, is also rejecting this version of herself. When she thinks about Jewishness she connects it with class: for her being a Jew is to be lower class, which, for her, signifies vulgarity. She associates being Jewish with the working class status of mother's family and extended family, of the small, cramped, bare-bones homes of the family members, of incessant worry about money and having to put practicality before aesthetics, with body language that signaled a lack of refinement that she dismissively labels "ethnic." This version—destructive, demoralizing, shameful, and ugly—must continue to be repudiated.

My Jewishness, which began as a form of ethnic identity, thus becomes part of a larger chain of signification including intense emotional ties to my mother and her lost worlds. It also resonates with issues of gender and class, within which nest themes of loss. Thus the ancient melodies in synagogue make me mourn not only for my own spiritual unrootedness and the loss of my mother but also for the losses of my mother and those of her parents, of generations of unspoken and unmourned loss, a lost sense of community and the world as you knew it, loss of your native language, loss of your parents, a sadness for which there are no words. It has implications for what I can and cannot know—Sara without the "h."

I often find myself wondering what was lost. What were my grandparents like? What was their life like in the "Old Country?" Where exactly did they live? What did they do? Why did they leave? Poverty? Pogroms? Did they have memories of wonderful sights, smells, and joys that had to be left behind? Did they have relatives who they missed? What was the journey to the United States like? What did they imagine their life would be like here? Was coming to the United States worth giving up everything they knew? Were they here illegally? Did they arrive hopeful, only to become disillusioned and bitter? What were my grandparents like as people? What was my mother's early life like? How did my grandparents' Jewishness become experienced here? Was my mother's repudiation of her orthodox roots more than an immigrant child's discomfort with her greenhorn parents? Did she have to disconnect from her religious roots as a way not to miss her parents? Should I see my mother's need for self-creation, the ultimate ideology of being an "American" as a way for her to deny longing and loss. She did name me Sara, without an "h." It sounds the same as Sarah with the "h," but something is missing.

In Jewish religious tradition there are particular rituals that mark and guide the grieving process. When a loved one dies, the family sits shivah; for an entire week the family suspends it usual activities in the outside world and remains at home. They are taken care of by family and friends who visit and provide food and emotional comfort; they grieve with the mourners and help them to talk about their loss. One aspect of the grieving process is the covering of mirrors. By blocking concern for vanity and the outside world it keeps the mourners centered on their inner experience and relationship with their loss. When I was about 16 I remember going into the bathroom and finding the mirror covered with a towel shortly after my mother had her first mastectomy. I was puzzled. Why is that here? But I asked no questions. I told myself that my mother must have placed it there because it was too excruciating to look at herself naked, too horrific to witness her mutilation and the loss of her breast. It was only years later that I learned covering mirrors were a part of the Jewish way to mourn. By reviving this ancient custom perhaps my mother was mourning not only a loss of the woman she was but also mourning again for her lost parents and calling forth, through that ritual, her needed connection with them.

How does all of this affect my work as a therapist? On the broadest level there is a continuing tension in my work, both my choice of profession and how I practice it, between needing to know/see/hear/remember and to avoiding such knowing. As a psychoanalyst, it is my job to help clients remember, yet I have a tendency to avoid asking clients certain incisive questions when their experience is too dangerous for me. While this has ameliorated some over the years, I well remember a supervisor pointing out that I often assumed I knew what a client's experience was without doing a detailed inquiry. Why was that? What comes to mind is my inhibition with my mother, how painful it was to her when I wanted to know about her life and how I felt that my questions were hurtful and intrusive. How could I remove the towel from the mirror? In one way, this reticence contrasts with the Jewish injunction to know and remember and with the personal part of my Jewish identity that values and pursues knowledge. In another way, however, it protects me/mother from facing the pain and rage of unspeakable loss. Not asking questions prevents exploration of trauma and loss and it re-creates the conditions of silence that have contributed to its very creation. It is Sara, without the "h."

My Jewish clients vary in their own understanding of their Jewishness. Some identify with Jewishness religiously, ethnically, and culturally. Others identify as Jews only ethnically and/or culturally. There are shades of identification in all of these ways. Part of my job is to help them understand who they are as people and to explore their multiple identities and identifications. That being said, with some clients, I use my Jewishness to create a sense of alikeness between us. Sometimes it feels like a way to further an alliance, especially if the client has difficulty negotiating the many overt differences between us (age, gender, physical appearance) at the outset of treatment. Other times, my Jewishness enters the treatment as part of my countertransference. In one case, I let a client know I was Jewish as a way to communicate to him how well I understood all of the work that had gone into his orchestrating a complicated Passover seder. Surely I could have mirrored his pride without my self-disclosure. Not having grown up with a father who presided over Passover nor a mother who prepared it, I no doubt unconsciously wished to be part of his seder; what chutzpah to invite myself!

I do not usually announce that I am Jewish; my name is not easily recognizable as Jewish, the spelling of my first name is not the Jewish spelling, and I don't look stereotypically Jewish. I do take off from work on the major Jewish holidays, which I spend with a community of friends. Because of these absences, clients often figure out that I must be Jewish, and if they ask I usually explore with them what it would mean if I were or weren't Jewish. With one client, who is Muslim, exploring the issue led to her complicated feelings about Jewishness and stirred up equally complicated feelings for me regarding her being Muslim. Her mother, she said, disliked Jews. My client herself proclaimed that she wasn't prejudiced and didn't care if I was or wasn't Jewish. However, her mother believed that Jews were greedy and self-centered. Why did she have to tell me this, and what then did it mean to choose a therapist who might be Jewish? Already there was a split for her, mother holding the client's own negative feelings, which paralleled my own dissociated racial devaluation, split off and given to my sister to hold. We looked at the meaning of my client's choice in various ways over the course of our work: as a rebellion against her mother, declaring herself separate, different and "better" than her mother; as a projection of her own feelings and fears of being a selfish and exploitative person; as a wish to both value and devalue me. In the countertransference I felt defensive, and it was a long time before I could ask for a fee increase without feeling like a greedy, exploitative Jew. I wanted to see her as a secular Muslim, a "good" Muslim, splitting Muslims into categories of good and bad depending on the extremity of their religiosity, and I wanted her to see me as a "good" Jew. I do not know if I would have been able to treat this client had her stance been more militant and had our religious differences been more in the forefront of the work. I could identify with my client's stated conscious perception of herself as humanistic and inclusive. I could identify with her respect for learning, in general, and literature in particular.

Over the course of treatment, themes and meanings of Jewishness have changed. There were times when my client actively wished to become Jewish and other times she embraced being Muslim. Sometimes discussions of religion were about religious differences; other times discussions of religious differences were a way to talk about her conflicts between her American versus Egyptian identity. Discussions of our religious differences also served as a vehicle to explore fundamental differences between her parents, conflicting self-representations as well as conflicting desires for merger and separation with me. As with any bit of clinical material, there is both revelation and concealment. Sara, without an "h."

For many years I have worked with deaf and hearing impaired people. Originally drawn to this population by what I thought was chance, I have come increasingly to understand its deep personal meaning for me. A major issue in working with the deaf is communication: what can be said, how it can be said, and who will understand it? Most deaf people have hearing parents. Although there are some deaf who are able to function well orally in the hearing world, the majority have great difficulty in navigating the hearing world via speaking and lip-reading. They prefer to communicate in American Sign Language (ASL), a totally different language from English that is "spoken" through the hands and body. When parents and children do not share a fluency in the same language together, neither parent nor child can know each other's thoughts, feelings, and experiences. You can imagine the sense of loss, disjunction, and continuing trauma felt by all. My attempts to build a bridge of understanding between myself as a hearing person and my client as deaf re-create my own wish to know my mother and the unspeakable nature of her/my/our loss. In my silent signing, I am desperately trying to scream connection. I am trying to heal my client's ruptured object world and to repair my own. I am Sara, without the silent "h."

I have realized, through writing this paper, that the psychoanalytic community has provided a secular Jewish home for me. Psychotherapy, and psychoanalysis in particular, is largely a Jewish endeavor. Despite Freud's proclaimed atheism, his development of psychoanalytic theory and technique is Talmudic in its insistence on radical questioning and multiple interpretation. A central idea for Freud was to help his patients struggle from intrapsychic slavery to freedom. The way to do this, at least in part, was to help patients remember the traumatic incidents that they had repressed yet were playing out and endlessly re-creating in their lives.[2]

Remembrance would bring liberation; one could think about painful experience and not have to continually reenact it. Yet this is also a central tenet of Judaism, marked by the annual Passover seder. The Passover celebration, to which you will recall I symbolically crashed, recounts the Jewish people's traumatic journey from slavery in Egypt to freedom. Jews from all over the world unite at Passover and share a special meal to remember the history of the Jewish people in their flight from slavery to liberation. The symbolic reenactment of this escape, this continual remembering and making concrete, unites Jews in their heritage, reconnects them with the pain and bitterness of slavery as well as with the joys and responsibilities of freedom. One must remember so as not to become enslaved again. Silence is anathema. How much one loses in Sara without the "h."

---

[2]It is ironic that Freud's early followers, with all of their insistence on the importance of remembering, did not directly address the issue of the Holocaust. Many of the post-Freudian early analysts were Jews, who themselves had lost family members to the Nazis and had to flee their homeland. Yet there was a striking absence of discussion about their trauma in their theoretical writing.

A Jewish Woman Who Celebrates Nature

BARBARA E. SANG

It had been a beautiful sunny day. My 91-year-old mother and I sat in the garden at her nursing home feeding the birds and counting the grasshoppers that hung on the window pane. We observed the unusual cloud formations above us—enormous, white, fluffy, and low hanging. Before we left this outdoor space my mother asked me to cut off some of the branches from a bright red bush to bring into her room. She handed me a sharp knife, carefully wrapped in a paper towel, which residents are forbidden to have.

Instead of taking a taxi to the nursing home when I arrive at the Princeton train station I rent a bicycle and then ride along the Delaware and Raritan Canal towpath followed by a back road. On my return trip on this particular day I was just about to enter the bike path when out of nowhere a thunderstorm came up. I quickly ran for cover in the bushes under some trees. The rain came down in torrents and I became drenched. It was as though I had taken a shower with my clothes on. As I hovered over my backpack to shield my favorite camera inside from getting wet, I recalled that today was one of the Jewish High Holy days. Was it Rosh Hashanah or Yom Kippur? I never can remember which is which or what they mean. I chuckled to myself while thinking that if I had been an observant Jew I would have been in the shelter of some synagogue and not out here suffering from the wet and cold. A half hour later, as I rode through the deep puddles on the towpath splattering mud all over myself, I knew that I was practicing the "religion" I grew up with: Nature, with a capital N. Despite the physical hardship I had experienced, it was through this kind of interaction with nature and the out-of-doors that I feel a spiritual connection. A few days after this experience Beverly Greene asked me to contribute to an anthology on Jewish women. It took me by surprise because I don't think that any of my Jewish colleagues would have ever thought of me for such a project. This assignment made me think about in exactly what way I had a Jewish identity if I didn't practice my religion and knew very little about it.

My mother was born into an orthodox Jewish family who came to New York from Odessa, Russia, around 1900. She was given the name Sidney, the same name as a dead brother. I do know that Jews never use the full name of the dead person but only his or her initials. My mother married a Jewish man whose family did not practice the religion and who believed that religion was on the golf course. According to my mother, she never practiced her faith because her mother told her that it was her wifely duty to follow her husband's beliefs. Knowing my mother's stubborn ways, I am sure she would have followed Jewish customs if she had chosen to do so. Instead, she created for herself a nontraditional life for women of her time that included her own spiritual rituals. As a child my mother had been a tomboy who played football with the boys. She had wanted to be an athlete or gym teacher, but these were not acceptable careers for "nice Jewish" girls. For a short time my mother had been an elementary school teacher and a piano teacher, as she had been an accomplished pianist. Thereafter, she became a high diver, swimming instructor, ice skater, and excellent in many other sports. In the mid-1940s my mother was one of the first women to become a professional photographer, and she received recognition for her work. She developed her own black and white film and was adept at using an enlarger and other technical photographic equipment. She was a portrait photographer, sports photographer, and photojournalist, traveling all over the world to take pictures of people from other cultures. One of her ongoing series was how women in different countries held their young. She also taught basic darkroom techniques in the local community. Mother had considered taking flying lessons to become an airplane pilot but fortunately gave this up. She was a dyslexic who had considerable orientation difficulties and was able to drive a car under only very controlled circumstances. Later in life my mother remarked, "I was one of the boys." My mother's three sisters also did not practice the Jewish religion. It is possible that for these women Judaism was experienced as Old World. Two of the sisters aspired to be artists, once again defying Jewish orthodox tradition.

I grew up in a mostly all Jewish neighborhood in Brooklyn. I felt left out on Jewish holidays when everyone got dressed up and went to synagogue but us. I wished to be part of all this, to be part of the Jewish community. I do recall the one time we did go to a synagogue when I was a child. Sitting still was an ordeal for me and I didn't feel comfortable in the solemn atmosphere. I did, however, enjoy the ceramics class held afterward for the children but we never went back. I also didn't like going to the movies because I had to give up being physically active.

As a child there were so many other ways that I was different from my peers that made me feel like I didn't belong: I had to wear homemade clothes that were a different style from the store-bought ones worn by my peers, I was much smaller and thinner than my classmates who didn't want to play with me because I looked like a "baby," and I was forbidden to read comics or have the same toys as the other children because they were not "educational." I was constantly getting into trouble because of my mother's refusal to go along with "rules" she felt were unjustified. I got yelled at for not having the proper (official) camp uniform because my mother did not feel it was necessary to pay extra money for a stripe down the side of my shorts. Similarly, as part of the practice of "good hygiene," each child had to show a clean handkerchief in school everyday. Since my mother thought handkerchiefs were unsanitary, I had none and therefore had to bear the humiliation of failing hygiene. Unknown to me at the time was that I was also dyslexic. I was ridiculed for my reversals, slow reading, and my bad spelling and grammar. I also reversed numbers so I was a poor math student. They considered leaving me back.

Another way our family was not like the other Jewish families was that we were not permitted to eat most "Jewish" foods, such as lox, corned beef, hot dogs, bagels, etc. My mother seems to have transferred the strict observance of the kosher diet of her childhood to the strict observance of what she thought was healthy—no soda, no food with dyes, no smoked food, no spicy food, no ice pops, etc. Other people could eat these things; why couldn't I?

My mother's favorite question, which I must have heard several times a day was, "What do you care if you don't have what everyone else has?" Or, a variation on it, "Why do you have to be like everyone else?" I think that my mother's challenging me to question things as they are later became part to my own life philosophy. It served to enable me to stand up for what I believed, even if it went against accepted norms. In my late 20s I became one of the first female psychologists to challenge the notion that homosexuality was an illness. Those were the days when colleagues feared being seen with me lest others make assumptions about them. To this day I tend to trust my own instincts, and I am not as concerned with conforming to what others think as compared to women of my generation. My early training to think for myself and to be driven by my own internal curiosity has led me to prefer a more eclectic, more fluid model of psychotherapy. I don't feel comfortable being locked into one particular theoretical orientation with its own worldview and its own language. It feels too mechanical to me. It seems to me that I can hear what clients are saying better when I don't listen with preconceived ideas. This is not easy to accomplish because we all have biases. Over the years I have been developing my own theoretical orientation, but I try continually to keep my words and concepts fresh and not get caught up in my own rhetoric.

I associate the quest for knowledge and education with Jewish values. Unlike other Jewish parents whom I know, however, my parents were not concerned about my getting good grades or even if I went to school. My mother strongly believed people learn because *they* want the knowledge; they do it for themselves. Neither parent was supportive of my desire to attend college. My father, who had a limited education partly because of dyslexia and attention deficit/hyperactivity disorder, feared I would turn into an intellectual snob who would have no respect for persons less fortunate than myself. Although my parents' position on formal education was extreme, it had the effect of freeing me from the pressure to perform. It created in me a passion to learn and explore. Since childhood and adolescence I have had many interests (art, science, sports), including a desire to understand the creative process itself. I try to help my clients free themselves from the external and internal constraints that inhibit self-expression. Based on my work with artists over the years I have found that preconceived ideas of what *should* be, comparison of oneself with other artists, and overconcern with what others think are sure ingredients for paralysis.

Although my home life centered around sports, which was certainly not typical of a Jewish family at that time period, reading and art making were also an integral part of our daily life. Since my mother's father had been a teacher and scholar in Russia, the valuing of good scholarship probably filtered down to me indirectly through my mother and aunt. My official initiation into the world of knowledge occurred at age six when my mother took me to the library to get my first library card. Getting new books and returning old books was a weekly ritual that I looked forward to. At this time I was also given my first encyclopedia, *The Book of Knowledge*, which made me feel very grown up. My aunt Sarah (called Sally) also had a significant influence on my intellectual development. She was a painter, poet, and clothes designer. Once a week she would take me to a museum and lecture me on such painters as Rembrandt and Turner, their use of lighting and painting techniques. My aunt made it clear that her favorite artists were those who painted the poor and the working class, such as Daumier, Goya, and Lautrec. It was through my aunt that I first became conscious of class differences and prejudice against the poor and people of color. My aunt also loved books, and she introduced me to such authors as Walt Whitman, Amy Lowell, and Willa Cather. She took me to concerts and introduced me to Rosalyn Tureck, one of the greatest interpreters of Bach. My aunt and I would frequently go on sketching trips around the city, under the Williamsburg Bridge or on the platform of the Third Avenue El. She was an incredible drawer. When I was 13 years old I was permitted finally to work in oil paints just like my aunt, and she got me started.

Aunt Sarah the artist was schizophrenic, as were several other of my mother's siblings and cousins. Sarah had been hospitalized several times before I was born. In my possession are many detailed, intricate portraits that she did of the other inmates during her many hospital stays. Despite her artistic talents, Sarah was never able to function in the everyday world, but she continued to draw, paint, write poetry, and sew in her railroad flat in Williamsburg, Brooklyn. She lived at the poverty level but refused help. Aunt June, the youngest of the four sisters, would send us postcards with neologisms written in circles. I date my interest in psycholinguistics to her idiosyncratic use of words. As a psychology student I wondered why people became schizophrenic; the prevailing belief of poor parenting didn't seem to fit. Recent evidence shows that schizophrenia has a significant genetic component that interacts with such external factors as head trauma and the use of certain drugs. Cognitive dysfunction is related to changes in brain structure and chemistry. The close relationship I had with my aunt Sarah has enabled me to see people with severe mental illness as persons to be respected in their own right. My curiosity about why there was so much mental illness in my family was certainly a factor in attracting me to the field of psychology, both as a helper and a problem solver.

My mother was also an avid reader when she was not taking photographs, playing sports, or doing household chores. We often had heated debates with one another on a variety of subjects, such as politics, religion, food, etc. Many years later she would say, "Remember you said _____ ? I now see what you mean. You were ahead of your time." I don't know if this kind of intellectual sparring with my mother is part of a Jewish tradition of questioning things, of not taking things at face value. This kind of questioning and openness to other possibilities has become part of my own way of thinking and gets translated into the way I work with clients. I help people to see themselves in ways that don't necessarily conform to the expectations of our society, be this in the area of gender roles, sexual orientation, or the way you live your everyday life. Since the intellectual climate in our family was "women centered," I grew up with the notion that women were more competent than men. In my early years I had no direct male influences. It was not until college that I discovered that men may have something to contribute. My experiences seem to have been the reverse of most women my age who saw men as the "experts." My attraction to a feminist orientation was a natural outcome of my background.

A good part of my Jewish identity comes from knowing my family history: My grandfather on my father's side was an atheist who came to this country in 1898 from Russia/Poland. His mother owned a bakery. He had a choice between learning dairy farming or architecture. He chose architecture. It was my grandfather who designed and built the first Jewish theater in New York, which was in Brooklyn. He was also one of the first designers of the split-level home. In my midadolescence my grandfather came to live with us, and he would tell us stories about his homeland at the dinner table. Our family members were pacifists and refused to go to war. In order not to bring disgrace to the family they had to change their names. On riding through the wheat fields to make the name change, Zang, which means wheat, was chosen. On arrival in the United States my grandfather was told that he didn't want his name to be the last letter in the alphabet, so the Z was changed to an S. My grandmother's father was the sheriff of a village outside of Vilna. He was responsible for helping the Jews in the area with their passports so that they could escape to America. According to an aunt who recently died at the age of 102, my grandfather was also a violinist who wrote songs that made fun of the gentiles. They loved it. Why our family was spared the cruel treatment given to other Jews in the area is unclear. As I get older I realize that so many questions I could have asked remain unanswered. I am not even clear why these grandparents migrated to this country.

My mother's parents came to this country from Odessa, Russia, to escape the pogroms and anti-Semitism. Circumstances were so awful that they did not want to talk about it, which is probably why I know so little about their lives in Russia. My grandmother was trained as a tailor to earn a dowry for her two older sisters. Girls also learned a trade in order to support their family if necessary or if they became widows. My mother has always emphasized how important it was for me to be able to take care of myself financially. My grandfather, who had been a teacher and scholar in Russia, was taught by my grandmother to use a sewing machine so that he could work in the United States. Subsequently they bought property in Williamsburg, Brooklyn, and also had a large dry goods store. My grandmother ran the store, waited on the customers, and took charge of the family while my grandfather went to auctions and spent his time sorting the goods that he didn't want to sell. My grandfather was a true patriarch, reading his books all day and then having a tantrum if his tea was not on time or made the correct way. Although my mother was close to her father, she saw the way her mother was oppressed and did not want to repeat the pattern. From what I understand, the occupation of tailor was a common one for Jewish men who were forbidden to enter other trades and professions. I was not aware that women were also trained as tailors. Sewing and clothes designing were another significant part of our home life. My mother called herself a "sewaholic" as she was constantly cutting out patterns or making alterations. Being able to sew freed my mother from having to wear fashions she did not like or clothing that didn't fit. She preferred to wear overalls, which were not in style at the time. Aunt Sarah could design clothes without a pattern and would make us our clothes for the season. I recall the pink wool suit with the taffeta lining that I got one Easter when I was nine. Our family paid her for her services. My mother was disappointed that I didn't follow family tradition and learn to make my own clothes, but I was never good at it. At least I can do most of my own repairs. Sewing was like a social event in our family; we would all sit around for hours having in-depth conversations on a variety of subjects and sew.

At the age of seven my Aunt Sarah sat me down and showed me a large group photograph. She pointed to three women relatives who had been scientists who had been killed by the Russians. She also informed me that many of our relatives held high positions in the Russian government despite their being Jewish. This interchange had a profound effect on me. It was my first introduction to the fact that being Jewish was a stigma and that not everyone accepted us. I always find myself feeling pride when I hear that a Jewish person has been successful in a particular field, especially if it is an area that Jews have been traditionally excluded from.

We moved from our rented brownstone in Brooklyn to an upper middle class suburban neighborhood in Queens when I was in the sixth grade. My grandfather designed and built most of our "California ranch house." It was World War II and the able-bodied men were away fighting. The girls in my new elementary school class had already formed tight bonds with one another and I was once again not included. I played punch ball with the boys and became a skilled tree climber, to the neighbors' dismay. It had been an all-Christian neighborhood when we moved in, and a few years later other Jewish families arrived. I felt out of sync with the Jewish girls my age who were obsessed with makeup, fashion, and boys. Many of these girls had nose jobs in order to look less Jewish, clearly a manifestation of oppression that, unfortunately, continues to this day. I felt alienated by the values and behavior of my peers and started looking outside of my neighborhood for companionship. I would travel to Manhattan to find others who shared my interests in art and politics. I discovered the International Students' League and made friends with people from different countries and different ethnic backgrounds.

For the most part, our family was quite different from other families in its neighborhood. The fact that my mother and I did heavy duty gardening was frowned on. Gardening was "man's work," or you hired a professional gardener. My father was rarely home as he was either working or out with the "boys." My mother, with her athletic muscles and long blond hair, was like a single parent and therefore was threatening to the more traditional women around us. My mother also stood out from her neighbors because she spoke out against injustice. For example, she wrote an article for the local paper questioning why people admired her sun tan yet showed prejudice toward people born with color. I grew up believing that if you didn't like the way things were that speaking out was a good way to make change.

Although my grandfather was not too fond of my boisterous table manners and had to be told that if he didn't like it he could leave, he nevertheless taught me many skills that were useful to artists. I would come to my grandfather to saw off a piece of wood for me, but he would insist that I learn how to use a saw myself. He taught me how to do electrical wiring, how to make fake brownstone, and how to prepare plaster of Paris for my sculptures. Using tools and construction type materials is what boys learned. My grandfather also tried to teach me how to read and make architectural blueprints, but it never interested me, to his disappointment. I guess it was because of my art projects that I became the one to learn my grandfather's trade rather than my brother. These were certainly nontraditional skills for a girl of my time period and made me aware of how gender roles were imposed on us by society. It also made me in just one more way different from other girls my age.

Around the mid-1950s Jews were for the first time being admitted into the fashionable country clubs for a select group of Christians only. Since my father was a serious golfer he joined one of these clubs on Long Island. Neither my mother nor I had any interest in going, but my father insisted that the family come so he could show us off. As a Jew there was a lot of anxiety about fitting in and "looking right" so *they* would accept us. The women were expected to wear the latest elegant fashions, and it was unacceptable to wear the same outfit more than once. I found the values of the country club to be alienating, and I was quite outspoken about the many contradictions I saw. Why did I have to spend money on a dress I didn't want when this money could be spent on more food or art materials?

Growing up I didn't personally experience overt oppression as a Jew. I did, however, live through World War II. Even if I was eight when the war ended I had some awareness that Jews were being killed en masse. The summer before I started college (1954) I attended an art camp in East Brewster, Cape Cod. This was my first actual experience with anti-Semitism. We were told that Jews would not be served and we did not attempt to be served for that reason. My paternal aunt's husband was the first Jew to be admitted into MIT's engineering program. They warned him that he would not be able to get a job in this field after graduation. He did not get a job and instead became a successful junk dealer. I read *The Diary of Anne Frank* in late adolescence, which stirred up deep feelings in me. I identified with Anne Frank because I was also a diary keeper and a person around her age. The pain I feel about what happened to her is so overwhelming that I was unable to visit her place of hiding when I was in Holland as a young adult. I feel the same stabbing pain when I learn about other individuals who are persecuted for being Jewish, but I also feel the same way about persons of all nationalities who suffer from discrimination. In the pacifist tradition in which I was raised I am opposed to any form of violence of one person against another. We live in such a strange world. As a psychotherapist I help individuals lead more satisfactory lives. Doctors work to make individual patients well. Yet we kill masses of people at a time, as though their lives matter little. It makes no sense to me.

My mother seems to have redirected the orthodoxy of her upbringing to the celebration of Nature and the seasons. Observing Nature and rituals connected to the seasons took on a spiritual dimension. One of my earliest childhood memories was buying an assortment of seed packets in school for 2 cents each and then planting the seeds in small pots along the circumference of our Brooklyn brownstone porch. What a joy it was to see these seeds sprout and later bloom. Each season had its own special rituals: spring was a time I got real chicks, baby ducks, and, on one occasion, rabbits. On Passover we did have matzo as well as bread in the house (along with ham). In summer we collected shells and starfish on the beach, which were dried on shelves in an antechamber outside of the kitchen. In fall we did projects with leaves, acorns, pumpkins, and assorted fruits that fell off the trees. As a young child in Brooklyn I was mesmerized by a succah I could see from our back windows; it consisted of a straw hut with vegetables and fruits hanging from the ceiling and walls. People supposedly ate their meals in the hut, like a Jewish Thanksgiving. Succoth was the only Jewish holiday that made sense to me, as it fit in with our own family rituals of the fall season. Winter celebration centered around making pine cushions and observing the structure of snowflakes. In all seasons I was encouraged to keep a leaf and wildflower scrapbook. I would identify and label my specimens from books we had in the house. Unlike my mother's oldest sister's family, we were forbidden to have a Christmas tree. My mother made it clear that Jews did not celebrate Christmas. We did have the traditional Chanukah menorah and got a small gift each night. Strangely enough, we were also allowed to have Christmas stockings, which were hung on the fireplace and filled for Christmas day.

In my earlier days I had been a serious painter, but due to space constraints I turned to photography, something I never imagined I would do. I began as an underwater photographer and gradually found myself photographing nature and organizing my work around the seasons. I had an exhibit of my photographs, which was titled "Studies in Continuity and Change." My work has a strong spiritual component—it is the dealing with the mystery of life and death. I am especially drawn to places with water and try to capture their essence, such as Fire Island, Cape Cod, Sandy Hook, and the Delaware and Raritan Canal. Since my mother has been in a nursing home for the past five years I have started to keep a journal of the wildflowers, birds, and animals I have seen in these places.

I illustrate my finds with photographs, drawings, and pressed flowers, thus re-creating the Nature scrapbook ritual of my childhood. It is a meaningful way for me to deal with my mother's imminent death and probably my own. It is a way of marking the passage of time. I also continue to celebrate the seasons in my own apartment just as we did when I was growing up. I usually have two "appreciation" corners where I display seasonal objects such as plants, flowers, leaves, pumpkins, wood carvings of birds, etc. These changing scenes keep me in touch with the rhythms of life.

When my mother was in her late 30s and early 40s she worked as a librarian in the local Jewish center and served as a lifeguard in their pool. She went through what I call her "Jewish period," reading endless books on Jewish history, Jewish novelists such as Israel Zangwill, Isaac Bahevis Singer and Sholom Aleichem, and Jewish philosophers such as Martin Buber. She never became interested in practicing the religion. My mother would tell me about what she was reading and would try to encourage me to read the same books, but by that time I was already in college and had other interests. When I was in my late 30s and early 40s I discovered Eastern philosophy. It felt very familiar to me; it articulated what I already discovered as an artist and someone connected to Nature. The belief that humans are both good *and* bad, compassionate *and* cruel, that things are neither all black nor all white presents a challenge to the polarized thinking of Western thought. In 1975 I presented a paper at the American Psychological Association's first panel on homosexuality. It dealt with a theory of interpersonal oppression developed by a former classmate of mine, Lila Lowenherz, and myself. Essentially it outlined how polarized thinking or "judgmental dichotomies" are a source of oppression in our relationships to self and others. Many other of the concepts expressed in Eastern philosophy are also useful to me as a psychotherapist, such as "letting go"—being at one with what you are doing, and "no mind"—not having preconceived ideas but being open to other possibilities. I have written a paper for artists on Zen, creativity, and psychotherapy.

Looking back on my life I realize that I have spent most of it in the company of Jews. I went to Bard College, which attracted mainly Jewish students from the New York City area, and for graduate school I attended Yeshiva University, which also had a predominantly Jewish student body. Since I have little basis for comparison I am not sure exactly what about my experience was "Jewish." What both of these schools had in common was that they were "process" oriented; that is, they were concerned with the underlying mechanisms of how things worked. More traditional schools in psychology were, in our view, more reductionistic in their attempt to be "scientific." Both schools did not conform to the thinking of the times as they took into account "social context." If Jews share a certain way of thinking it is probably so much a part of me that I take it for granted. I have noted, however, that Jews tend to be socially conscious and are concerned with social justice and the welfare of others in the "community," not just Jewish persons. Jews have been active in labor unions and charitable organizations. This, the giving back to others, the caring about others, is a part of Jewish values. I would say that this description fits my own value system.

When I am with secular Jews I assume that they are more "Jewish" than I because they at least know the history of the Jewish people and the significance of the holidays. I am currently working with a client who is a Polish Christian engaged to a Jewish man. She has chosen to convert to Judaism and is attending special classes. We laugh about her knowing more about Judaism than I do. This client is, however, in considerable conflict because she does not want to totally negate her own heritage. Why should she have to give up attending a church mass because she loves the music or have to give up having a Christmas tree, which holds many special childhood memories? I try to help her find some kind of balance that fits her own needs. During the Christmas holidays she reported first becoming aware of what it feels like to be a "minority." There is evidence of the Christian religion all around to the exclusion of other religious groups. At work she spoke up and insisted they have both Christmas and Chanukah cookies.

Because my last name is Sang I have tended to attract a large number of Asian clients over the years who assumed that I was Chinese or hoped I was. If a client clearly wants to work with an Asian therapist I refer them to a Chinese colleague and former classmate. I feel I work well with Asian clients because of some kind of intangible overlaps between my background and philosophy and Asian culture. Nevertheless, I am always cautious about imposing my own values and experiences on another person. I try to see each person as a unique individual in the context of their culture. It always surprises me when Jewish clients contact me as they have no way of knowing I am Jewish. These clients don't seem to have a preference about the ethnicity of their therapist but are often pleased when they find out I am Jewish, that we share this in common. A similar dynamic occurs for me with gay and lesbian clients. Given what I have said about myself in this paper one might not expect me to prefer working with a Jewish therapist but I must confess that I would definitely want a Jewish therapist. Whether true or not, I feel a Jewish person would understand better how different my family was from other Jewish families and would therefore have a better understanding of who I was. I am assuming that this person would also be a feminist.

I am most conscious of being Jewish when I am in the company of non-Jews. At my first cousin's funeral in Lowell, Massachusetts, I realized that my aunt, my father, and I were the only full-blooded Jews in the funeral parlor. My aunt had decided on an open casket to accommodate the large numbers of Christians who would be coming to pay their respects to my cousin who had been a well known golfer in the state. I do know that Jews do not believe in open caskets. At the funeral I got to know my cousin's son, his wife, and their two sons, who subsequently became important "family" to me. The two younger cousins are only one quarter Jewish and have had almost no exposure to Jews. When I attend my younger cousin's piano recitals in New Hampshire and look around me I know that I am probably the only Jewish person in the room. This is a new experience for me. Last year I received a Chanukah card from the 12-year-old cousin with a knish on it and she wanted to know what it was. I had some vague idea; most likely it was on my mother's forbidden food list. I have other family members who have married people from other religious backgrounds or ethnic groups. My first cousin's son is married to a Japanese woman. My cousin tells me that such intermarriages are quite common in that area of California.

Prejudice occurs not only between different ethnic groups, religions, countries, etc., but within families. I am not "mainstream" enough to be exposed to my younger sister's children. Is this because I am a feminist, a lesbian, or allow people of color in my home? I have had to make "family" outside my immediate family. What and who is family? This is a reoccurring issue for myself and many of my clients. Over the years I have worked with people whose parents are of a different religion, ethnic background, class, etc. There are many variations on their conflicts that center around "belonging" and fitting in. If one parent is Jewish and the other Christian (Black/White, religious/nonreligious) their children may find themselves not accepted by either religious community. A client of mine who is Black was sent to an all White private elementary school and college to ensure she got a good education. She is too "White" for her Black friends yet constantly faces prejudice from her White peers. She struggles to find a place where she can be accepted for who she is. Another client whose father is a minister in the Midwest has been rejected because she is living with her boyfriend and not upholding "Christian values." Based on my experience with my own siblings I understand how it feels to be devalued and rejected because you don't conform to someone else's belief system. Feeling like an "outsider" can contribute to all kinds of emotional distress. Clearly we all need to learn ways to counter this kind of oppression and feel good about ourselves. But, in order to accomplish this I feel we need to make changes on a very basic level: we need to change the way we use language ("labels") to deal with differences. It is easy to get into positions which invalidate someone else's reality and see our way as the "right" way or only way. Paradoxically, sometimes the more similar we are, the more small differences between us become magnified and alienate us from one another. I see psychotherapy as part of this process of change; we have learned to be adept at putting ourselves down as well as others. Making changes in our use of language won't happen quickly or easily but is worth the effort.

In keeping with my insatiable curiosity and tendency to be pulled in many directions, the last five years have been a time of revisiting old interests in a new way. First, I wrote a paper on the lesbian relationships of the well known French animal painter Rosa Bonheur (1822–1899). I challenged the popular belief that Rosa saw herself as a "man" and that she had a traditional heterosexual relationship with her lifetime partner Nathalie Micas. Rosa, Nathalie, and Mrs. Micas created an all women's world for themselves in which each contributed what they did best. Both Nathalie and her mother were successful businesswomen. The interaction of these women raises questions about what is "success" and "power" for women. Rosa, who was most likely dyslexic, had considerable insight into the creative process. She saw Nature as a spiritual practice. Rosa was very concerned about the future of the environment and our destruction of one another by war and violence. I recently discovered accidentally the memoirs of Emilie Carles, another French pacifist (1900–1979) who grew up a peasant in the French Alps. Against all odds she became a schoolteacher who dedicated her life to educating the poor and talking out against war and destruction of the natural environment. Like Rosa Bonheur, Carles found spirituality in Nature.

In summary, it is difficult for me to tease apart just how my minority status as a Jewish person influences my feminist orientation from the many other ways I am a minority—I am dyslexic, lesbian, and have a nonconventional upbringing. I have attempted to show how my different experiences have contributed to my ideas in such areas as gender roles, power dynamics, and oppression. Being Jewish is only one part of the whole. Writing this paper has inspired me to make a more deliberate effort to explore my Jewish roots. With this goal in mind I recently bought a book, *The Jewish World, Revelation, Prophecy, and History*. Will I have time to read it?

Being Jewish and Being a Psychotherapist

HANNAH LERMAN

The worst version of a stereotype that anyone can believe is that all of the individuals inside of a group are the same, whether the stereotype is negative or positive. No group of people is monolithic along any dimension of traits you could name, whatever people outside that particular group think. People within one group are as diverse as people within any other group. In my experience, whatever the group, there are cliques, interest groups, groups with common backgrounds, and/or warring factions that demonstrate that its members differ in significant ways from one another and whose ideologies battle for ascendancy. The Jewish people are not an exception. They, like other peoples, hold their own stereotypes about themselves as well. Over the millennia, there are many different ways in which Jews have sorted themselves into groups.

The most obvious way is according to their type of Jewish religious observance. Along these dimensions, the groups are the Orthodox, Conservative, and Reform Jews (also, in Israel now, the Reconstructionists about which I know nothing). Orthodoxy is, of course, the most extreme form of observance. Its adherents wear traditional clothing and maintain habits of observance that go back thousands of years. Men wear beards and side curls and married women cover their heads whenever they are outside the home. These people adhere to the most traditional forms for choosing and serving food according to religious principles and observing holy days. The Conservatives are less conspicuous in clothing, habits, and manners in our modern society. Men and women still sit separately during religious services, and women can perform religious rituals only in the home, most notably lighting the candles on Friday night to usher in the Sabbath. The Reform Jews have modernized most of the observances to more contemporary forms and have even ordained women as Rabbis. One probably should also include atheists and agnostics as groupings, for, among Jews, it was not necessary to be religious or practicing to be accepted as Jewish; one only had to come from a Jewish family background (technically, according to Halachic law, to be born of a Jewish mother). That this happens seems to be different from most other groupings that are based on religious orientation. There are and have been varying degrees of tolerance and intolerance among and between these various groupings over time.

When I was growing up, I also heard about classification of Jews according to the regions of Europe from which they came. Most Jews in the United States were from or were descendants of people who came from Europe. My own knowledge of these was very vague and incomplete. I have later learned much more about the significance of being members of these particular groups holds. I heard originally about the Litvaks and the Galicianas. The Galicianas were peasants from Eastern Europe, the Litvaks were more cultured and educated. Technically, the former term refers to those who lived under Lithuanian rule in the sixteenth and seventeenth centuries and not citizens of Lithuania as one might expect. Lithuania in those years was a center of Jewish political and cultural influence. In the present, the distinction between the two terms includes class differences, with the Galicianas being looked down on.

Later I learned about Jews from yet other portions of Europe (and eventually about African and Asian Jews as well). Those Jews who migrated to Germany, especially the Rhine Valley, became known as Ashkenazi, while those who settled In the Spanish peninsula were called Sephardic. These last were the most systematically hunted during the years of the Inquisition. To avoid being exterminated, many families overtly became Catholics and practiced their Judaism only secretly in their homes. The baptized Jews became known as Marranos (which is Spanish for swine) and, among other places, have descendants today in the Spanish southwestern states of the United States. I heard a moving story once about a young woman who approached a woman rabbi in one of these states and told her that she must be Jewish because of rites that she saw her mother perform at home. She had been raised as a practicing Catholic.

When I look back on my childhood and my family, I have come to identify yet another way of separating Jews into groups. I saw two types within my own family. My mother and her family were Conservatives whose main practice of religion was to attend synagogue on holy days and for the women to maintain kosher (religiously clean) kitchens. They were not very concerned with ethnic background, although most of them came from either Poland or Russia. They were, however, quite clannish about being Jewish and wanted only Jews to marry into the family (to some extent, this has changed somewhat within my family since my childhood). In my teens, long before I even thought about marriage, I argued with my mother, who wanted me to marry "my own kind," meaning someone who was Jewish. I would say that I would marry "my own kind," meaning someone whose beliefs and feelings accorded with mine but not necessarily someone who was Jewish. The argument went on endlessly for many years.

My father, on the other hand, personified the political intellectual who was usually atheist in religious belief and socialist in worldview. Although culturally Jewish, his worldview was above religion and he strove to accept people as they were, although his deeds did not always fully accord with his words. He had grown up in an Orthodox Russian Jewish family but had repudiated this way of life by the time he reached the United States. His sister, who had retained her Jewish upbringing, was more similar to my mother's family, but her children were more in tune with my father. He had been an itinerant labor organizer for the radical union, the International Workers of the World (IWW or Wooblies) before marrying and settling in New York City. During his organizing days he had met many different kinds of people and, thus, had a broader view of the world and intellectual ideas.

Although both types of Jews within my family respected and promoted education, I came to identify with my father and, indeed, met more and more Jews like him as I progressed through my own education. They were the free thinkers. They were Marxists. They argued intellectual issues, often (at least in New York City) at the tops of their voices. They thought about people as members of the human race rather than identifying with Jews only. I remember arguments with my father about the relative importance of heredity versus environment in the development of human beings. My father was adamantly on the side of environment, believing that how children were raised was the major determinant in the development of their personality. Although I mostly believed similarly, I was less definite in my beliefs and argued with him as I learned more about the theories of psychology, some of which supported his view and some of which did not. My running argument with my mother was highly emotional while, at least overtly, my main argument with my father was intellectual.

I was never a practicing Jew in a religious sense, but Jewish culture was all around me. I lived in a mostly Jewish neighborhood, ate Jewish food, and socialized with other Jews for the most part. In later times, I have been almost apologetic about what I do not know about Jewish religion and culture. Although I was not at all familiar with Jewish religious law, I did learn somehow that Jews had a special ethical sense of fairness and that this was a part of our culture. As I learned more, I learned that the Jewish religion taught that all humans were children of God and not just the Jews. I really do not know just how I inhaled this atmosphere, but I did. This positive view of Jews, as much of a stereotype as any negative view, remains with me to this day. I still feel personally hurt whenever I see a Jewish person act in any way that I judge not to be upholding this ethic. In personal matters, since Jews and Jewishness is not particularly a part of my everyday life and Jews are not easily visually recognizable apart from those who visually espouse orthodoxy in their clothing, it has mostly been religious Jews whom I have identified as acting against my stereotype. On a larger scale, my stereotype includes a view of the state of Israel that makes me want to cry inside when I hear about how Palestinians are treated by Israelis. I want to shout "Jews don't act this way."

My personal interest in ethical practice and even in the formation of psychology's ethical code comes to me, I think, as a legacy of this background. I remember being very impressed by the idea from Jewish mythology that the morality of the world can be maintained only by the presence of a particular number of righteous moral and ethical men (*sic*) who are alive at any given moment. It was thus a part of both religious heritage as well as my socialist background that brought me to the idea that my purpose (anyone's purpose) in life was to leave the world as at least a little better place than it was before.

Despite being nonreligious, I have experienced the isolation of Jews from the mainstream. One vivid recollection of my childhood are the feelings of being left out during the Christmas season. Everywhere except in my family I saw the decorations, preparations, and gaiety and heard the allusions to Christian teachings. I knew, however, that it wasn't for me. Never mind the Hanukkah programs that the school put on (I lived in a predominantly Jewish neighborhood after all), that was not enough to invite inclusion because the radio, newspapers, and department stores all emphasized Christmas spirit, whatever that was, and Jesus Christ. One advantage to marginality, I have discovered, is the ability to observe. For both personal as well as cultural reasons, I was an observer rather than a participant in much of culture for many years. I think that this has contributed mightily to my ability to work as a psychotherapist. One negative effect of my separation on my professional work was, however, that, for years, I had great difficulty responding in any way whatever when clients spoke in any way whatever about their Christian faith in psychotherapy sessions. I was not a Christian and had no emotional core from which to respond to these comments. I never initiated the discussion of religious faith and have only come after many years to be able to respond neutrally if not empathetically when the topic comes up. Jews customarily do not talk much about faith and instead focus on religious practices for the most part.

I came of age during the beatnik era (for those younger than me, I do not mean the era of the Beats—that came later). I frequented the Greenwich Village scene in New York where it was happening, but I remained, as always until later, an observer, not a participant. My peripheral stance lasted through the Civil Rights era and the Vietnam War protests. I recall my father writing me when I was in graduate school and chiding me for not marching against the Vietnam war. Although I was a sympathizer, I did not act politically until the Feminist movement arrived. I think that I was (passively) looking for something but hadn't found it until then. To me, my introduction to the Feminist movement felt like the new ideas reached down into my guts, grabbed onto my then vaguely socialist principles, pulled them out of me, and reintegrated me into a whole with my background and my present intertwined. Years later, in a Jungian workshop, I wrote a dialogue with my inner wisdom figure, who was my father (he had died by then). In it, I reminded him of his disappointment with me for my nonparticipation and seemingly bourgeois ideas and I tried to show him then that I was living his ideas, although in my own way. I said that I had things to teach him now and offered him books to read.

Psychoanalysis at the time I entered the field of psychology was the major clinical theory of personality development and influenced how many did therapy even if they were not psychoanalytically trained. Not only had Sigmund Freud been Jewish but so were most of his early disciples. Freud, a nonreligious Jew, was, moreover, culturally Jewish in many ways. As I maintained in my book *A Mote in Freud's Eye*, the idea of the Oedipus complex is closely related to Jewish cultural beliefs. One prominent idea, held implicitly if not overtly in many families, is that any male child could grow up to be the long awaited Messiah and is viewed in that light, as Freud was, by his mother. Boys' relationships to their mothers are therefore special in the Jewish culture. The boy grows up, however, and disappoints the holders of this hope so he is never as important to his wife as he was to his mother. I see these ideas as encompassing the germ of Freud's concept of the Oedipus complex, although he ostensibly used Greek mythology as its base. Also, Judaism was a minority and definitely prosecuted faith during the time of Freud's Vienna. I think that this made it easier for Freud to isolate himself and his theory from the mainstream and to harden his views in the face of potential and actual attack. Other people have pointed out many other aspects of psychoanalytical theory that relate closely to Freud's Jewish background, but these have always been the most salient for me. I also found very strong antiwoman bias in psychoanalysis, as it also exists in traditional Jewish thinking and practice.

Despite my critique of Freud's theories, particularly as they relate to women, I do believe that people act with unconscious motives at times. I adamantly do not believe in the content that Freud put into his version of the Unconscious, namely the id, ego, and superego, nor do I believe that the stages of physical development accord with the oral, anal, phallic, and genital phases of psychosexual development. Although I think that the adults mainly have their psychological origin in childhood, I also think that people can continue to develop psychologically into adult life. Freud discarded trauma as a cause of developmental problems; I think he was flat wrong in this. There are many theories of why he shifted his views. I indicated my own view in my book: it involved personal feelings that he had trouble facing.

In my years of practice, it has become apparent to me that there are many kinds of traumatic stress that most individuals experience in many different phases of their lives, and I believe that these experiences are all, alas, very influential in human personality development. I have come to think that post-traumatic stress disorder (PTSD) is the most significant, diagnostic category in the *Diagnostic and Statistical Manual of Mental Disorders*, apart from the purely organic syndromes and perhaps inherited psychosis. I think that traumatic stress of one kind or another can be found behind almost all psychological problems of living. Because I was not personally a Holocaust survivor nor was I related closely to anyone who was, I do not think that my ideas about trauma come directly from the experiences of Jews, although it may have been influenced by this. I have learned how pervasive traumatic experiences, often unacknowledged by others, are in the individual lives of most women, but I do not leave out the cultural, racial, ethnic, and other socially accepted traumas that are also so prevalent for so many people.

Because my overt orientation is nonreligious, it is only after the passage of much time that I have come to recognize how being Jewish is even a part of my being. At an earlier stage, I would have said that the fact that I was born Jewish had little if any significance either in my life or in my professional practice. Some wisdom anyway seems to come with age.

The Jewish Nonsheep as Lesbian Feminist Therapist

LAURA S. BROWN

Two Jews, three schuls.

—various Jews

Don't be a sheep and follow the flock.
        —Sandy Brown (aka "Dad"), personal communication,
                                all of my childhood

If I'm not for myself, who am I for.

—Rav Hillel

This chapter has wandered, like a good Jew, for what feels like 40 years in the desert. Sitting in a hotel room 12 stories above the city of Beer Sheva, Israel, looking out at that desert, I seem to finally be able to bring it to its fruition. When I began to write this four years ago, I began by saying that if brevity were truly the soul of wit, then my contribution to this volume would be summarized in the three short sayings with which I began. How I am a Jew—deeply, completely, argumentatively, contrarily—can be discerned in and between those quotations. I am a Jew as my family are Jews and not as some of my family are Jews, because in my family flocks are not followed, including flocks headed by parents. But because of how my family lives out being Jewish, I am a Jew to the bone, to the marrow, to the mitochondria of my cells. Deeply, in other words. How I am a Jew distinctly influences how I am a therapist, a feminist, a lesbian, just about everything—the outsider, the critical thinker, the loyal, connected person, the expert in interpersonal violence, all of these are about my Jewish family. My Jewishness permeates my work and my theory and informs ways of relating to knowledge, which in turn have shaped my professional directions.

Each time I draw a genogram I tell a new truth about my family of origin. I am an eldest daughter of two eldest children of four eldest children. Violence, physical and emotional, marked my family. My mother's father drank, beat her mother, and beat her. My father was an angry man who emotionally terrorized his three children while never laying a hand on me, although one of my brothers was not so lucky. Everyone pretended that these violent men were not violent. In fact, each spoke the cliché about how wonderful Jewish husbands were because they would never beat their wives. So I also grew up in a family full of secrets. I know about confidentiality because ours was ironclad (for all of the wrong reasons, of course, but there it was).

Cutoffs are a hallmark of my father's family of origin. His parents stopped speaking to him for his last two years in college while he, still living at home like the good Jewish son that he was, was engaged to my mother, of whose parents his parents disapproved. Fourteen years later my father cut off his parents when he perceived a slight to my mother. Luckily they were speaking again when his father died of a sudden heart attack.

Three years later it was my turn, cut off when my father became aware of my attempts to behave heterosexually in a responsible manner via the presence of a pack of birth control pills in the dresser drawers that he searched. I was invited out of the family and later accused of being the cause of my younger brothers' own adolescent acting out. The cutoff extended when I came out as a lesbian two years later—talk about the irony. He has done his best to continue to avoid communication, walking out of the room when my partner walks into it, although as my mother ages he once again seeks to have a daughter. So we know how to have boundaries in my family, high, hard, impermeable ones. I am attracted to ambiguity after growing up in the presence of rigidity, which makes for some skill as a psychotherapist.

Yiddishkeit, that indefinable quality of Jewishness, is central to my family. We were raised joyously celebrating the Jewish holidays, no Chanukah bushes in our household, but long, loud seders presided over by my Zeide (the one who did the cutoffs). I attended afternoon Hebrew classes from elementary through high school. My parents met in a college Zionist youth group; in 1982 they made aliyah and have lived in Israel ever since. Jewish books and art were in our home; Jewish thought colored our understandings of the world. In a neighborhood where we were the first Jewish family and few other Jews ever lived, Jewishness was my foreground identity among my peers. As a Jew, I was deeply *other*. Since I was supposed to not be a sheep and follow the flock, this otherness made it near impossible to join the flocks around me. Thus, I escaped, through exclusion, full indoctrination into the norms of American femininity, which allowed me the experience the truths of feminism more easily when I encountered them.

With such an interesting family (and I say this with no irony intended), and one that was so emphatically Jewish, one might think that I would find any excuse to flee my culture of origin as a strategy for distancing myself from the whole *mishugass*. But here I am, still and always very much Jewish.

While I struggled for a few years after my initial feminist awakening with the whole problem of Judaism as a patriarchal religion, I quickly came to the conclusion that there were no patriarchy-free meaning-making systems and that I was at least familiar with, and in a position to be a feminist critic of, this one.

Doing a cutoff from Judaism is something I didn't want to do because cutting off, while a family tradition, is one that I have set myself against. My powerful intention to stray from this family norm of disconnection is, as it turns out, the enactment of another family norm, which is to never go along with norms. In a flock that cuts off I refuse to disconnect—and so I am a Jew, still. Browns are loyal critters, and my loyalty to my culture has been powerful. While it is not an uncritical loyalty, it is there nonetheless; because I am loyal, I feel I can also be honest in my critiques, knowing that they stem from love and the desire for my family and my culture to be whole and healed rather than from a desire to destroy. As we say at Passover, only the wicked child says "this has nothing to do with me." This has everything to do with me, "this" meaning my family, and *K'lal Yisrael*, the community of the Jewish people.

A proud contrarian stance is equally central to my family of origin's values, unlike the history of violations, problematic yet full of potential. In my family of origin the easiest way to be forbidden something was to argue its usualness among one's peers; the sheep and flock metaphor would be invoked, and there we three siblings would stand, stopped in our tracks. I, somewhat slowly, and my brothers, younger, wiser, and quicker to catch on, began to figure out that being countercultural in some way, any way, was a strategy to gain parental support and approval, until it didn't (until Laura comes out as a lesbian, apparently too non-flock-following even for my contrarian parents).

In my age cohort of baby boomer Jews, the fashion was to hate Hebrew school and plan to exit as soon as the last bar or bat mitzvah gifts had been opened. My contrarian path was to become the obnoxious kid in the Hebrew school class who cozied up to the teacher, behaved well, and kept on pursuing Jewish education well past the bat mitzvah. I was in Hebrew school one way or another until the day I graduated from college; I earned my living and paid my bills while in college teaching it and supplemented my paltry stipend in graduate school coaching a famous behaviorist's two sons for their bar mitzvahs thanks to all of those years being contrary to my peers. My contrarian family values gave me an unusual opportunity for a girl of my generation who did not go to Hebrew day school. I received a truly excellent Jewish education from some talented, knowledgeable teachers, many of whom were women. Our synagogue, long before the active embrace of women's leadership by the Conservative movement, had powerful women all over its educational system. They supported one another, and the few girls who made it through the filters imposed on our progress by the sex discrimination that was still the norm in Judaism. I still treasure the inscription in a copy of *Sefer N'viim*, the Book of Prophets, given to me by Leah Levin, my bat mitzvah teacher, in which she refers to me as *talmidah metzuyetnet*, an excellent student, because I treasure what she was to me. Being a Jew pointed me at being a feminist because it foregrounded my being female. At schul, I was the Other, a girl who wished to lead services, and was told she could not because her sex was a barrier to doing so, a student who wished to be excellent, not rebellious in class.

Those teachers were able to make the connections for me between Jewish teachings and the movements for social justice with which I was becoming increasingly involved as a young adolescent. Jews make choices, I was told, look at this line in *Shmot* (Exodus) where G-d tells the Jewish people that they have to choose to follow Torah. Jews run after justice, here in *Vayikra* (Leviticus), and oh, yes, check out those prophets while you're at it preaching against the rich and powerful and calling for more of that justice for the poor and oppressed. Jews were slaves and the stranger, the "other," in the land of Egypt, so we have a obligation to be the friend and ally of the stranger among us. While Jewish education could, and sometimes did, focus on the laws of *kashrut* and *sniut* (modesty), my teachers for the most part grasped their audience well and found ways to engage us around the things that mattered to us—*tikkun olam*, the healing of the world, a concept that has motivated me for my entire adult life in both personal and professional realms (Brown, 1997).

Of course, as a good Brown, I also could not follow my parents' flock. I have already discussed my rejection of rejection (although I suppose that one could see my stance here as a cutting off of cutoffs, but that's a level of analysis that may be of the reductio ad absurdum variety, so let's leave it alone). My parents have also assisted me to pursue my Jewishness more by attempting to lead the family flock in a direction in which I clearly did not wish to go. As they edged further into strict Orthodox observance during the 1970s, becoming *Baal'ei Tshuvah* (Jews who return to strict observance), I became more interested in how Judaism could integrate with feminism and with other, heart-opening forms of spiritual practice. I do not think that I ever overtly rebelled against their newly rigidifying stance or even rejected it. I simply found myself being drawn more to Jewish Renewal ideas and writers and to the places where my Jewish and feminist values met. My initial critiques of patriarchy in Judaism, now echoed in scholarly fashion by the first generations of lesbian rabbis took me further into being a Jew my way. Like a good Brown, I was not a sheep. In my parents' home, I am an Other, the child who belongs to no organized synagogue, who may not keep every holy day or holiday but who infuses her work and her life with the spirit of being a Jew.

So I have to thank my contrarian family structure for making it easy for me to be a Jew and a feminist and a lesbian all wrapped in one package. Being a Jew was at first another way to be different from the other kids at my mostly Protestant elementary school: get on the Hebrew school bus, skip after-school athletic events and social get-togethers, go study for another two hours. Then it was a way for me to be different from the kids in the Hebrew school class: be a devoted scholar of all things Jewish, win the Bible contest, come back to the old school and teach. And while I wasn't looking, Jewishness stuck to me, so that when I grew up it was all tangled up in the rest of me. It created the platform for doing theory, for debate and argument, for taking ideas seriously, and for knowing the value of interpretation.

Browns are, in addition to being contrarian, stubborn. "*Achshanim*," as my *Zeide*, my father's father would say, the Yiddish word for stubborn people. "We're *achshanim*, we Browns." This is a remarkably stable family personality trait that extends out in all directions and is now manifesting itself in the youngest member of my immediate family, my seven-year-old nephew. I sense that a part of my continuing connection to and identification with being a Jew has something to do with that stubborn streak. I will not give up on my culture, no matter how much it angers me. I will not give up on my parents no matter how much they anger me. I do not give up on clients, no matter how frustrating (okay, occasionally I have, but maybe 3 in 30 years). Loyal, stubborn, two aspects of the same attachment strategy. I have had to learn how to leave before I am thrown out; like a good Jew, I remain and risk expulsion rather than simply flee.

Jews have persisted through all kinds of creative attempts to kill us for two millennia and more. I will not cooperate with annihilation. Although my parents fault me bitterly for not birthing children, seeing that choice as "as bad as Hitler" to quote my mother, I believe that my strong, visible presence as a Jew in the world of feminist psychology has been of value, not in passing along the biological material of Jewishness but in passing along the intellectual genetics of Jewishness in the DNA of feminist practice. I ask questions, think critically, engage in the Jewish practice of pilpul (argument about scholarship), except that rather than doing it at Torah study I do it with feminist scholarship. My writing about feminist psychology has been replete with references to Jewish constructs as I make transparent the Jewish roots of my feminist identity. My stubbornness, which is a part of being in my family, has manifested in my insistence that my important identities cannot and will not be set up as in opposition to one another but rather as interwoven and feeding one another (Brown, 2006).

So how is this therapist informed by all of these themes? As a Jew I know that getting what you want takes time; exile can be long, return is never simple. The process of psychotherapy with the people I work with, survivors in many instances of long-term, chronic trauma, is a long exile from self and safety, and I know that time must be taken for the healing process, the process of return to self, to occur. I know that asking difficult questions is necessary and that life contains pain and loss but that pain and loss can be transformed through connection into joy. So, as a therapist, I ask difficult questions, create spaces where I invite people to feel their younger selves' pain in their adult selves' bodies and time frames, knowing that this is a route to empowerment and contact. My family has taught me the value of standing in the outsider position, to prize that place in the social ecology and to know that anyone can become an Other. As a therapist I seem constitutionally unable to otherize my clients, rather I see us standing together in alliance, both of us on the outside looking in. By doing so, we create an inside in which therapy can happen.

Here in Israel, where I am surrounded by people who talk as I do, eat as I do, move through the world in familiar patterns, I am at home and still the other, a visiting American with rusty and inadequate Hebrew. Yet I feel completely comfortable in this place of contradiction. I know, here, precisely how I am a Jew and thus I know precisely how I am a human being in all of the intersectionality of my identities. I know, and thus can be for, myself; I am for the other. I am apart, in no one's flock, but have created a flock for other sheep of a different color. I argue, I dispute, and I thrill in the diversity of epistemologies and methodologies that have emerged in the fields of feminist practice. And now this article can stop wandering in the wilderness.

REFERENCES

Brown, L. S. (1997). The private practice of subversion: Psychology as tikkun olam. *American Psychologist, 52.*

Brown, L. S. (2006). Still subversive after all these years: The relevance of feminist therapy in the age of evidence-based practice. *Psychology of Women Quarterly, 30,* 15–24.

From Hidden Child to Godless Jew:
A Personal Journey

SOPHIA RICHMAN

I was born into the Holocaust, a Jewish child marked for death. As far as I know, my parents, Leon and Dorota Reichman, did not think much about their Jewish heritage until World War II when Hitler came into power and suddenly their Jewish identity was thrust on them like the Star of David that they were forced to wear.

My father came from a shtetl in Poland. I believe that his parents were comfortable with their Jewish identities and followed the customs and traditions of their religion, but when my father reached adulthood he was drawn to communism and its antireligious stance. My mother hailed from Lwow, the big city in the province of Galicia, in southeast Poland, where all of my ancestors came from. Lwow, known as the Vienna of the East, was the third largest city in Poland and had a large Jewish population. My mother's middle class family had lived there for many generations and was well assimilated into Polish culture. If they considered themselves Jews, it was only in a secular sense. Two of her three brothers had married Polish Catholics. One of them went so far as to convert in the 1920s, to move away from his family of origin, and to hide his Jewish identity from his children for the rest of his life. Not surprisingly, he was the only one of her five siblings to survive the Holocaust. To this day his branch of the family does not recognize their Jewish roots.

With a combination of ingenuity and good fortune, my parents and I survived the Holocaust, all three of us in hiding. My mother and I assumed a Christian identity and my father was hidden by my mother in the tiny attic in the house where we rented rooms after his escape from a concentration camp. Taking on a Christian identity was a reasonable choice for my mother. She spoke fluent Polish and was more familiar with Christian traditions than with Jewish ones.

As a toddler during the years in hiding, I of course had no idea about the fact that I was a Jewish child whose life was in constant danger, but nevertheless I expect that I had some awareness of the terror around me. It was in the air that I breathed during my waking moments, and it was reflected in the vigilant terrified faces and the hushed tones of my parents. I have a few fragments of memory from those years in hiding. The most vivid relate to my discovery of my father as he emerged from the attic, and the injunction against revealing the secret of his existence to the outside world (Richman, 2002, 2006a, 2006b).

Mother had been fortunate to obtain false identity papers that were real and not simply forged. One of her good friends, a musician whom she had studied with at the conservatory in Lwow had an uncle who was a priest. This uncle provided my mother with the birth, marriage, and baptismal certificate of one of his deceased parishioners whose date of birth was similar to my mother's. Dorota assumed this woman's identity, taking her name and creating a story that would explain why she was without a husband.

With these papers in hand, Mother turned to another friend from childhood, a convert who found her a place to live in a small village on the outskirts of Lwow where no one knew her. When we went into hiding I was about a year old. Mother arranged to have me baptized. Because my name Zofia or Zosia (as I was called) was a common Polish name it did not have to be changed. Mother considered herself lucky to have a baby who did not yet talk and who did not look Jewish. With my fair skin, blonde hair, and blue/green eyes I could easily pass for a Polish child. She was more "Jewish" looking; her large, sad brown eyes and brown hair could have given her away, but with me as her cover she was safer.

With her new name, Maria, my mother played her role of a devout Catholic well. She placed a religious medal around her neck as well as mine and took me to the local church regularly. Many years later she described these experiences to me. She spoke about her positive feelings about the church, which was one of the few places where she could feel relatively safe. She loved the ceremony, the music, and the scents and described it as akin to a theater experience.

Apparently even after the war, Mother held on to her Catholic identity for a while. Lwow, where we returned after liberation, was now annexed to Ukraine. At war's end, there was an opportunity for survivors to either remain in Ukrainian territory or move to Poland. We chose the latter. There we took up residence in the home of a Catholic couple. I learned recently that during our stay in the town of Chorzow, Mother continued to pass as a Catholic. She created a cover story about the fact that she had been persecuted because her husband was a Jew and that she had hidden him during the German occupation.

Unfortunately, I learned of this only after her death and I could not ask her about her motivation to deceive the landlords who had become our friends. I presume that she did not feel safe in Poland even after the Holocaust. In fact some of the incidents that took place in Poland shortly after the war suggest that her concerns were not totally irrational. It is also possible that her ambivalence about her Jewish identity influenced her as well. Perhaps she felt that my father, who could never pass because of his looks, had endangered her life.

My father's ambivalence about Judaism took a different form. I was not aware of it until I read his memoir (Richman, 1975). This account of his life in the concentration camp was written while he was in hiding and translated and published 30 years later. I had always assumed that he had clearly rejected Judaism, at least the religious aspects of it. The story in my family was that my father had required my mother to publicly give up her religion as a condition for their marriage. Before their wedding in 1937, she took out an advertisement in the local Jewish paper announcing that from that day forth she was no longer a practicing Jew.

After the war, Leon had very little patience for anything connected with religion and often expressed feelings of contempt for those who preached it. For all the years of my childhood, both parents seemed to share a strong conviction that religion was a divisive force in society and God was a construction. Yet from my father's memoir I learned that during the war, when he was persecuted because of his Jewish blood and imprisoned at Janowska (the notorious concentration camp in Galicia), he seemed to find meaning and consolation in religious ritual. In what was probably his favorite and most meaningful chapter of the book, he describes the commemoration of Yom Kippur by the inmates of the camp. It is surprising that this man, who identified himself as an agnostic, and who to my knowledge never set foot in a synagogue as an adult—before or after the war—would write such a moving, powerful piece and include it in its entirety in the book proposal that he submitted for publication. Apparently he believed that this piece more than any other represented his best writing and was the most significant. On that day in September 1942, Leon seemed to reconnect briefly with his religion as he participated in collective mourning with his Jewish brethren. Perhaps the ritual observance of this most holy day gave him a chance to express his blocked emotions and for a brief moment in time find some solace in the religion of his childhood.

When we arrived in France in 1946, I tried very hard to become a little French girl. I began kindergarten immediately and learned the language quickly. Like my mother, I had a gift for making friends. My parents managed to find a few survivors from Poland, and we spent some time with these Jewish families, but I was not as comfortable with their children as with my little French friends from the neighborhood and school.

I felt at home in postwar Paris where everyone seemed to be as poor and struggling as we were. Once again I was living in a Catholic environment and it felt natural. Perhaps it resonated with my earliest years in the little village when I went to church with my mother. All of my playmates were Catholic. I remember trading and collecting pictures of the Virgin Mary with baby Jesus and assorted saints. I cherished these colorful images and sometimes prayed to them.

By the age of eight or nine my little schoolmates were preparing for their First Communion and they were all excited about the big event. When I spoke to my parents about it, they simply said that we were Jewish, and that we did not celebrate this event. I was deeply disappointed. I think it was the first time that I realized that we were different from others and that difference was called "Jewish." I determined to convert as soon as I would be old enough to do so. My neighbors applauded the idea, while my parents remained silent on the subject.

In 1951 we arrived in America. That had been our goal from the beginning of our journey out of Eastern Europe, but the quotas had made it very difficult, even for those of us who had a relative in America working hard to bring us over. We had remained in Paris on a temporary visa for the five years that it took to finally obtain the much coveted visa to the United States.

Once we became American citizens my parents bought a cemetery plot. We had finally arrived to the place where we would remain forever. The plot was in a Jewish cemetery. Now that we were in America my parents seemed to become more Jewish. All of their friends were Jewish, most of them survivors who had arrived after the war. They became part of a community united by common experiences of persecution.

Yet the synagogue was never a part of my parents' life. They remained staunch atheists and attended temple only during functions like the bar mitzvahs of their friends' children, weddings, and funerals. Jewish holidays were not celebrated except as occasions for family dinners. I think my mother fasted on Yom Kippur, probably more out of a sense that all of her friends were doing it than from any religious feelings. Occasionally a friend would invite us to a Passover Seder and we attended. For me it was an interesting performance, like the theater analogy my mother had used to describe her experience in Catholic Church during our hiding years.

Chanukah was never celebrated in our house; there was no menorah, no gifts, barely an acknowledgment of the holiday. I wanted to celebrate Christmas like the majority of Americans but my parents refused to let me have a Christmas tree. So I purchased tree ornaments anyway and hung them on the branches of a rather tall potted plant in my room. I exchanged gifts with my friends.

For a brief period of time, my parents sent me to a Zionist summer camp. They had never been Zionists and to this day it is unclear how I ended up at Camp Ein Harod sponsored by the Zionist organization Hehalutz Hatzair. My fellow campers idealized Israel, and many planned to emigrate there in the future. As for me, I was only interested in Israeli music, dancing, and the boys. When camp was over, I continued to attend weekly meetings in the organization until my parents heard rumors that this organization had communist affiliations and promptly took me out.

A MINYAN OF WOMEN

During the college years I flirted with Buddhism. It was a philosophy that made sense to me. But the part of me that was uncomfortable with organized religion won out. I was coming to believe that religions divided people and created conflict among them. I had had a firsthand experience with the horrors committed in the name of religion. My attitude toward organized religion was reinforced when I read Freud's (1927/1961) treatise on the subject *The Future of an Illusion*. Freud's formulation of religion as a construction meant to deal with man's helplessness and powerlessness in the face of the harshness of nature and of civilization made sense to me, as did his concept of God as a projection of the powerful parent. Freud's designation for himself—"a Godless Jew"—described me as well. At this point in my life I could accept my ethnic identity, but it was not a significant part of my self-concept. It was merely a fact, something that described me, the way that my physical characteristics identified me.

My friends were always of diverse backgrounds and ethnicity. I was interested in different cultures and traditions. When it came to dating, my parents were insistent on my dating Jewish boys. Deep down I think they had a mistrust of those who were not Jewish. Their years of exposure to anti-Semitism made them readily suspicious. Whenever I met a new guy, their first question was always, "Is he Jewish?" I found myself irritated by that question because it was not my criterion for a relationship.

When I married at the age of 22, I did pick a nonpracticing Jew. Still my parents were not especially pleased with my choice of husband despite the fact that he was of the same ethnicity. They were also critical of the way we chose to marry. Our decision was pretty impulsive; we did not plan a wedding, and we were married by a rabbi in his chambers. I think it was my in-laws' idea. My father refused to attend the ceremony. His major complaint was that we were not married by a justice of the peace, as he had been, and that he did not approve of a religious ceremony.

The second time that I married my father had the same complaint but reluctantly came to the wedding. The circumstances of my second marriage were quite different. I had fallen in love with a young Greek American whose family was Greek Orthodox. They were churchgoing people and my husband was the only one in his family who had rejected his religious upbringing. Like my father, he was an atheist with strong antireligious feelings. Our wedding ceremony, however, was a unique affair, an unconventional celebration of our union. We were married in the apartment that we shared by a good friend, a psychoanalyst, who was ordained as a Protestant minister. We wrote our own vows and asked her to omit the word God from the ceremony.

At first my in-laws had great difficulty with my husband's choice of mate—an older woman, non-Greek, Jewish, divorced, hardly a match for their first born. My only asset in their eyes was that my name was "Sophia," a name they could pronounce, a Greek name. Over the years I took some pleasure in knowing that I could "pass" with that name. Once I had passed as a Christian child, now I could fit into the Greek community, at least superficially.

When our daughter Lina was born the relationship between our families solidified. Everyone cherished the baby who was the first grandchild on both sides. We even found some similarities between our diverse cultures. For instance, we were amused to see that both grandmothers made the same little magical gesture over the body of our newborn. They pursed their lips, and spit three times—*Pu, Pu, Pu*—an ancient incantation to keep the evil spirits away. Even though they did not speak the same language (my mother-in-law never learned English), these two women loved the same grandchild passionately and came to appreciate each other as well.

Both grandmothers were determined to pass on their culture and/or religion to our child. They worried that we would not do the job adequately. My mother-in-law, who always had a prominent cross dangling from her neck, decided that Lina, her grandchild and namesake, should not be deprived of this important religious symbol. I in turn made sure that every gold cross given to Lina as a gift ended up in the top drawer of my dresser rather than on Lina's neck. My mother was not going to be outdone by the Greek side of the family. She took every opportunity to send cards noting the Jewish holidays and even gave her a menorah as a gift one Chanukah.

The grandmothers had good reason to be concerned that our child was not going to get a religious education from us. On the subject of religion, my husband and I were perfectly compatible. As a child, my husband had been given a religious education. Besides parochial school, he also attended church regularly and was proud to be the head alter boy, until adolescence when he vehemently rejected religion. He too had read Freud's *Future of an Illusion* with the same enthusiasm as I had years before. So when our daughter was born, it seemed natural that the subject of religion was never even broached. Unlike many interfaith couples who are faced with the decision of how to bring up their first child, we never considered it an issue. Cultural exposure was another matter however. We wanted her to be exposed to both of our heritages. We celebrated all holidays as if they were secular events and enjoyed the traditions of our separate cultures.

Our daughter, however, did express some of her struggle to integrate the diverse experiences which she was exposed to. When she was four or five, during the Chanukah/Christmas holiday she drew an interesting picture that revealed some of her conflicts. The colored pencil drawing featured a large anthropomorphic heart, with eyes and a smiling face. Inside this heart face she boldly printed the word "LOVE" in large block letters. Above it she printed her own full name conveying the message that this heart/face was a self-representation. At either side of the heart in the lower right and left quadrants of the page respectively, she drew the symbols of Chanukah and Christmas, a menorah on one side and a carefully decorated Christmas tree on the other. The drawing appeared to be a perfect integration of her separate identities. After its completion, however, something seemed to trouble her. She proceeded to rip off the lower right hand corner, the one with the menorah, then Scotch-taped it back on. I wondered if this artwork symbolically expressed her ambivalence about her Jewish side. And did her ambivalence reflect my own confusion about my Jewish identity?

My Jewish identity had been figuratively ripped off and then subsequently reattached in an awkward way with the result that I never felt like a real Jew. The first menorah I ever owned was the one that my mother bought for my daughter when she was a toddler. After my father's death, my mother seemed to more readily accept her own Jewish identity. She joined Hadassah, the women's Zionist organization, and became an active devoted member. She found a purpose and a sense of community in the organization dedicated to the development of Israel. She was recognized as a leader and honored with an award for her service and when she died she left a substantial contribution to this organization. She had come a long way since the day in 1937 when she had renounced her Jewish identity to meet my father's condition for marriage.

As I entered middle age, I too experienced a shift in my sense of myself as a Jew. As with my mother it was a gradual process. For me it was part of accepting my past, facing the Holocaust and acknowledging its impact on my life. For many years after World War II, the subject of the Holocaust was avoided by survivors whose energies were focused on creating a new life and by a society that was unreceptive to their tales of horror. Some psycho-historians have referred to this period of history as a "curtain of silence," a "conspiracy of silence" or a "latency period" and conceptualized it as the common reaction to psychological trauma, "intense individual and collective defense mechanisms functioned to ward off preoccupation with, and memories of, traumatic experiences" (Bergmann & Jucovy, 1982).

The curtain of silence began to lift in the 1970s, and by the 1980s and 1990s, society was flooded with Holocaust related literature, art, and psychological research. With dwindling numbers of survivors, there was a sense of urgency about getting the story from the last witnesses. Survivors who had been discouraged during the postwar years from talking about their wartime experiences were now encouraged to share details of their wartime trauma.

Thirty years after the Holocaust, my father Leon Richman published a memoir of his experiences in Janowska, the concentration camp where he was imprisoned for about a year. He had written the manuscript while he was in hiding after his escape from the camp, but as with so many other survivors, it took many years before he was ready to share it with the world. His "coming out" was a major event for him as well as for me; it gave me permission to face my own demons. For so many years I had been given the message by my parents that since I was so young during the war years that I was not affected by those events. They desperately wanted to believe if I didn't understand what was going on around me, and I didn't remember the details, then I would be spared the suffering. I complied with their injunction to forget the past, and did not even consider myself a survivor until the late 1980s.

Gradually and slowly I began to reconstruct my journey out of the Holocaust. Therapy in my 20s had not been especially helpful in dealing with that part of my past. The analyst, as so many other professionals of his day, was not sensitive to Holocaust issues and colluded with my avoidance. Jewish psychoanalysts with roots in Eastern Europe were particularly vulnerable to countertransference problems when working with survivors who could bring the horrors of the Shoah into the consulting room (Danieli, 1984).

Eventually, during my own psychoanalytic training, I found an analyst who was more tuned in and we began to explore the complexity of the impact of the early traumatic experiences on my life and my choices. When analysis was over, I continued the process and my self-analysis culminated in the decision to write a memoir (Richman, 2002).

Once the decision was made, the process took over. The writing flowed with unexpected ease and within a year I had created a narrative that integrated the fragments of memory and experience into a coherent whole. The memoir went beyond the war years and dealt with the reverberations of the Holocaust throughout the life span. I was surprised to discover that recording the narrative on paper provided me with a depth of understanding richer than what I had learned in years of analysis. By examining my life in its totality, I was able to recognize the intricate patterns in its fabric.

One of the most interesting discoveries related to a reenactment of a childhood experience when I turned 30. Although I had been in therapy at the time, I had no insight to connect the present with my past. That insight came as I wrote my life story.

After the dissolution of my first marriage, I became romantically involved with a Roman Catholic priest. We met while he was training to become a psychoanalyst. He had decided to leave the Church but while he waited for dispensation from the Vatican he functioned as a part-time parish priest and moved in with me. On Sundays, we would attend his church together, I hanging back a few yards while parishioners kissed his hand reverently. Occasionally I helped him write his sermons. What a charade! A Godless Jew writing Roman Catholic sermons. It made me smile, and at the same time it made me uncomfortable to think that we were deceiving his devout parishioners.

It was only many years later, when I was writing my memoir that I became aware of the significance of that relationship in the context of my early history. I came to see it as a reenactment of my wartime experience. Catholicism had been an important part of my life at that time; in fact, it had been instrumental in saving it. Faithfully and regularly my mother had brought me to church in the little village where we lived in hiding. There she relaxed and enjoyed the "show" as she later referred to it. I became as familiar with the sounds and scents of the Catholic Church as with the air that I breathed. In the present of my life, in that small parish church where my lover/priest presided, I found myself in hiding once again. I blended in with the other parishioners who did not know my secret. He and I played our roles carefully so as not to be discovered, only this time without the punishment of death hanging over us.

Another insight that emerged as I wrote the story of my life was the connection between my speaking inhibition and the injunction of childhood to be silent and to keep the secret of my father's existence from the world outside of our little apartment. Throughout my life I have experienced difficulties expressing myself orally in group situations or when I am examined by authority figures. Under those conditions I have felt inarticulate and blocked, unable to formulate my thoughts or find the right words to express myself. What seemed like a public speaking anxiety, a common anxiety, was actually less about speaking in public and more about saying the wrong thing. In fact, I have been comfortable in front of audiences, no matter how large, as long as I have a written text in front of me. Presumably, in those circumstances, I can totally control what comes out of my mouth; there is no danger of something regrettable slipping by my internal censor. The past and present are merged in my reaction. I learned my childhood lesson well for it was taught under penalty of death. Be careful what you say, for it can have dangerous consequences.

In contrast to speaking, writing has always come easily for me. With speech so problematic, writing became a wonderful means to self-expression. Writing the story of my life also represented a way to come out of hiding, another major theme. It was immensely gratifying to write my story and then to receive the positive feedback that followed. One surprise was that people began to relate to me as "Jewish" in a way that I was not used to. My publisher sent out promotional material describing me as a "Jewish analyst," Barnes & Noble put my book in the "Judaica" section, and I began to get invitations to speak about the memoir in synagogues. The book received an award from the Jewish Women's Caucus of the Association for Women in Psychology. Even a friend from childhood, an African-American woman started to send me greeting cards for Passover and the Jewish New Year after I sent her a copy of my book. I did not feel any more Jewish, but somehow, the world now perceived me that way.

One of the repercussions of my publication was the dramatic reaction from what was left of my extended family. It has been the only negative reaction to the memoir to date and took me by surprise. Perhaps it should not have. My mother's brother who had converted to Catholicism when he was a young man in the 1920s had kept his Jewish roots secret from the family he created. He had converted, as so many other Jews had, in order to have a better life in anti-Semitic prewar Poland, and although Hitler did not honor such conversions, my uncle managed to escape to England during the war. After the war he returned to Poland and had two more children, one of them born in Oswiecim (Auschwitz) where he settled immediately after the war, a rather strange and ironic choice of locale for someone whose entire family of origin was practically wiped out by the Nazis.

Uncle Manek and my mother had stayed in touch. Despite her ambivalent feelings about him, she was determined to maintain a relationship with him and his family. He was her only surviving sibling, a fact that took precedence over whatever awkwardness there remained between them. When he came to visit her in America in 1971, I met him for the first time. During that visit, Uncle Manek went to the local Catholic Church daily. One by one I met his children, my cousins. Two had remained in Poland, two had emigrated to the United States, and one had found his way to Australia. After my uncle's death, one by one the children learned the family secret. Somehow it leaked out, as secrets often do.

I was unaware that my first cousins maintained the secret from the next generation. Apparently their children did not know that their grandfather was born a Jew. My book exposed this fact and all of the dissembling around it. My cousins reacted swiftly and with rage. They were very upset that I had not changed their names in the book in order to protect them. I promised that when the book was reprinted I would give them all new names, which I did. Subsequently, there have been some attempts at reconciliation with this branch of the family. The wedding of my cousin's daughter brought us all together in October of 2004. The ceremony was a very "Catholic affair." I was no doubt the only Jew among the several hundred guests. Prior to the event, my cousin had written to me asking me to please refrain from discussing the past with the younger generation. I reluctantly agreed to respect his request but let him know that if asked a direct question, I would not lie. It had taken me too long, and I had struggled too hard to come to terms with my past to now lie about it.

Keeping secrets has always been somewhat problematic for me. The impulse to expose is very strong and in conflict with the need to honor another's right to hide. I have chosen a profession where my core issues take center stage. Psychoanalysts are the keepers of secrets. We are legally and ethically bound to keep from revealing what we are told in our consulting rooms. Patients trust us with their secrets knowing that we will respect their confidentiality.

Furthermore, psychoanalysis has always been concerned with issues of hiding. Most people go into psychoanalysis for greater self-understanding, but at the same time they struggle against knowing certain things about themselves. In our relations with others a similar dilemma exists, namely the need to be known and the desire to remain private. These conflicting needs are universal. But in the case of survivors of trauma, the dialectic between the wish to be known and the wish to remain hidden is heightened and complicated. Elsewhere, I have written, "Typically survivors face the past with great ambivalence. The responsibility to preserve the memories coexists with the impulse to forget; we are perpetually suspended between concealment and disclosure" (Richman, 2002, Preface, p. *xiv*).

As a psychoanalyst who has written a memoir disclosing the most private details of my life, I face the issues of self-disclosure in a profound way. Disclosure on the part of the analyst/therapist is of particular interest in the mental health field. Currently there is much literature on this controversial subject (Aron, 1996; Ehrenberg, 1995; Jacobs, 1999; Pizer, 1997; Renik, 1999). The impact of the memoir on my practice has been of great interest to professionals struggling with these issues, and I have written about it (Richman, 2006a, 2006b).

I believe that my decision to become a psychologist/psychoanalyst was profoundly influenced by the experiences of childhood. Memories of a hidden childhood are fragile and easily challenged, particularly when the adults around are eager to protect these children from such memories. My parents were intent on perpetuating the myth that I would not remember what I was too young to understand, and they never attempted to explain anything to me. As a young child, surrounded by death and destruction I was left on my own to make sense of the chaos around me. The profound confusion of my childhood had long-term effects. The need to understand turned out to be a pervasive theme in my life. I believe that it was one of the main reasons that I chose my profession. I am committed to understanding human behavior and motivation; it is my job to help people make sense of what is puzzling in them and in their interpersonal relationships.

Also, I am certain that it is not an accident that I have chosen to dedicate myself to a healing profession. It is striking that so many child survivors of the Holocaust and second generation have entered the mental health field (Kestenberg & Kestenberg, 1988); we have transferred our concern with our traumatized parents to our patients. We are programmed to be rescuers and caretakers and have found a vicarious way to heal ourselves as well. Our dedication to a healing profession is also an opportunity to give back because we feel grateful to have been spared.

My profession has been a tremendous source of gratification and healing for me. It is immensely satisfying to feel deeply connected to others, to feel that the work that I am engaged in is meaningful as well as intellectually and emotionally fulfilling. For me, one of the most exciting aspects of my work is that it gives me an opportunity to come into intimate contact with people whose lives are totally different from mine. It feels like a great privilege to be able to enter and learn about the world of another in such detail. At the same time it is sometimes challenging to be able to relate to those who are so different. Nowhere is this as evident for me as when I am working with people who are highly religious, regardless of their particular religion. It is in those situations that I worry about my countertransference.

My concern is that because of my personal bias, I may miss some significant aspects of an individual's values and belief system. Religion plays an influential role in the lives of many. According to a recent Gallup Poll, 88% of the population surveyed reported that religion is important in their lives, and 96% reported a belief in God or a universal spirit (Aten & Hernandez, 2004). If such a large proportion of the population is religiously committed, then it behooves us as therapists to be sensitive to those issues as they emerge in our work (Aron, 2004). Yet I find that the subject of religion does not come up very often, and I wonder if that is because I am not as attuned to it. Perhaps I don't inquire about this aspect of an individual's life in a way that I do about other areas of their experience.

With that concern in mind, I recently raised the subject with a patient whom I had been working with for many years. She is an African American Protestant minister who is a pastor at a local church. In our analytic work we have explored many areas of her life, including her feelings about her work and her calling, but not much had been said on the subject of what it's like for her to be in analysis with someone who knows very little about her religion. In fact, it seemed easier for us to address issues of racial difference than to talk about our religious differences. When I asked her if she felt reluctant to bring up certain thoughts and feelings on the subject of religion because she felt that I might not understand, she denied it and said that she preferred keeping her religion out of psychotherapy. She then reminded me that prior to her work with me she had had a negative therapeutic experience. She had been in crisis and had consulted a pastoral counselor who had suggested that they pray together. In that context, my secular position was experienced as neutral and safe.

In contrast, I have encountered situations when my being a secular Jew was experienced as threatening to the treatment. Two situations come to mind, both that involved Jewish orthodox women, one who chose me as a therapist because she knew that I was Jewish, the other because she assumed that I was not. As a result of inadvertent self-disclosure each of these women discovered aspects of my religious beliefs that disturbed them and led to complicated transference/countertransference enactments.

The following vignette illustrates some of the complications. Sarah, who identified herself as an Orthodox Jew, had very strong and complex feelings about her Judaism. Her parents had not been religious and in her youth she had been attracted only to non-Jewish boys and ended up marrying one of them. After her first child was born, Sarah became very interested in her religion. Her husband had been raised as a Catholic but had always had an interest in Judaism. He was happy to comply with her wish for him to convert, even if it meant undergoing circumcision. He embraced his new religion with great dedication and became an active member of their synagogue. The practice of their religion was an important part of their family life.

A MINYAN OF WOMEN

I saw Sarah in my home office. The office was attached to the house and had a separate entrance on the side. As she parked in front of my house one December morning around the holidays she noticed from the corner of her eye the Christmas wreath on the front door. When I ushered her into the consulting room she told me how angry it made her to see this wreath. She went into an elaborate explanation of its meaning. She found it offensive that a therapist would display a symbol that had such negative connotations. At the very least, she said, a therapist should be neutral. She had chosen me as a therapist because she had assumed that we had the same background and now, after many years of working together, she was suddenly faced with an aspect of me that was new and disturbing.

Because we came from the same small community, she was no doubt aware that my husband like hers was a non-Jew by birth. The fact that I had handled religious differences in my own marriage so differently from how she had chosen to deal with them in hers was apparently quite threatening. Ultimately, we were able to make good therapeutic use of this event and the relationship survived the confrontation and was enriched by it.

Another patient learned about my Jewish identity accidentally, and it was then that I realized that she had assumed that I was not Jewish and apparently had chosen me precisely for that supposed fact. When we examined her disappointment, she revealed that she was more comfortable with someone who had no knowledge of her religion. She felt that a therapist with her background would be less objective and more likely to judge her.

The fact that she assumed that I am not Jewish may seem puzzling, yet it is understandable in the context of both her wish for me not to be and certain characteristics of mine. I have often heard the comment "you don't look Jewish," a fact that of course saved my life. Also, it is evident to patients that I don't observe the holidays since they often have to remind me about them.

My complicated personal history has had a powerful impact on my ethnic identity, a situation that is typical for child survivors of the Holocaust who were hidden in plain sight with a Christian identity. Hogman (1988) has written about the long-term effect of exposure to a Catholic environment in the early years on identity formation. Her research based on interviews of Jewish children raised as Catholics during the Second World War makes it clear that their Catholic experiences caused identity confusion and necessitated a continuing effort to find a way to integrate the Jewish and Catholic aspects of their identities.

My personal struggle to reconcile these mutually exclusive identifications in order to have a coherent sense of identity was also probably complicated by my parents' ambivalence about their own Jewish identities. Only when I faced how I had been uprooted from my Jewish roots could I own them as a part of me—not as a religious but as a cultural identity. My Jewish heritage is a fact of life, but religion is a matter of choice. While at this point in my life, I am comfortable with myself and the choices that I have made, still I am aware that the thread that connects me with my ancestors is frayed and barely visible, and I feel sadness about the potential loss of that connection.

REFERENCES

Aron, L. (1996). *A meeting of minds: Mutuality in psychoanalysis*. Hillsdale, NJ: The Analytic Press.

Aten, J. D., & Hernandez, B. C. (2004). Addressing religion in clinical supervision: A model. *Psychotherapy: Theory, Research, Practice, Training, 41*, 152–160.

Bergmann, M., & Jucovy, M. (Eds.). (1982). *Generation of the holocaust*. New York: Basic Books.

Danieli, Y. (1984). Psychotherapists' participation in the conspiracy of silence about the Holocaust. *Psychoanalytic Psychology, 1*, 23–42.

Ehrenberg, D. (1995). Self-disclosure: Therapeutic tool or indulgence? *Contemporary Psychoanalysis, 31*, 213–229.

Freud, S. (1961). *The future of an illusion*. New York: W. W. Norton. (Originally published in 1927).

Hogman, F. (1988). The experience of catholicism for jewish children during world war II. *The Psychoanalytic Review, 75*, 511–532.

Jacobs, T. (1999). On the question of self-disclosure by the analyst: Error or advance intechnique? *The Psychoanalytic Quarterly, 68*, 159–183.

Kestenberg, M., & Kestenberg, J. S. (1988). The sense of belonging and altruism in children who survived the Holocaust. *The Psychoanalytic Review, 75*, 533–560.

Pizer, B. (1997). When the analyst is ill: Dimensions of self-disclosure. *The Psychoanalytic Quarterly, 67*, 450–469.

Renik, O. (1999). Playing one's cards face up in analysis: An approach to the problem of self-disclosure. *The Psychoanalytic Quarterly, 68*, 521–539.

Richman, L. (1975). *Why?: Extermination camp lwow (Lemberg) 134 janowska street, poland*. New York: Vantage Press.

Richman, S. (2002). *A wolf in the attic: The legacy of a hidden child of the Holocaust*. New York: Routledge.

Richman, S. (2006a). Finding one's voice: Transforming trauma into autobiographical narrative. *Contemporary Psychoanalysis, 42*(4), 639–650.

Richman, S. (2006b). When the analyst writes a memoir: Clinical implications of biographic Disclosure. *Contemporary Psychoanalysis, 42*(3), 367–392.

Nu! You Make a Living at This?

SARI DWORKIN

Judaism has played an important part in my life. The religious aspect of being Jewish has waxed and waned over the course of my life, but everything I have done and continue to do is connected to my Jewish identity. Although had I been asked just a couple of years ago what part Judaism plays in my professional life I would have said that it is a part of my political activism, academic activism, and my activism in professional organizations like the American Psychological Association and the American Counseling Association, but it doesn't play a part in my therapy practice as a psychologist. Now I recognize that my Jewish identity is central to all I am and all I do. All other parts of my identity flow from that solid Jewish trunk. I probably would not have chosen to be an academic and a therapist if not for my Jewish core.

My father was born in what now is the Ukraine but in 1906 was Russia. My mother was born in the United States on the Lower East Side of New York. In 1916 the lower east side of New York was considered the Jewish ghetto of New York. Whenever I teach multicultural counseling and tell my students that on my father's side I am a first generation "American" and on my mother's side I am second generation, they are surprised since I look and act (at least according to them) very White and very mainstream (that is, until I disclose my bisexual identity). It is true that there is very little of the "Old World" in me, but I still occasionally throw in a Yiddish word or phrase, speak with a New York accent that grew out of Jewish immigrants speaking English with a Yiddish accent, and behave in a manner considered rude and vulgar by many a WASP friend. My childhood was similar to that of many first and second-generation children of immigrants. My parents struggled between wanting me to keep some of the old cultural traditions and wanting me to fully assimilate into the mainstream culture. A major difference between immigrant cultures when I grew up and immigrant cultures today is that there wasn't a multicultural movement that valued diversity and the celebration of all cultures when I was growing up. My mother having been born here was more willing to see me shed Jewish mannerisms than my father was. This conflict between my mother and father about how my brother and I were to be raised was a source of confusion for me as I struggled to define my own identity.

My father came from an Orthodox Jewish family and his father was a cantor (the person who leads the congregation in the chanting of the prayers) in Russia. They lived in a small shtetel that was often subject to pogroms. The family, along with many other families, decided to emigrate to the United States to escape persecution and to be able to freely practice their religion. My father was proud of being a Jew, and had it not been for the depression he would have become a rabbi. During the depression my father felt he had to work to support his family of origin who were quite poor. While his work caused him to stop practicing one of the most important religious traditions in Judaism, the observance of Shabbat (Sabbath), the day of complete rest, he wanted his children to fully live the Jewish tradition. Whenever possible he would attend religious services on the Shabbat.

My mother came from an observant Polish family, but their major emphasis was education and to live the American dream. The depression did not hit her family hard and she was one of the few women of her generation to go to college and on for a master's degree. (Her brothers all obtained doctoral degrees.) My mother shed many of the Jewish observances of her family while still remaining religiously Jewish. In addition to shedding some of her Jewish identity she also embraced the socialist and communist ideas of her day. While my mother rarely spoke about this "communist" period in her life (understandable since she lived though the McCarthy era), her liberal ideas were passed on to me. The Holocaust, a defining period in history for most Jews no matter where in the world they lived, claimed the lives of some of my mother's extended family that had not left Poland in time. Her fears for the safety of the Jewish people manifested in a strong belief that Jews should never emphasize their Jewishness or any difference. Jews should avoid being too Jewish and too much in the public eye. My mother and father's differing Jewish values impacted my childhood upbringing.

The first time my parents disagreed about what their children should learn was over the Yiddish language. (I didn't learn about this conflict until later on in life.) Both my parents and my mother's mother (the only grandparent alive when my brother and I were born) spoke Yiddish fluently. My father wanted the children to also speak Yiddish, but my mother perceived this language as the language of the lower classes, of poor Jews. My mother won (as she almost always did), and Yiddish was used only when the adults didn't want the children to understand what they were saying. I have a sense of loss about this and am very sentimental when I listen to Yiddish music, as I often do. The next conflict was over my education. (It is important for the reader to know that my brother was the child of my mother's first husband who died young. My parents' religious conflicts were more about me than about my brother.) My father wanted to send me to a yeshiva, a Jewish parochial school. My mother was horrified. She taught physical education at a New York City Public School, and while most NYC public schools had a majority of Jewish teachers and students (Jewish holidays were official holidays when the public schools were closed) there was some diversity. Yeshivas were private schools, and half of the day was spent on secular studies and the other half of a much longer school day consisted of Jewish religious studies and the study of Hebrew. To my mother yeshivas emphasized Jewish separation and difference. I did not go to a yeshiva.

The next conflict I remember clearly was not about me but did affect me. Having come from observant families both my parents grew up in kosher homes. Up until I was about seven years old our house also was kosher. This meant not eating milk and meat at the same time and buying products certified kosher by a rabbi. It also meant having four sets of dishes, pots, and silverware. One set of each was for every day (one for meat and one for milk products) and one set of each was for the holiday of Passover. My mother decided that this was nonsense and too much trouble for a working mom. She began mixing up the dishes and buying any products she wanted at the supermarket. Since my father worked long hours he didn't even notice what my mother was doing. Eventually she told him, and slowly he began to accept the new circumstances. In fact by the time I was about 10 years old my father was eating bacon (pork is not kosher) for breakfast.

Then came the battle over my learning Hebrew. At first I enthusiastically went to Hebrew school every day after my public school day. But few of my friends were doing this, and while I was quite good at Hebrew, I hated going. Mother said, "Fine, don't go." Dad was furious, but I stopped going to Hebrew school. This was after my brother's bar mitzvah, and I was keenly aware that no such big event and marker of change from childhood to adulthood was going to happen for me. Girls didn't get bat mitzvahed at that time. This was my first awakening of a feminist consciousness, although I wouldn't have been able to verbalize that at the time.

The positive impact my father's love of religion held for me consisted of prayer and holidays. Every night my father and I said the Shema prayer together (this is a central prayer of the Jewish religion). Every High Holy day we went to the synagogue and sat together. (It was a conservative synagogue that did not separate men from women. Another point in favor of my feminist beliefs.) Every Passover my father led a seder, the Passover holiday meal retelling the Jewish exodus from slavery and from Egypt, and had me invite a friend who either was not Jewish or was Jewish but from a nonreligious family. Also on Friday night, the beginning of the Shabbat, not only did we light candles (which I loved and still love) but each member of the family put a little bit of money into the Tzadaka box, a box for money for charity. My donation came from my allowance. This is where I learned that it is required of us to give to those who are less fortunate. A lesson I've carried to the present day. Perhaps this practice began my desire for a career that improves the lives of others.

From my father I learned the love of God and the religious tenets to care for those less fortunate, to pursue justice, and to mend or repair the world (tikkun o'lam). From my mother I learned that women should have a career and be able to take care of themselves, to value diversity and the principles of socialistic democracy, and on the less positive side to not be too different from others or too visible. When my mother recounted to me that she failed the teacher's exam the first time she took it because she pronounced a hard "g" in the word *long*, I saw anti-Semitism. (This pronunciation stemmed from speaking Yiddish, her first language.) My mother saw the expectation for assimilation and accepted the fact that she needed to take speech lessons prior to retaking the teaching exam. My mother supported my efforts to get rid of curly hair. I used to go to Harlem, and together with many Black women had my hair straightened. For me hair straightening was an attempt to look White and WASP. Often my mother would comment that I was lucky not to have a Jewish nose and therefore did not need to experience the pain of a nose job. (Most of my girlfriends in high school had nose jobs.)

Toward the end of high school and through my first few years of college the United States was engaged in the Vietnam War. I became an antiwar activist and began my progressive activist career. While my mother was sympathetic with my antiwar beliefs, burgeoning feminism, and understanding of racism, classism, and heterosexism, she was frightened by how public I was. This fear carried over to when I came out as a lesbian. "Can't you be a more quiet activist? Must you tell the whole world?" My father wavered between believing in my sense of social justice and his own patriotism having been a sergeant in the United States Army during WWII. During this period my father passed away, and the loss was devastating, but it increased my sense of needing to repair the world and also my sense of a need to support my Jewish identity as well as to support Israel. Both my father and my mother believed that Israel was essential for Jewish survival.

Israel became and continues to be one of the difficult issues for my activism. The conflict in Israel also added to my struggle between my desire to be visible as a Jew and my mother's desire for me to be invisible as a Jew, an activist, and a lesbian. I quickly learned that the "left," while heavily populated with people of Jewish extraction, was not a place where the visibility of Jewish issues or where the push to recognize anti-Semitism was welcomed. The Israeli/Palestinian conflict was viewed only through the eyes of the oppression of the Palestinian people. My problem with that was not over supporting the Palestinian people but over the lack of understanding that Israelis also have a need for security, and given the history of the Jewish people, Israel must survive. Part of participation in leftist causes included participation in women's liberation. While the women's movement allowed for the presence of lesbian activism, there was ambivalence here about the "pushiness" of lesbians advocating for lesbian issues and, also, the "pushiness" of Jews was not welcomed. Sometimes I could be a lesbian and sometimes I could be a Jew (primarily within the progressive Jewish community), but rarely could I be both. Judaism was invisible in the lesbian community and lesbianism was invisible in the mainstream Jewish community.

Developmentally these struggles were happening at a time that I was also considering the type of work I wanted to do. This also was a struggle for me as I tried on various majors and occupations. Becoming wealthy was never a goal. Helping people in some way was primary for me (tikkun o'lam). Mother wanted me to be a public school teacher (as she was) since this career was the easiest career for combining with raising children. My rebellious streak ruled that out. Also mother always emphasized that eventually a man would take care of me. My feminist, lesbian identity told me that wasn't going to happen. Since my favorite subject was psychology, becoming a counselor or psychologist was the career I finally settled on.

Post undergraduate I entered a master's program in school counseling. Mother was happy since this would put me into the public schools. Also, she understood this profession. School counselors did academic guidance, worked with students who were discipline problems, helped with record keeping, and administered tests. I was not satisfied. I wanted to work with people's emotional, couple, and family problems. This is what I had studied as part of my psychology undergraduate degree, and this is where I needed to focus. I was beginning to become strongly interested in sexual identity and gay and lesbian issues and wanted to work more with people struggling with this.

Eventually after a number of twists and turns including a stint in VISTA (Volunteers in Service to America) on an Indian reservation (pursue justice, mend/repair the world), I entered a doctoral program in counseling psychology. For four years every time I telephoned my mother she asked, "What is it you're studying? What is it you want to be?" I would then begin a discourse on humanistic psychology, creating an environment in which clients could grow and self-actualize while I listened to and focused all of my attention on them.

"So people pay you to listen to them? Nu, you make a living at this? Jews do this type of work?" "Yes, Mother, I make a living at this, and Freud was a Jew!"

Of course life rarely goes as planned. I ended up as a full-time professor and part-time psychologist. My sexual identity changed from lesbian to bisexual (although I still am actively pursuing the end of oppression for all people, not just bisexual people), and my Jewish identity changed from Reform Judaism (a progressive branch of the Jewish religion) to Jewish Secular Humanism, where God does not play a part (but the ethical and social underpinnings as well as ethnic traditions remain important).

Combining my Jewish values with academia was easy. The instructors for our multicultural counseling classes had me come in to explore anti-Semitism as well as gay, lesbian, and bisexual issues. The university often scheduled important meetings at the beginning of the academic year that invariably fell on my highest holy days, Rosh Hashanah and/or Yom Kippur. I joined with other Jewish faculty to protest the scheduling of these meetings. Student groups were often protesting one societal injustice or another, and it was easy to publicly express my values by attending these rallies and meetings. My sympathies with the Palestinians and outrage at the Israeli government sometimes met with criticism from other Jewish faculty, but there were Jewish and non-Jewish people at the university and in the community who shared my views. Recognizing how Judaism impacted my therapy practice in more ways than helping those in need took more awareness.

One of my clients was a Japanese American lesbian woman. I always make explicit the differences between my client and myself when those differences seem relevant. I asked her how it felt to be working with a White therapist. She said, "You're not White, you're Jewish, and that's why I chose you." Upon further exploration my client pointed out the similarities between the oppression that she and her family often experienced and the oppression that my ancestors faced. This client–therapist relationship brought me to a deeper understanding of the delicate balance Jewish Americans face between having White privilege (for those Jews who are White) and yet still facing discrimination as Jews.

Religious practices and spiritual beliefs often come up within my therapy practice. In spite of the fact that few of my clients are Jewish the beliefs and rituals I practice sometimes are helpful to clients. I have often explained the shivah practice where Jews grieve deeply for a loss for seven days. (Actually, the grief process covers a year with increasing movement from self-absorbed grief to once again being part of the world at large.) Clients experiencing loss welcome hearing about the Jewish practice that truly recognizes how grief impacts one's daily functioning. Sometimes my clients and I can develop a meaningful ritual emphasizing their beliefs while incorporating portions of the Jewish shivah process.

Because I take the Jewish holidays off from work, those clients who need to be rescheduled want to know why. My feminist practices allow me to be more transparent than therapists from other theoretical frameworks, so I tell my clients that it is a holiday for me. If they ask questions about my religion I will answer them, of course keeping my answers short so as not to interfere with their time. This not only satisfies their curiosity, but it gives them the freedom to discuss the place religion and spirituality has in their lives. I've come a long way from my early fears that Jews should not be visible about their Judaism. (The events of 9/11 brought some of my fears back, but this did not last.)

Some of my clients have been both Jewish and lesbian. My visibility as a Jewish and as a nonheterosexual (bisexual) woman helps these women explore ways to combine these two identities and these two communities. As I have stated elsewhere Jewish lesbian and bisexual women often are pressured to hide their lesbian/bisexual identity within the Jewish community and to hide their Jewish identity within the lesbian/bisexual communities. I serve as a role model for bridging these communities when possible. (None of the Jewish lesbian women I have worked with have been Orthodox Jews. Had that been the case I would have worked with them about how to continue within the Orthodox community while hiding their lesbian identity and still feeling good about themselves. Fortunately, now I would be able to refer these women to the videotape *Trembling Before God*, which covers Orthodox Jewish gay/lesbian individuals.)

It's been a difficult and yet exciting journey exploring my Judaism from childhood to the present moment. For many people their religious beliefs inform everything they do. While I no longer hold strong Jewish religious beliefs I recognize how I have been impacted by the ethical principles of Judaism. I also am very aware of how the ethnic and religious traditions still function for me. Judaism impacts my professional as well as my personal life. In teaching, research, and therapy practice I am a Jew. "Nu! You make a living at this?" "Yes, Mother, I make a living at this."

A Journey From the Big Apple to the South and Beyond

JULIE R. ANCIS

I was born in Brooklyn, New York. When I was six years old, my parents, brother, and I moved to Manhattan. I attended the local public school from 3rd to 6th grade and a private school from 7th to 12th grade. I attended undergraduate and graduate school in upstate New York and completed my doctoral internship in Maryland, right outside of Washington, DC. In all of these settings, Jews surrounded me. New York has a history, a particular flavor, that makes being Jewish perfectly fine and in fact is often celebrated. This is the case even with the great diversity that exists in New York. Thus, while two out of three of my closest friends in grade school were not Jewish—one was born in Pakistan and one in Burma, and my best friend in high school was perhaps one-eighth Jewish—I felt surrounded by people who accepted and/or "understood" Jews. They understood Jewish cultural expressions and Yiddish words; they knew the major holidays, history, experiences, and perspectives of Jews. Being Jewish is not some unknown, foreign experience to most non-Jews who grew up or spent significant time in New York City. The feeling of being "the other" did not occur until I moved south for my first academic position. It was then that I felt almost compelled to seek out other Jews.

My mother, born Helen Friendenreich, grew up in what she described as an Orthodox family. Her father was American born, with Austrian roots, and her mother was born in Austria/Poland. My mother had one sibling, a younger sister, my aunt Lily. My mother had a strong Jewish identity, growing up surrounded by aunts and cousins and living in a predominantly Jewish neighborhood, first on the lower east side of Manhattan and later Brooklyn. The message my mother conveyed was that being Jewish was significant.

It was my mother who passed down the traditions associated with so-called major Jewish holidays. From her, I inherited an appreciation of these holidays and related rituals. She told me that her mother kept a kosher home and was a real "balabust" in the kitchen. Yet, it seems that my mother grew up in a time when girls were not particularly educated in their Judaism beyond the home and kitchen. Thus, she did not know how to read Hebrew and did not know the prayers. Later in life, she traveled to Israel on a Volunteers for Israel trip and learned to read Hebrew by attending classes. Yet, I think it was difficult for my mother to carry out the religious traditions with my father being a self-declared atheist and not having a strong religious background himself. His parents fled from Tsarist Russia, the Ukraine, or Pale, where Jews were forced to live. My paternal grandfather told me the story of his own father who was beheaded by the Cosaks. As a young man, my paternal grandfather apparently met Karl Marx, as his older brother was engaged in revolutionary endeavors. Any family that remained behind and did not emigrate was killed either during the time of the Tsar or in the Holocaust.

My father, Joe Ancis, was a comic genius, well known among comedians and those in the business. He is an underground legend known as the "man behind Lenny Bruce." Despite being a self-described atheist, he was always searching for an answer, the meaning of life, trying to understand how others could believe in God. He once told me the story of how he approached some young boys in a religious section of New York who were playing basketball. He asked them if they knew of Michael Jordan and other great players. The boys indicated that they did not watch television because their Rebbe told them not to. My father then asked if their Rebbe told them to jump off a ledge, would they then do this? He could not understand this blind obedience, what he described as cultlike. I spent the summer of 1984 in Israel learning Hebrew and traveling. My father and brother came to visit me and I checked out of the Tel Aviv University dorm and into the King David Hotel to be with them. There was a convention taking place for Jewish scientists from Ivy League universities, most of whom were Orthodox. My father approached these men and inquired as to how they could be scientists at Princeton, Harvard, and the like and actually believe in God. My father had a way that enabled him to readily connect with others who quickly adored him and wanted to be in his presence as much as possible, no matter their background. One scientist offered to sit down and meet with my father to discuss how the Torah could be understood from a scientific perspective.

I think that my father desperately wanted to believe in God, but as he would say, he had a "hard time buying the story." Nonetheless, his identity was filled with a pride. When asked if he was Jewish, he would declare, "All my life." He would often relate that the three "greatest thinkers" who influenced the 20th century, Karl Marx, Sigmund Freud, and Albert Einstein, were all Jews. I received the message that this was a people and identity to be proud of, that I was part of this group of thinkers and achievers. I was taught that even though there were only 12 million Jews out of a world population of 5 billion, that Jews had received a disproportionate amount of Nobel

Prizes and had made incredible accomplishments. Despite attempts to eradicate us, the exiles, pogroms, the Holocaust, and persecution throughout the ages, we were not only here but also thriving.

Both of my parents were nonconformist. My mother was extremely creative and talented with her hands from painting to jewelry making, knitting, needlepoint, and even re-roping chairs. My father was a music, dance, and art lover who exposed me to the arts in the United States and abroad. They had my brother and me later in life, but were very youthful in terms of energy and perspective.

I received many messages about what it meant to be Jewish. One message was to be proud of my people, heritage, and related accomplishments. Another message revolved around being part of a people who experienced a history of persecution and Jew hating. My father said something to the effect that if 6 million dogs had been murdered versus Jews, in reference to the Holocaust, that there would have been more of a public outcry.

Messages about Judaism as a religion were more complicated. I have always felt as though I have been searching for my Judaism. I did not attend a religious school, we were not members of a synagogue growing up, I did not learn Hebrew as a child, I did not have a bat mitzvah ceremony, and my brother did not have a bar mitzvah ceremony. I have always felt a longing for a greater understanding of Judaism, a longing for a Jewish education, a longing to read Hebrew, to know the prayers, to connect with my religion.

In 1983, at the age of 17, I traveled to Israel with my friend from elementary school. Her stepfather had founded one of the first kibbutzim. It was an eye-opening experience. I remember seeing the Wailing/Western Wall in Jerusalem for the first time as the sun descended in the background, then standing in front of the wall with hundreds of other Jews at the start of shabbos. Approximately 30 of us, strangers, clasped hands as we stood in a circle and started singing melodies. I did not know the words of the tune. Feeling a mixture of longing, loss, joy, and reconnection, I started to cry. I was determined to learn to at least read Hebrew like so many of my Jewish peers. I took Hebrew classes in college and went back to Israel in 1984 to study the language at Tel Aviv University.

While I have often felt great longing and loss related to not having a deeper understanding and knowledge of Judaism, I always felt grounded in my strong Jewish identity. This remained solid, despite situations where I felt like "the other" or felt that I could not be open about my identity. I never not wanted to be a Jew.

Moving to the South propelled me to look deeper into my Judaism. In some ways, I was motivated by a desire to find and connect with fellow Jews. This was never an issue growing up in New York. I now found myself as the cultural other, the northerner, the "Jew" when I moved to Norfolk, Virginia, and then Atlanta, Georgia, for academic positions. I certainly felt this at other times in my travels in the United States and abroad, but these were for limited time periods, always secure in the knowledge that I would soon be returning home. In moving for prolonged periods to the South, which became my home, I was inspired to seek out other fellow Jews for comfort, camaraderie, a shared language. In addition, the longing to understand Judaism as a religious identity never waned.

Moving out of New York City resulted in an introduction to the synagogues and Jewish social networks of the South. I developed acquaintances and friends who were fellow Jews. However, these were mostly Jews who grew up with a greater religious background and were accustomed to the synagogue, who knew Hebrew and related prayers from a young age. Moreover, these were Jews who were primarily raised in the South, a cultural group different from the one I was accustomed and that took me some time to understand. In some ways, synagogue attendance and participation in Jewish related events in the south has required a certain amount of conforming, something I was not used to growing up given the nonconformist ways of my parents, upbringing in Manhattan, and particular personality. I have traveled extensively, have had friendships with people from diverse backgrounds, and was taught to appreciate the contributions of many people beyond those who were or are White and Jewish. So in some ways I felt part of and connected to this Jewish life in the south, and in other ways I felt like an outsider. Once, in a synagogue meeting where I was involved in coleading their learning institute, introductions were made around a table. Participants were mostly older congregants, and there was a great emphasis on introducing oneself by name and generational rank of membership. When it was my turn to introduce myself, I tongue in cheek proudly announced myself as first generation member from New York. My introduction did not seem to be particularly appreciated by those proud of their third, fourth, and fifth generational status. I just could not relate.

I have attended synagogues of many different denominations: Reform, Conservative, Reconstructionist, and Orthodox. Aspects of each appeal to me and others do not. I still often feel apprehensive about critiquing any one denomination as the more I learn, the more I realize how much I do not know. Orthodoxy in many ways provided me with an appreciation of Judaism for Judaism's sake. The Conservative movement has provided me with an alternative perspective to certain laws and behaviors. I have moved from a self-imposed pressure to find a place and stick with it to one where I have developed a greater appreciation of Judaism in its multiple expressions. And this has become increasingly "okay." I feel more grounded in my knowledge of Judaism, in prayers, in understanding that one's connection with Judaism may be expressed in a multitude of ways.

My daughter attends Jewish school, and I am comforted that she will know her heritage perhaps in a deeper and broader way, in some respects, than that which I was exposed to. In some ways, this is a returning to the Judaism of my ancestors. She will be able to make more informed choices regarding her Judaism and not grow up with a feeling of loss or disconnectedness from her history.

While moving to the South has resulted in perhaps a deeper search in terms of my Judaism, my fear of anti-Jewish sentiment has also revealed itself living in the South. I remember driving to a popular attraction outside of Atlanta with my daughter, who was four years old at the time. I inadvertently exited the highway too soon and found myself in a small town. I saw only White people and images associated with the lynching of Leo Frank, of Chaney, Goodman, and Schwartz, of the KKK, etc. sprang to my mind. I could feel it in my body. I was lost and needed to get out of the car and ask for directions. I recall feeling relieved that I was driving a German car, that my hair was pulled back straight instead of out in its natural curliness. I remember being very cognizant that when I talked that I did not sound like a Jew, Yankee. I was scared of being "found out." Again, this has occurred before in other places, but generally not where I "live."

TEACHING AND CLINICAL IMPLICATIONS

My experiences as a Jewish woman and the influences of gender, geographic location, socioeconomic status, sexual orientation, and life events, have translated into particular clinical sensibilities and perceptions. Much of my clinical work has occurred in the North, in Manhattan, Brooklyn, upstate New York, and the Washington, DC area. In clinical contexts, my being Jewish, for the most part, was not necessarily a salient issue. Several clinical settings in upstate New York were culturally different from my upbringing, especially in terms of the percentage of Jews as clients and supervisors. There was the Counseling Center of the Jesuit College where I completed a practicum. There was the anti-Semitic director of a substance abuse clinic where I conducted another practicum. Nevertheless, I was in my home state connected to like-minded individuals who supported my identity, and me, only a two and a half hour drive from New York City.

Teaching in the South has been a challenge to my Jewish identity and has forced me to look closer at what being Jewish means. The confluence of my northern and Jewish identity often makes me feel like a fish out of water. The majority of students I have taught are not Jewish and have had limited experiences with other Jews. In addition, the majority are from the South with relatively conservative upbringings. I have often felt very different as a Jew, as a northerner, as a feminist, as a world traveler, with a New Yorker's exposure to diversity.

The majority of the classes that I teach are in the area of multicultural counseling. I train both students studying to be master's level counselors as well as doctoral level psychologists. The challenges associated with teaching multicultural courses are sometimes compounded by internal struggles related to how my being Jewish will be understood. One area relates to whether, how, and when I self-disclose that I am Jewish. Identifying overtly as a Jew in class is still something that does not come naturally. It is a decision that involves much thinking beforehand if I should or I should not. There remains that anxiety associated with others knowing, others with limited experiences, others with stereotypes, others who harbor their own and their families' prejudices.

I often wonder to what degree the material, especially multicultural work, will be filtered through this newly acquired knowledge. Will this knowledge exacerbate students' already existing discomfort with the material and toward me? Will I serve as the target of projected negative sentiments toward Jews? Relatedly, I sometimes feel that for those resistant to multicultural material, my identity will serve as an additional excuse to dismiss the material. "Oh, what do you expect," they will say, "She is a liberal Jew from New York."

Even talking about the Holocaust, indicating that a particular theoretician was Jewish or discussing Judaism feels like I am outing myself. After all, I ask myself, how many of my non-Jewish peers are talking about issues related to this minority group in their classes? Beyond outing myself publicly as a Jew, I often feel that if I "let myself go" by expressing myself authentically via verbal and nonverbal behavior, along with talking about one or all of the aforementioned areas, students will pick up that I am a Jew. The messages I received growing up about past and present Jew hatred remain a part of my psyche, which find expression in particular contexts. These are not merely messages passed down from generation to generation. I have actually been privy to such sentiments and behavior, many times without the person's knowledge that I was Jewish. Witnessing internalized anti-Semitism among other Jews is another clue to its existence. These events have only served to validate the messages I grew up with: Be aware, it could happen again.

Relatively early in my current position, my teaching program had a relationship with another school that aims to train master's level students in Christian counseling. The focus of the other school was relatively fundamentalist in nature. Discussions about LGBT (lesbian, gay, bisexual, transgender) issues were difficult given the interpretation of such relations as sinful. Without openly disclosing my religious/ethnic identity, I always felt like the New York, liberal, feminist Jew who was trying to pollute their minds. The students were not particularly respectful, where I imagined they would be. One day I found a book titled *Jesus the Carpenter* in my mailbox. I assumed that one of the students put it in my box. I felt confused and taken aback. Could they tell I was Jewish? Was this an intentional insult? Did the person just think I needed a little Jesus in my life? What was the message?

So, anxiety related to holding an identity that is not always accepted and sometimes disdained is a personal experience, one that allows me to connect with the fears of others around their own identity. One privilege I hold is that

I can "hide" my Jewishness if need be, particularly since my last name does not reveal it. Nonetheless, the apprehension, the discomfort, the fear associated with the potentially negative sentiments of others around my identity is something I have felt in my guts. I understand what it feels like to be "the other" in terms of one's cultural identity, to not feel completely comfortable being oneself in public. This understanding allows me to empathize with clients who are or have been "the other."

The pain associated with others not understanding the historical persecution of a group to which one belongs is something I can relate to. My Jewish identity, related messages received, and readings by authors like Angela Davis and bell hooks have enabled me to see parallels in experiences of racism, sexism, heterosexism, anti-Semitism, and other social ills. I always have had difficulty understanding how those with a history of persecution are not sensitive to the plight of others who also have a history of persecution based on another identity. This realization and empathy with others enables me to encourage students to make parallels, to push them to imagine being in others' shoes, to understand the impact of discrimination and prejudice on the past and current lives of people. This is more than an intellectual exercise for me; this is a heartfelt understanding that forces me to challenge students around these issues. As a professor, I stress the relationships between an emotional and intellectual understanding, the development of clinical insight, and a therapeutic relationship.

At the same time, my experience as a Jewish woman allows me to be cautious around making interpretations about parallels between various oppressions. The ways in which Jewish women experience oppression, discrimination, and stereotyping may relate in some ways to how others experience isms. However, the prejudicial experiences they encounter are specific to their identities as Jewish women. That is, they have a particular flavor. The stereotypes of the overbearing, nagging, uncouth, in your face, obsessed about appearance and material goods Jewish woman is in many ways unique to Jewish women. Contending with these stereotypes and emotions they elicit in others is different from the stereotypes associated with other identities. Jewish women's struggles and related messages passed down from generation to generation about success, partnership, and overcoming obstacles are bound up in a particular history. While Jews are certainly not unique in their experience of oppression and discrimination, each group's oppression is unique to their own history. To proclaim to understand someone's experience because one has had similar challenges in some way is presumptuous. Again, this is relevant in a clinical setting. While I may have a degree of emotional insight into the lived experience of a Black woman as a function of my own challenges and struggles with stereotyping, I can never fully claim to "know" this experience in the core of my being as I have not lived it. Rollo May and other existential philosophers and practitioners communicated this concept on a broader level. I know how I feel when someone from a different religious/ethnic identity and/or gender claims to "know" my experience. I caution students and myself about being quick to make such a claim with the intent of "connecting" with their clients. It may in fact be perceived as a therapeutic miss, one the client may never directly communicate.

Being Jewish provides me with a particular sensitivity to differences in nonverbal and verbal expression. My expressions derive from being Jewish, growing up in New York, being raised in a upper middle socioeconomic lifestyle, having first generation American parents, having three grandparents who were born in Eastern Europe, etc. The resultant behaviors could be characterized as expressive, direct, relatively unrestrained, speaking with a singsongy intonation, in contrast to that of someone from a White Anglo-Saxon Protestant background which, from a Jewish perspective, could be seen as repressed or restricted. In addition, the concept of code switching, or adapting my speech and nonverbal gestures depending on context, is familiar to me on a personal level. I am able to provide examples in class of situations in which I have been the recipient of misinterpretations due to my cultural expressions. As such, I am able to communicate the importance of understanding cultural background and its connections to verbal and nonverbal behavior in a clinical setting. This often occurs in my counseling theories class when we watch videotapes of "master" therapists counseling culturally different clients and listen to their postsession interpretations. One session involved a White male therapist with an African American female client. The therapist labeled this seemingly very high functioning client who evidenced strong coping skills in handling life stressors as having histrionic and narcissistic features. It seemed that this diagnosis was mostly attributable to the client's culturally influenced style versus actual qualities associated with these personality disorders. My own expression and personal experiences enable me to understand such misses. As such I am able to speak about the dangers of misdiagnosis and the need for cultural competence along the lines of assessment and interpretation of behavior.

FUTURE

The longing for a more grounded understanding of Judaism has taken different forms as I have gained more life experience, sought related learning opportunities, and settle into myself as a more mature adult. Interestingly, I now have a greater understanding of the connection between practice of the religion, social justice, critical thinking, and challenge of self and others. The culture and related behaviors are intrinsically tied to religious practices, a connection that many Jews are not aware of and one that has been interesting to me.

This relative comfort with who I am is valuable in a teaching and clinical setting. The more authentic I am, the greater the ability to connect with others. I celebrate my love for the richness of Judaism. In addition, I retain my thrill at listening to a range of music from Klezmer to classical, Bob Marley, the Beatles, Led Zeppelin, Miles Davis, Aretha Franklin, Eddie Palmieri, and a multiplicity of other music and musicians. I love dancing salsa, classical and modern ballet, jazz, African styles, and other dance forms. I love paintings, sculpture, poetry, and literature. I have always appreciated the many rhythms of life as expressed in music, dance, language, paintings, food, nonverbal expression, perspective etc. I am a multicultural woman who loves the expressions of my own background and those of others. It is a wonderful feeling that I hope will continue to influence my teaching and clinical work.

Jewish in Alaska: Scanning the Room

ELLEN COLE

My mother died one month ago at the age of 89; it was her time to go. One would expect that this would be a religious or holy time for my Jewish family. Maybe a rabbi would be called on. Not so. The funeral home that arranged for her cremation (cremation, itself, not a Jewish practice) was run by the Gallaghers (not a Jewish name, I am quite sure). My father, brother, and I did not want any kind of religious service. Instead, we are going to have a party three days from now that we're envisioning as a "camp activity." My dad is calling it a "Jewish wake." My mother was a gym teacher, camp counselor, head counselor, and camp director. The family will gather in shorts and T-shirts, surrounded by photographs of this beautiful, energetic woman, and laugh and cry and share memories of her life.

Utterly secular, don't you think? Well, yes, but her camps were Jewish camps. They included Friday evening services. This is where I learned to recite the *baruchas* (*baruch atoi adenoi elohanu*). The campers and staff were all Jewish. We are asking guests to bring "Jewish camp food" to the memorial party.

I have three more short stories to tell. Then I will briefly describe my personal journey from New York to Massachusetts, Vermont, Arizona, and Alaska; explore the history and current status of Jews in Alaska; draw some conclusions from all this; and end with implications for therapists who work with Jewish clients.

Story number two: Yes, I was born and raised in New York City. I understand New York public schools are now closed for the Jewish High Holy days, but this was not so when I was a child. On Yom Kippur and Rosh Hashanah it seemed as though my brother and I were the only ones in school. You see my atheist parents didn't want to be hypocrites; we weren't going to temple, so we had to go to school. Utterly secular, but, with the notable exception of Aline Abramo, the Italian Catholic girl on the corner with whom I shared a birthday and who taught me to say "Hail Mary full of grace," my neighbors were Sheila Bernstein, Susan Kurtz, Linda Sirota, Stewie Weitzman, and Mark Train. These were Jewish kids. I thought everyone was Jewish (except for Aline). That's just how it was.

Story number three: My family celebrated Christmas. Santa came to our house through the chimney. We left cookies for him and he reciprocated with presents. We hung Christmas stockings and had a glorious Christmas tree topped with a Star of David. Never once did I think this was odd. No one in the neighborhood seemed to mind. It was quite a fun part of my childhood.

Story number four, more recent: I moved to Anchorage in 1995 at the age of 54. Just about my first week here I attended a meeting of Jews at the Fourth Avenue Theater. A couple of sociologists from Brandeis, Bernard and Joel Reisman, had just completed a study of Jews in Alaska (Reisman & Reisman, 1995). They were reporting on their findings and asking for feedback from the city's Jewish population. It was fascinating, but I felt like an imposter. I sat there wondering if I was even Jewish. How could I be? I didn't even know what Hanukkah was. At one point the facilitator did a go-round, asking for a statement from each of us. When it was my turn, I said I didn't think I could comment because I wasn't religious and I wasn't sure I could call myself a member of the Jewish community. Now there were two rabbis there. One was from Anchorage's Reform/Conservative Congregation and the other a Lubovitch. Ten years later it's still a bit of a shock to me to recall that the Lubovitch rabbi stood up (in his black hat and black suit, speaking with a heavy Eastern European accent) and said, most kindly, "Are your parents Jewish? Were your grandparents Jewish? Of course you're Jewish. Of course you can comment." And he was right.

CONTEXT MATTERS

In 1958 I graduated from New York City's Jamaica High School, where the majority of students seemed (at least from the vantage point of my memory now) to be either Jewish or Black. The Black kids were in the technical track and the Jewish kids were college prep, de facto segregation, really. We didn't share classes. I recall there being only one Black student in my classes, a very smart and handsome boy who I believe went on to Princeton. My pals had last names like Rosenberg, Wachsman, Shivak, and Schneider. Nevertheless, in this context, I didn't feel Jewish, and it wasn't important to me. I never gave it a thought. Later I moved to Boston where I attended college and graduate school. My roommates and most of my friends were still Jewish, none of us observant, and again, I didn't think much if at all of myself as Jewish.

While I was still in college I married a Jewish boy from Harvard who was the son of one of my mother's friends. In some ways, looking back, it was an arranged marriage. He was the man I was supposed to marry. The marriage lasted less than five years. By that time I had a son and was living in Vermont. I think this was really the first time that I realized—really realized—that I was Jewish and not everyone else was. It wouldn't have occurred to me to go to temple, even on the High Holy days, but I tended to gravitate toward the other Jews in my small town. We spoke the same language. We were well-educated, politically liberal, even radical in those back-to-the-land, early hippie, anti-Vietnam War days. We spoke rapidly, loudly, waving around our hands. We didn't mind talking at the same time, interrupting one another. We were, you might say, Jewish expats originally from New York.

Several decades later, married now to a wonderful non-Jewish man, we moved to Prescott, Arizona, home of over 50 churches and no temple or synagogue in sight. (Note: Since I moved to Alaska, a synagogue has been built in Prescott.) The lack of a temple wasn't an issue for me; I probably wouldn't have gone there anyway. But not having a Jewish community, pals who talked my language, felt uncomfortable. Eventually, three other Jewish women and I began to meet together about once a month. We shared our histories and drank tequila. We called ourselves the "Oy Luck Club" (*The Joy Luck Club* was a popular book at the time). Even our partners gathered together occasionally. None was Jewish, and they began to call themselves the "Goy Luck Club." We had a lot of fun. I began to realize that there was something about being Jewish that was very important to me. It was something about camaraderie, and deeper than that, a value system. Even though we were born in different parts of the country, one of us was a lesbian and a rabbi, another a heterosexual Jewish woman from a famous Jewish family who had become Buddhist, and two of us considered ourselves atheists, we came together as Jewish women. We had known since birth that we were on this earth to make it a better place, to live true to the spirit of *tikkun olam*. We were Jewish, and we were social activists; there was never a doubt about this.

Over the years it has become clear to me that as I moved further away from Jewish population centers I have identified myself more and more as Jewish. On the one hand this can be seen as maturity, self-acceptance, coming into my own, or perhaps reflecting the eighth Ericksonian stage of wisdom. On the other hand, I believe it may be more a question of the comfort that comes from the familiar, of feeling safe among "my own kind," and feeling just a tiny bit on edge when that's not the case. At my university there is only one other Jewish faculty member right now, and there is one Jewish staff member. When I am in a crowd I find myself scanning the room for a Jewish face, and I smile when I find one (even though I may of course be wrong). I smile when I hear a distinctively Jewish name. I find myself, and this has been true for a long time, gravitating toward my ethnic minority colleagues, toward the lesbians and gays on my campus, the international students (one of whom is a young Palestinian male). We have a usually unspoken common denominator. We're not really outsiders, and I wouldn't use words like "oppressed" or "nondominant," but we share a recognition that a threat or a slur or some kind of tension may be right around the next corner. We seem to have an innate desire to champion the underdog. We share a certain zest for life that may come from being that underdog. I feel these things more strongly in Alaska than I ever did in New York or Boston. Context matters.

JEWS IN ALASKA

Alaska is called "the Last Frontier," and Alaskan Jews have referred to themselves as "The Frozen Chosen." Note the inherent pride of being hearty, living on the edge, adventurous. A census of Alaskan Jews (Reisman & Reisman, 1995, p. 91) identified a "state population of 2,940 Jews, representing 1,240 Jewish households." This is "less than half of 1% of [Alaska's] general population" (p. 7). Interestingly, like most Alaskans who are not Alaska Native, "Sixty-nine percent of Alaskan Jews moved to Alaska since 1975" (p. 34), drawn not only by the frontier spirit but by the oil industry and the pipeline. One of the major findings about Alaska Jews, observant or not, from this excellent study, is "the importance they attach to being Jewish" (p. 95). Needless to say, this comes as no surprise to me. The authors speculate that this may be attributed to the difficult Alaska environment—the harsh climate causing people with similar backgrounds to band together for mutual support. This may be true to some extent. However, I believe, based on my personal experience, that wherever there is a very small Jewish population, a Jewish identity will become much more important than it might otherwise be.

If another Alaska Jew were to be writing this, he or she might be discussing the new rabbi, or the old one who was forced to leave. They might be discussing how much money was raised for the temple renovation or the United Jewish Appeal. They might be bemoaning the numbers of Jews (like me) who don't attend Friday evening services. Many Jews, even in Alaska, have and enjoy a support system that I do not. But I do not relate to Judaism through religious observance. I relate to it through culture. It's the bedrock of who I am.

IMPLICATIONS FOR THERAPY

I want to discuss here issues related to the nonobservant Jew in therapy, particularly one who lives in a community, like Alaska, with a very small Jewish population. Most important, the therapist should not wait for the client to initiate a discussion about Jewishness. Always ask. And do not assume that being Jewish means the same thing to one client as it might to the next.

Recognize that being Jewish is a religious identity to some and a cultural or ethnic identity to others. My non-Jewish friends are invariably perplexed when I say something like, "My father is a Jewish atheist." Or, "I'm Jewish, but I don't really know much about Moses, or the destruction of the temple by the Romans, or even Zionism and the Promised Land."

Some issues that *might* concern Jews like me (and do, in fact, concern me) are an occasional longing for the familiar and comfortable, a desire to know more about my religion and culture but having too many other interests to really put forth the effort to learn more, and guilt about being married to a non-Jew and not providing my children with a Jewish education. From my readings and conversations with friends, I know that this last issue is a huge problem for many, many of us. When I read Alan Dershowitz's (1997) *The Vanishing American Jew*, I thought, *Guilty as charged.* I have four grown children, not one has married a Jew, not one will raise my grandchildren as Jewish, and it's my fault. I have single-handedly killed American Jewry. Dershowitz has my number.

If it were not for the writing of this article, I do not think I would ever have even imagined bringing these issues into a therapy session. They are not the thoughts that occupy much of my consciousness. But when I stop and reflect, I realize that some of them have brought me a great deal of emotional pain. Another example: Until my husband and I visited Israel and Palestine two years ago, we could not discuss this part of the world, or anti-Semitism for that matter, without my getting extremely emotional. At a very deep level, I didn't "trust" his responses; I felt threatened and afraid, in a way I would not have if he were Jewish.

And a final example: My women friends are and have always been extremely important to me. I currently have six different groups of women with whom I associate regularly: my tennis pals, a weekly summertime hiking group, a monthly bookgroup, a small singing circle, a group of feminist faculty colleagues, and friends who gather monthly to "whine and dine." At the present time there are no other Jewish women in any of these groups (the one other Jew recently moved out-of-state). I feel sad about this, yet I truly love my friends.

I would feel fortunate to be able to explore any of the previously mentioned issues in therapy. They all relate to my being Jewish. They are all important to me. And yet none would have brought me to a therapist's door.

In 1990 I coedited, with Rachel Josefowitz Siegel, a special issue of the journal *Women & Therapy* that was a year later published as a separate book. The title was *Seen but Not Heard: Jewish Women in Therapy* (Siegel & Cole, 1991). We stated in the preface, "When Jewish women are seen in therapy, the significance of their Jewishness is not often recognized. Even Jewish clients themselves may not be aware of its impact on their lives" (p. xiii). The articles in this volume were primarily theoretical and conceptual. I did not tell my own story in this book and am grateful for the opportunity to do so here. It makes the original message ring even truer for me.

This narrative is a call to therapists to be proactive in eliciting deeper truths from Jewish clients than those that may appear on the surface, particularly for Jews who do not realize the depth of their Jewish identity. They may not be observant. They may have few Jewish friends and a non-Jewish partner and appear to be fine about this. They may live in a community with a very small Jewish population. But they may, even unwittingly, be scanning the room.

REFERENCES

Dershowitz, A. M. (1997). *The vanishing American Jew: In search of Jewish identity for the next century*. Boston: Little, Brown.

Reisman, B., & Reisman, J. I. (1995). *Life on the frontier: The Jews of Alaska*. Waltham, MA: Brandeis University.

Siegel, R. J., & Cole, E. (Eds.). (1991). *Seen but not heard: Jewish women in therapy*. Binghamton, NY: The Haworth Press.

Somewhere Else: The Geography of a Life

ELLYN KASCHAK

I was just trying to get home.
—Rosa Parks

Ben Kornetsky and Sonia Weingart met in 1918 and began "keeping company," as they called it. It meant that they would have a brief series of dates and, if nothing went wrong, become engaged to be married. It was a simple courtship, somewhere between the old country custom of arranged marriage and the American custom of choosing one's own mate. They came from a group of people at a time when mating was for life and was more about survival than romance or personal gratification.

Sonia was no greenhorn, having sailed past the Statue of Liberty with her mother, Slova, and younger brother, Gidelie, some 12 years earlier. I know nothing of the trip in steerage across the Atlantic except what I can imagine, having read numerous such accounts. Were they eager, frightened, sick, confused? I can only guess. Mine is not a family that talks about these things.

In an effort, some years ago, to affirm my own heritage, to assure myself that I did have a history and a people to whom I belonged, I was able to track down a copy of their certificate of entry into the United States. It hangs over my desk now as I write these words, material proof that I come from somewhere.

She arrived on Ellis Island, little Sonia Weingart, and left it as Sarah, undoubtedly the result of the indifferent pen of a bureaucrat who was not familiar with the name Sonia but only with Sarah, at least for a Jewish girl. She was young enough to have attended only American schools and to speak unaccented American English, although at home she spoke Yiddish, as did the rest of her family.

The three of them were met at the dock by her father, who had come first to America to escape conscription into the Czar's Army. They had all come to start a new life in America, where they were not, as Jews, confined to shtetls and subjected to the drunken whims of Cossacks and other citizens of a nation that had been practicing anti-Semitism, albeit not as efficiently, long before Hitler ever thought of the idea.

Several months before, they had walked across the border of Russia in the protection of dark night, the same way that many of today's immigrants cross from Mexico. The journey really began a year before when Sonia had held her baby brother David in her arms, silently hiding in a cellar as a drunken group of men burned and pillaged their home and the homes of all of the other Jews in the vicinity. It was a simple, but satisfying, Saturday night sport to them. To David, it was the end of his short life, as he suffocated and died in her arms. These days, we would worry about the family's post-traumatic stress. Some of us have that luxury. My ancestors worried only about escaping to a place where they could live a quiet ordinary life in peace, where the trauma had a chance of becoming "post." For them, the name of that place was America.

Once in New York, they went to live in one of the tenements on Hester Street with Aunt Etel, for whom I am named. I know nothing more about Aunt Etel, although I have asked many times. Seemingly there is nothing to tell, no more particular reason for the name I was given, no hopes or expectations connected to it. Yet mine was an American name and that was enough.

In New York, Sarah was permitted to attend school, and she completed junior high school before she was needed by her family to assume the tasks of her mother who had died, I imagine, in some form of epidemic that raged through the teeming tenements of the Lower East Side. Sarah raised her younger brothers and sisters and soon also went to work in one of the sweatshops of the garment industry, where Jewish and Irish girls sat hunched over rows and rows of identical sewing machines, selling their labor for an American dollar.

My grandfather's story was just a little different. He came from Poland by himself at the age of 14 after his father was murdered in the street outside of his small clothing shop. He was to find work and save enough money to bring his mother and sisters out of the danger of the Polish streets. He did so, but he was not able to get them all out before the Nazis, supported by the modern inventions of Henry Ford and IBM, were able to develop a smoothly running assembly line for the purpose of exterminating Jews in larger numbers. He arrived at Ellis Island as Benjamin Kornetsky and emerged as Ben Cohen, a greenhorn now easily marked as a Jew. On Ellis Island the Americans manufactured more Cohens than the entire tribe of Jews could produce in centuries, such was American efficiency.

I imagine that they were eventually introduced to each other by a relative or the local shadchan. At any rate, they married and soon moved to a small apartment in Brooklyn, which was the next stop for many of the Jews of their generation. There are no wedding photographs, no documents to give me even a hint about their early life together. In Brooklyn they raised three children: my mother, the oldest, and her two younger brothers. Eventually the whole family on both sides was living in Brooklyn and was able to maintain an extended family through that one generation, a kind of American shtetl. By the next generation, a more American pattern of suburban migration, combined with the many nurtured wounds and feuds of a Jewish family, led to separation and fragmentation.

Ben had gone right to work as a peddler and eventually in the sweat-shops, where he spent an entire lifetime sewing collars onto men's jackets. They called his assembly line *piecework* and he called his short subway ride from Brooklyn "going to the place." Ben never was able to attend school or learn to read or write in English. His speech remained forever accented by his native Yiddish. When he finally was eligible to become an American citizen, it took his wife, Sarah, and my mother three months to teach him to sign his name.

Although I know only this much about my mother's side, shards of information, of my father's family, I know even less. His parents were Charlotte Friedlander (this is close, but not exactly the right name, as my mother claims not to remember her name) and Samuel Uram. I assume that they arrived here in much the same way and also as young children. I do not remember this grandfather very well, but my grandmother, who lived into my adult years, also spoke unaccented English. I have been able to trace Samuel's arrival on Ellis Island with his parents, but not Charlotte's, if that was her name.

My father was the youngest of their five children and the only male to survive into adulthood. His older brother, whom he idolized as many younger brothers do, died at 17. My father kept a framed photo of his brother on his night table for the entire rest of his life. We children were not permitted to mention this photo of our young uncle, as it might upset his brother. Yet that boy inside the picture frame watched the entire life of our family day by day until his baby brother became an old man.

My mother, a woman exquisitely sensitive to actual or imagined slights, which then blossomed and grew under her careful nurturance, sustained an unknown injury from my father's parents on her wedding day and harbored a growing resentment as the years passed. As she felt that they did not like her, she decided to like them even less and kept her children from them as much as possible. I grew up addressing them by their last name, Grandma and Grandpa Uram. My mother's parents were Nana and Grandpa.

My own parents, Celia and Bernie, were the first generation to come by their American names naturally. They both were able to finish high school before "going to business" in the city. I do not know what business it was, but I do know that, with their high school diplomas in hand, they were able to find work in the offices of Manhattan and not on the assembly line. These were the offices of small firms, as the large corporations all had formal policies against hiring Jews. You could get one of those jobs only if you had the inclination and the ability to pass. Celia and Bernie did not, although one of my uncles changed his name to Corbin for that very purpose.

They met at a union organizing meeting when they were both 19. I cannot imagine either of them at a remotely political event and, if this story is true, they certainly never again associated themselves with politics in any way. Once, as a child, I asked my mother if she was going to vote for Eisenhower or Stevenson, and she replied that, as an American, she had the right not to tell me. And she never has. She exercised her family's hard-earned rights with determination.

Bernie proposed on their first date and they soon were married, despite my Nana's objections. He apparently was too skinny and "funny looking," too sarcastic, and had no financial prospects. I am told that he wore a long topcoat well out of fashion and would not wear his glasses so that he snubbed everyone he knew when he passed them on the street. As for the sarcasm, I have no doubts that he and Nana must have battled it out, as this was also one of her talents (I come by it honestly on both sides.). Nevertheless, my mother again exercised her American right to decide for herself and married this boy. I can hardly imagine them at 19, two children deciding to spend their lives together. And they did, until he died 54 years later of the same disease that had taken his brother.

To me, they became "Mommy" and "Daddy," these two children. Two years after their marriage, in the middle of WWII, I was born. My father had been unexpectedly drafted into the army despite his severe nearsightedness. The war had reached a point where they were taking everyone. As a result, he and I did not meet until I was five months old. My mother felt that, with no husband in sight, she was being silently accused of carrying an illegitimate child. I was that illegitimate child. I do not know exactly what kind of child they wanted, but I do know, from an entire childhood of hearing it, that I was not it. A boy instead of a girl. Of course, but this was not all. An obedient child. One who would grow up and live next door, never leave the shtetl, never rebel and never question authority. Did they ever get the wrong child! Some delivery service went out of business after filling that order.

Celia returned to work in order to save money for the time when she would be reunited with her husband and Nana quit her job to stay home with me. She had raised her brothers and sisters and her own children and started over once again with me. She was a young 42 at the time but kept her old country ways throughout her life, as did Grandpa. This and my very new, young eyes always made them look like little old people to me. I am well beyond their age now and I often wonder, if I could see them now, whether they would look like youngsters to me or like the little old immigrants that they were all their lives. In fact, I am already close to the age when Nana died, but I am getting ahead of myself by at least half a century.

I was raised by Nana for the first two years of my life with the woman called "Mommy" a visitor on nights and weekends. Grandpa took me for walks from time to time and to the neighborhood park, where "he put me on the swings," but the function of a man in those days and in my family did not extend any further. Raising children was women's work and women's business. Especially girl children. So the family lineage of oldest daughters extended from Slova to Nana to Mommy to me.

One day, the war ended and Bernie returned home to Celia and to their new daughter, Ellyn. Of his return I know only this much. He came by train to Penn Station, where he got on the subway and took the train to 18th Avenue in Brooklyn. From there, he walked to Nana and Grandpa's apartment on 53rd Street and knocked on the door to claim his wife and child. I do not know why no one met his train.

We all lived in that small Brooklyn apartment until one day, when, as it was told to me, he had had enough of battling with Nana for control of her terrain. Daddy went out and rented an apartment for the three of us. It was just a little further down 18th Avenue, a third floor walkup at a monthly rent of $40. Suddenly I was alone with these two strangers.

I remember that apartment well because we lived there for many years, for most of my childhood, in fact. It was a one bedroom apartment. Mommy and Daddy slept in the bedroom and Ellyn slept on a cot in the living room at night. The room was painted a fashionably dark maroon, the furniture covered in large tropical flower prints, retro styles that are much sought after today. During the day, I played in the courtyard where all of the mothers hung their laundry out to dry on clotheslines that extended from one kitchen window to another and supervised their young children out of those same windows. At supper time, the mothers, one by one, hung themselves out the windows and called for their children. When the ice cream man came by on summer days, the children called up to their mothers to throw down a coin or two for ice cream. Commerce was conducted at a high and insistent volume through these windows. Finally at about five or so, I was old enough to escape to the streets on my own, to the endless games of punch ball and the adventure of roaming our neighborhood, which was about three blocks long and two wide. But those blocks contained within themselves an empty lot, three candy stores, and several friends of the same age—an entire universe, in other words.

In that Brooklyn neighborhood I soon found my best friend, Bruce, right next door. He was two years younger than I and when his mother brought him home for the first time I knocked on the door or "called for him" to ask if he could come out to play. I was ever eager. Eventually he was able to, but not just yet. Once he could, we became inseparable adventurers of the streets until adolescence finally separated us by gender. In that decade, it was not possible for a teenage boy and girl to be close friends, but only to date, which was not what our relationship was. So we both moved on and away from each other to friends of the same gender. That was permitted.

Shortly thereafter, my sister Cheryl was born, looking nothing like me or my parents. She looked instead like a Chinese baby. If it were anyone but my mother, I would be suspicious and sometimes, even now, I joke with Cheryl about having had different fathers. But Nana had Asian features and my mother's brother Marty had a Mongolian-looking face. The Cossacks, the rapists from the old country, had followed us to the new world hidden in our genes.

Yet Cheryl was only alien *looking*; I was the true alien to my particular family. I could have been from the Williamsburg section of Mars for all they understood about my intellectual ambitions, my love for school and for learning and for reading and the world of ideas. This was no better and no worse than my love of sports and of adventure on the streets of New York. None of this was, in their minds, proper for a young girl, and they discouraged it all or, at best, tried to ignore it.

I resisted captivity. My mother rarely knew where I was as I got old enough to be somewhere else. I felt happiest and safest on the streets. She began to call me the Wandering Jew with a mixture of pride, puzzlement and dismay. But if I came home even five minutes late I was met with uncontrolled screaming and arms flailing wildly, release for her own terror: "You could have been lying dead in the street." Two lifetimes away, the Cossacks of her mother's childhood pursued her own daughter down the streets of Brooklyn.

Yet I would not be deterred; they could not break my spirit. I was, after all, an American girl. I lived as much of my life as I could on the streets of Brooklyn with my friends. I passed the rest of my time in the delicious world of books, where people led interesting and satisfying lives, had real talks about real things instead of complaining about and accusing one another, instead of keeping everything secret. I was content, at least for the time being, with the weekly bus ride to the library and the punch ball games in the street. And soon I had school to add to the list. I loved it from the first. There I got attention for my intelligence and humor that I did not get at home. Yet there I was also a problem child, would not sit still, would not be quiet, and would never do my homework, as I considered it boring and a waste of my precious time. I guess I was showing off. Causing trouble was my destiny.

Repeated cultural wounds eventually turn to individual suffering, as context becomes self. I can only imagine the wounds sustained, the centuries of terror and vulnerability that finally lodge themselves in the psyche, in the hearts and in the cells of an entire group and so an individual. Turned eventually into what psychology names individual pathology, passed down from mother to child, in my family, oldest daughter to oldest daughter as part of the mamaloshen. Be careful. Trust no one, especially yourself. Like so many African-American mothers who have had to warn their children and who wait anxiously every time they go out to see whether they arrive home that day intact.

And so I grew up on the streets of Brooklyn, in a neighborhood where everyone was either Jewish or Italian. It did not matter to any of us children except on Saturdays, when our walk home from the matinee included a mandatory stop at the local Catholic Church, where the Catholics among us would go to confession while the Jews waited outside on the steps guiltily, sure that we would be struck down if we so much as entered a church. For that time, on those steps, I was first and foremost a Jew, and, of course, on Christmas. I was also a Jew on what we called the Jewish holidays, when the Jewish students got an extra few days off from school. No big deal. Many years later I found myself in Israel on Christmas day and was amazed at how moved I was by the fact that it was just another day, December 25th. It was not a day to watch from outside as Americans celebrated, as if our 4th of July was to be celebrated on the 5th.

One more moment of acknowledged difference: At the beginning of each assembly in P.S. 180, all of the students recited the Lord's Prayer. I did not really know what it was, but was told with the other Jewish students not to recite it, to stand silent. This was a lot like music class, where the teacher went around listening to each voice and then told me and some others not to sing again but to "mouth" the words. Yet I did not think I was "mouthing the words" to "I am an American." These were only details.

Many years later, when I went to Costa Rica for the first time, someone asked me if I was a Jew or an American. I did not understand the question at first, but now, after 40 years of living part time in Costa Rica, I do. There you cannot be both. I had a slight feeling of superiority. In the United States we do not make these distinctions, I thought. I am glad that my grandparents came here and not to Costa Rica, as did the grandparents of many of my friends. Not that they were given a choice. They were lucky to be accepted anywhere and not to have their ship turned back to Europe.

I remember the Jewish holidays in Brooklyn. The family gathered in Nana and Grandpa's apartment. The table that folded up to stand against the wall was opened and filled the entire living room. My aunt and uncles and cousins were all there. This was before my parents stopped talking to them. The steam heat that was controlled only in the basement of the building almost always made the apartment too hot and even more so with all the food cooking in the oven. In the kitchen, the women all cooked. In the living room, the men watched football or any other sport that was being televised. If there was no game on television, they played pinochle. There was nothing of interest to me in either room. I longed to escape to the streets. But these were not my streets nor were my friends in this neighborhood. So instead I would wait for grandpa to put on his gray topcoat and hat and to set out on the five block walk to his shul, his prayer book in a blue velvet container under his arm. Only grandpa went to do this old-fashioned and foreign activity, yet I found it intriguing and always went with him to this small storefront shul. At this age, I was still permitted to sit among the men. Later on I would be required to sit behind the curtain in the women's section, an impediment to the concentrated holiness of the men.

A MINYAN OF WOMEN

A few years later, my parents followed the rest of their generation to the newly minted suburbs of Long Island, a 30 minute ride on the Belt Parkway and a world away. We moved to Valley Stream, which I once saw described in the newspaper, and rightfully, as a bleak working class suburb. It looked and felt like a desert to me, row upon row of identical little houses with identical stick trees in front of each, where shortly before an ancient forest had stood. Everything was 1950's modern, stark symbols of upward mobility. Yet I wanted only the horizontal mobility of the neighborhood. I longed for my old friends, for the streets and alleys of Brooklyn, for the corner candy stores and the street games. I was from somewhere else, back where Nana and Grandpa still walked those familiar streets without me.

Yet I was resilient enough. I made new friends on these new streets and I even eventually made friends with the streets themselves. But in the beginning, they only looked empty and too new to me.

I tried to continue going to shul without Grandpa. In the suburbs, it was a big fancy building and was called a temple. For about a year, when I was eleven years old, I got up every Saturday morning and walked the two miles to temple by myself. Once there, I sat in the back row through the entire service. Although the women and girls were not separated from the men by a curtain in this conservative temple, I was separate enough to be completely invisible to them. At the end of each service, there would be a gathering for wine, grape juice, and food. No one ever spoke to this little girl, trying so hard to belong somewhere, to find...what? At the end of this year, she became a secular Jew, no longer interested in religion.

Still today I consider being Jewish my ethnicity, my culture. I do not practice the religion, at least in a systematic way. Somehow, in my mind, it still belongs to the men. Once in a while, I might light a candle or attend a service, particularly those focused on social justice. I do, however, finally have a serious spiritual practice. It is fairly eclectic, but based mainly in Buddhism. This is so for many Jews of my generation. I see Buddhism as an antidote, as soothing, quiet, a way to reduce our inherited terror and sorrow.

I lived for the time I could leave the confinement of the suburbs with their carefully enforced and reinforced 1950's rules about gender. My way out would be through education. For generations of my ancestors, it was a way in, but they were not girls. No one supported this aim, but neither did they try to stop me. By this time they were exhausted by my insistence on my own life and could only yield and hope that I did not ruin my eligibility for marriage with too much education. I found a scholarship and won it; I found a job to pay for the rest, and I went to college. For me it was not ordinary, but a triumph.

I was on my way to somewhere else, somewhere larger, more interesting, and no longer forbidden to me. It was my own form of freedom and of surreptitiously crossing the border. I found a way to study and learn, although I had to give up punch ball and the streets to do it.

A MINYAN OF WOMEN

As a student, I was interested in the largest questions about human life, and they could have led me to the study of literature, philosophy, or psychology. In fact, they did. I did not like having to choose, to turn my back on one for the other. (I am more this way than I like to admit in many relationships outside of the academic disciplines.) As an undergraduate, I studied languages and literature, specializing in the work of Chekhov. I consider him, along with Dostoevsky, my first supervisor. I finally made a commitment to psychology in graduate school but never swore to forsake all others.

I wanted to study and understand individuals and cultures, to speak many languages, and to walk many foreign streets to hear them spoken. It was my Brooklyn writ large. If I was thinking about gender at all, I was thinking about how to escape it or, at least, circumvent it so that I could have the life I had dreamt for myself. Gender had long since been invented, but not yet discovered. It was that discovery that would change my life and occupy the women of my own generation. We were about to begin a struggle of our own for full citizenship in our own America.

I became a psychologist and a feminist at the same time and they intertwined irrevocably for me and my generation. It came as a shock, came at us with the force of a tsunami, that second wave of feminism. It touched our lives, our studies, and our work. So much that had seemed objective was slowly revealed to be imbued with gender bias, cultural bias, and racial bias. Why hadn't we seen it? A culture too can keep its secrets.

As a therapist, I was finally in a position to insist on hearing the real story. (This is not the moment to indulge my philosophical bent and discuss this complex issue, but I am a true believer in material reality, although not to the exclusion of other realities. That is, whatever the meanings involved, if someone's fist hits someone else's face, that is the material truth of the event). It was a lot better than secrets or no story at all. I was captivated by the questions and the sense, at last, that I had not only the right, but the obligation to ask and to keep asking questions until I got some answers that felt true and that proved true. And the social justice folded into feminist therapy also captured my heart and not just my mind. The personal application, the societal application, and the passion did not have to be separated. I did not have to forsake any of them.

Each life is lived on a multidimensional, living, breathing map much like a beating heart or a functioning brain. This map is always in motion and morphing, as certain feelings or concerns become more central and more salient for an individual, a community, or an entire culture. It is never static, and it is a representation of what matters in that person's life or that society's focus. It is a mattering map (Goldstein, 1993; Kaschak, 1992). On this map, contextual influences do not so much intersect as they combine and separate, meld together seamlessly with different vectors or gravitational pull.

Being Jewish was centrally located on my grandparents' maps and even on those of my parents, albeit in a different way. But on the map of my own generation and particularly on my own individual mattering map, this was not the case. My life was to be marked more intensely and clearly by the rigidly gendered world of the 1950s and the liberation movement that we founded to free ourselves. As my grandparents walked out of Eastern Europe at night, I walked right out of the gendered world of my upbringing in the light of day. My America was as much a time as a place.

This is a very ordinary story, yet one by which I am haunted. My mattering map is adorned with question marks, rendering these ghostly presences even more ephemeral. There are no simple answers; I can be sure of nothing but the questions.

And yet, as I was wondering how to end this story, since it has not actually ended yet, these ancestors expressed their opinions, albeit in dream form. In this dream, they are all hiding for their own safety deep in a cellar in an unidentifiable foreign country. They do not speak to me or to one another. On the wall of the cavelike room are written two Yiddish words: *Mitten drinnen*. As I awaken, I try to recall what these words mean. I remember hearing the phrase and my impression is that it was used when I was interrupting or annoying them. "Stop bothering me." Am I bothering them yet again?

In the 21st century, the definition is a keystroke away on Google. *Mitten drinnen* means "in the middle of everything." So my impression from childhood that I was bothering them in the middle of something more important was correct. It meant "Stop bothering me," the message clear from the tone if not the words themselves. In a slightly different tone, the dream also suggests that they were in the middle of hiding as a way to find safety and that, in their minds, silence ensured that safety. While I understand that approach, I am taking the risk of telling, as we used to say on those Brooklyn streets. Here I am telling on them. Yet here I am, also in the middle of everything, more than halfway through a complicated and rich life, stopping to look back and to find that they are not just secreted back in my early memories, but, at the very same time, here, there, and everywhere. *Mitten drinnen*.

REFERENCES

Goldstein, R. (1993). *The mind–body problem*. New York: Penguin Books.
Kaschak, E. (1992). *Engendered lives: A new psychology of women's experience*. New York: Basic Books.

Beyond Silence and Survival

DORITH BRODBAR

I was born in Tel-Aviv, Israel, where being Jewish was my right at birth. When I was three years old I came to New York City speaking only Hebrew and with little explanation from my family about where we were or what was happening. Initially we lived with my maternal aunt and her family in their Bronx apartment; however, within a month of our arrival we moved into our own apartment in a building across the street. My mother's parents, eldest sister, and her family soon followed. In a short period of time we all lived within a one block radius of one another in what was then a predominantly Jewish neighborhood in the West Bronx. Our family was close, and we came together at least once every week. It was common for us to frequent the neighborhood synagogues during Jewish holidays where my father and brother sang in the choir. I attended a day camp and after school activities with one of my cousins. Interaction with family and the broader community of immigrants from Israel was constant.

Hanukkah was joyously celebrated. We all huddled together to light candles, sing the blessing in harmony, and then gleefully open our presents. On Purim we dressed in costumes. Simchas Torah was spent at my grandfather's one room orthodox synagogue. We circled in front of the alter that held the Torahs, holding paper Israeli flags with apples stuck on top. The Passover seder was conducted in its entirety. The Haggadah, which tells the story of the enslavement of the Jewish people in Egypt and their long journey to freedom, was recited in Hebrew. My grandfather sat at the head of the table leading the recitation. All the other males followed closely and the rest of us joined in to sing the songs. My mother was always the most fluent and proudly held her own as the songs would increase in complexity and speed. There was a childlike enthusiasm and competitive quality to her singing. I suspect that when she sang those songs she was taken back to a time in her childhood in Germany when her relatives from Poland would come to join the family at their seder table. My mother always spoke fondly of this family, especially her cousins, Ignaz and Kaszik. All of her Polish family, including her beloved Ignaz and Kaszik, were lost during the Holocaust.

Now, during our seders, she sometimes appears as if transported back to that time in memory, exuding the same joy and passion she once shared with her now forever lost cousins singing those same Hebrew verses. It is as if reality is momentarily suspended, allowing her to be in their presence once more. Paradoxically, the enormity of the sorrow that she must have experienced having lost so many significant people in her life never seemed to surface at these moments. It was as though any hint of sadness may have threatened the moment. The enormity of her loss and pain was always very far removed. She has been so successful at concealing that pain that only in recent years did I become aware of just how close she came to annihilation and of the terror that was an everyday occurrence in her life for her childhood and for many years after that.

My mother was born, Erna Bakel in Berlin, Germany, in 1926. When I asked my mother about her life in Germany, the first thing she recalled was being ostracized by classmates who refused to shower with a Jewish girl. She was six years old when this happened, now 75 years ago. Despite how painful this recollection must have been there was no outward expression of pain on her face or in her voice as she recollected it. She might just as well have been telling a story about something mundane. The pain associated with this memory and many others were buried deep within her long ago and came to be expressed only in silence and in the form of the physical ailments that constantly plague her. I remember when I was growing up my mother constantly complained about the great pain that many physical ailments caused her. She expressed great sadness, hopelessness, and power-lessness over this pain. Now, in her older years, when bodily aches and pains that are a consequence of aging become more frequent, she has been able to acknowledge feeling emotional pain and owns feelings of depression. How-ever, she attributes feeling depressed to her physical pain and the limitations it imposes. She often says "Who wouldn't be depressed living with this pain!" She has experimented with antidepressants that she refers to as "mood enhancers" and for a time seemed to feel somewhat better. However, she never attributed her improvement to the medication and often abruptly stops taking it exclaiming, "They weren't doing anything." Following this, she would complain about her physical pain, and the pattern continues.

In Berlin, when mother was growing up, verbal and physical assaults on Jewish school children were common. Boys were especially targeted. Some, like my uncle, had to simply endure, but many, like my mother's family, moved so that she and her two elder sisters and brother could attend the "Jewish school." She was seven when they moved to an apartment on Muenz Strasse, "the only apartment with a balcony," she boasted. They were sur-rounded by Grenadier Strasse where there were many Jewish merchants with prostitutes soliciting business only one block away. She recalled that there were many different kinds of people living in their building. One of her neighbors was a communist man whom she later discovered joined the Nazi party. Another neighbor was a "Rebbe" who survived because he was a war hero from WWI. By the mid-1930s, her family was barred from going to their summer rental by the lake because "Jews were no longer allowed to swim." Jews could not sit on the bus stop benches. My mother and her siblings joined Zionist organizations, and her house became the place where all of their friends would gather to sing their Zionist songs. She recalls stopping on a street corner during this time to hear a charismatic man speaking to a large gathering of people. She quickly realized that the man was Adolf Hitler speaking from a platform on Unter Den Linden, a broad and expansive street that she described as analogous to the Champs Elysee in Paris. She recalled feeling drawn to his powerful oration but suddenly realized that being Jewish placed her in imminent danger. She briskly moved on. As a young girl entering adolescence, my mother was an excellent student and avid reader. It is hard to know how, as a Jew, she made sense of what was happening at that time in Nazi Germany.

During this period there were quotas on the number of Jews who could leave Germany and enter Palestine. As anti-Semitism grew worse and the climate for Jews became more ominous, many Jews wanted to flee Germany. My mother and her family dreamt of the day that they could leave for Palestine. Her brother escaped with some friends. Her eldest sister studied to become a "baby nurse" and was able to go to Palestine with her classmates. My mother, her parents, and older sister waited anxiously behind. Two weeks before "Kristallnacht" her family was granted permission to leave Germany for Palestine. "Kristallnacht," translated as the "Night of Broken Glass," has been regarded as the beginning of Hitler's "Final Solution," the plan to exterminate all Jews. Another family was originally selected to leave Germany but had already been sent to the concentration camps. This created an opportunity for my mother's family to leave in their place. My mother always jokes that this was her lucky moment in life and that she has never won anything since. Mother's family left Germany with virtually none of their belongings. They watched as the non-Jewish family contentedly examined and took over their apartment, with their furnishings, their belongings, and the piano that her sister played while my mother danced. They had to leave everything behind. In addition to their belongings they also lost the yearly winter and summer family visits with her close extended family in Kalish, Poland, and the cousin's visits to my mother's home in Berlin for the Passover holidays.

My mother, her parents and her sister went to a facility in Trieste, Italy, where Jews were sent to await their departure to Palestine by ship. Leaving her country of birth, her family, and all of her possessions when barely 12 years old, she developed an anger that remained with her for the rest of her life. At this time she changed her name from Erna to Esther during her passage from Germany to Palestine. The name Erna was German; Esther was Hebrew. In rejecting her German name I suspect that she was also rejecting the country that she had loved but that had come to betray her. It was an assertion of her Hebraic, Jewish identity and pride. Hebrew, with its new alphabet, was difficult to master, making reading a challenge. School, once a haven for her, was no longer enjoyable. Money was sparse and the family was forced to separate for a time. My mother and her sister slept in the book binding shop that belonged to their grandfather and smelled of glue. My mother was able to read English while still in Germany and now, surrounded by books, quickly escaped into the world of reading that continues to this day. Forced to begin working when she was 13, she was never able to continue her academic studies, yet another loss for her.

My mother's life in Israel was happy and memorable despite the fact that she and her friends all shared an unspoken and painful past and an unstable present. She describes being popular among her friends and was an excellent gymnast. It was this carefree and happy image of life that my mother always presented whenever I would ask about what her early life was like. The wonderful memories of her popularity among young men, her active social life, and competitions as a gymnast in the "Macabia," comparable to the Olympics in Israel, would be the focus of her response. She never discussed her childhood in Germany. It was not until I visited the Holocaust Museum in Washington, DC, that I realized that the time frame of the events on display was the time my mother was growing up in Germany. I also realized that the reality of my mother's early life could not have been as carefree as she depicted. Rather, they were years of progressive loss of rights and status. When I asked her why she never revealed the true nature of her past she replied that whenever she has done so she was told that because she had never been in a concentration camp, she was not a real Holocaust survivor, thus minimizing her experience of pain, degradation, and loss. There was no one who would validate the pain these experiences caused her, and it became easier to remain silent. I am convinced that her anguish came to be expressed in the agony of recurrent, distressing bodily pains. However these intense emotions and disconnected, displaced affects remained buried deep inside her, literally causing her body to hurt.

It was ironic to me that my mother's survival from so much danger and loss would be used to minimize her pain. It was as if her survival negated the trauma that she suffered in the course of her survival. That minimization in some ways retraumatized her and even taught her to minimize the impact of her own experiences. Like many people for whom somatization is a way of carrying in one's body that which you are not permitted to express psychically or emotionally, she was forced to suffer in silence, speaking of her pain only if it could be located in her body. To do otherwise would mean having that pain ignored altogether. I came to understand her silence and need to put a positive spin on so many of her early experiences.

My father, Salm, was 10 years older than my mother, born in Vienna, Austria, in 1916. His father was a very religious man who some described as an ultra orthodox "fanatic." What little I recall of him was that he was a scary bearded man who frightened me. I don't remember his mother but I am told that she was a sweet woman who worked very hard in the dairy restaurant they owned while my grandfather went to Suhl every day, where he studied the Torah. My father was the next to the youngest child of four. He had two older brothers and a sister just a year younger than him. His middle brother died of measles, and much of his mother's attention then focused on his older brother and younger sister. Like the typical middle child he got little attention from his parents and experienced his father as mean to him. Of the few occasions that I recall seeing my father cry, he did so when his mother died, his father having passed on long before. The other time was when my brother left home to go to college.

I am told that my father's original family name was Breitbart. The name was associated with someone in Jewish history who was a strong man, who would lie on a bed of nails or engage in other feats of strength. The problem was that he did these things on the Sabbath, violating an important observance of Jewish law. I am also told that my grandfather and others who shared this last name did not want to be associated with someone who did not observe the Sabbath and changed their name to Brodbar. When my father was barely five years old, my grandfather would send him out to other Jewish homes to teach them to read the Bible in Hebrew. He was very proud of his ability to do this and wanted desperately to please his taciturn father. According to my father, his relationship with my grandfather deteriorated when as a small boy he took himself to get a haircut hoping it would please his father. He did not know that it was forbidden to do this on the Sabbath. He was only a child trying to please his father. He recalls that his father was furious and that their relationship was never the same. He always maintained that his father never forgave him this childhood transgression and was always mean to him after this. My mother and other family members support this perception allowing that his father always treated him badly.

When my father was 13 and it was time for his bar mitzvah he looked forward to being presented with his first pair of long pants. This was the custom for all Jewish boys as long pants symbolized their entrance into manhood. My father never received his long pants. He was forced to endure the humiliation of reciting his Havtorah passage from the Bible in short pants. Dad became a soccer player, requiring him to attend games on the Sabbath. I have always felt that his failure to observe the Sabbath, by playing soccer, was his way of rebelling against his rigid and rejecting father. Even decades later as an older man and a father himself I could hear the hurt and disappointment in his voice whenever he recalled this important milestone. I often felt that a sense of humiliation was always with him and that he never felt wholly successful. I have also sensed that his own disappointment in his ability to gain his father's pride and love left him conflicted about the success of his children. As he grew older conflict gave way to a capacity to encourage me in my education and career, which made it easier to pursue my graduate study. Although he died long before I completed my doctoral studies, I do feel that he would have been happy for me and proud of what I had accomplished.

Despite my grandfather's rigid, unforgiving orthodoxy, it does seem that my father developed a sense of fondness for religious belief. Later in my life when I would complain about my difficulty relating to the Jewish community in our neighborhood in Queens and express bewilderment at what kind of Jews they were, he would tell me that if I wanted to find nice Jews, I should read the Bible. After his death in the mid-1980s, I recall clinging to the Bible searching for some comfort in the words but not making it past the "begats." Still, this was an important connection to my father, and I held on.

My father joined the British army and was actively involved in helping Jews escape persecution, transporting them into Palestine on a motorcycle. Later he joined the Israeli army and ironically fought against the British to gain Israel's independence in 1948. My father fought in a number of wars and received numerous medals, but never talked about them or his service. He implied that he spent some time with the Israeli underground but would provide us with no details, and he never spoke of his medals as something to be proud of. During the years that my father was in the army and before my parents were married, he saved his money and purchased land in the countryside in a town called Ramat Hasharon. My mother recalled that my father, who loved nature, would lie under the trees and dream about the house that he would eventually build on this land. My parents were married in 1948, the same year of Israel's independence. My mother described their wedding day as one where they traveled to the synagogue lying on the floor of my father's taxi in order to avoid the crossfire of bullets. They moved in with her parents, sleeping in the living room where they stayed until my brother was five months old. My father eventually had a house built on his land in Ramat Hasharon, where my parents moved with my brother for a short time. My mother felt very isolated in the countryside, so they sold the house for an apartment in Tel-Aviv. It was in this apartment, in the heart of the city, that I spent the first three years of my life.

My father's younger sister immigrated to London from Vienna and brought their parents with her. In London his sister was a famous actress, Riki Barr, but she eventually left the stage to marry an obstetrician who did not approve of her career. At that time the entire family joined my parents in Israel.

In 1957, my family left Israel, because my father was constantly being called to serve in the army reserves, leaving very little opportunity to earn an income from his taxi. He was obliged to pay taxes on his taxi business even though he was rarely at home long enough to earn a living from it. My father was a skilled mechanic in the aviation industry and had hopes of being promoted, but his politics at the time interfered. My parents decided to apply to emigrate to the United States, sponsored by one of my mother's sisters. They thought the process would take a few years and were unprepared when they were notified in two weeks after applying that they could come to America. Once again my mother had to quickly pack to leave the place that had become her home. The emotional reverberations of unspoken separations and losses of the past seemed to have intensified her sadness. Her unhappiness lingered for the first eight years that we lived in New York until she could finally return to Israel for a visit. I was keenly aware of her unhappiness and vividly recall the time she left for this visit. I was 11 and thought that I would never see her again. I was convinced that she would never return. At the same time my brother and I were being sent off to a Zionist sleep away camp. I recall feeling filled with sadness the night before our departure and openly weeping. My family assumed that I was crying because I did not want to go to camp. No one understood that I was weeping for the anticipated loss of my mother. In some ways I suppose I had actually lost her a long time before. Perhaps the abrupt departure from Israel was just one more in a painful accumulation of losses that she simply could not overcome.

My father was somewhat of a character in his own right. He would later regale us with stories about growing up on the same street as the Freud's in Vienna. He often maintained that he asked Anna Freud out on dates but that she thought he was beneath her. Our father could tell stories like this and leave you wondering how much was true and how much was a part of his inventive imagination. My brother and I once determined that Anna Freud would have been 21 years older than our father, which, if his story was true, might explain her not taking him seriously. Despite deciding that this tale was probably not true, there was a way that he could tell such a tale that always left us wondering if it actually did happen as he said.

During the time we lived in the Bronx my father was busy with his friends organizing a club called "The Israelis of New York." This was a group of Israeli immigrants and their families who gathered to celebrate holidays, and go on Sunday outings to various parks in the New York/New Jersey vicinity. I recall these excursions beginning in Gimbels' parking lot, all of the cars displaying Israeli flags attached to antennas. My father would always lead the procession to their destination where families would enjoy a day of picnicking and play. The air buzzed with the languages of these refugees sometimes flowing together in one sentence. The children, Americans in the making, conversed in English and played baseball and football, sports that were foreign to their parents. On the one hand I identified with the image of Israeli pride and my Jewish heritage. Being Jewish meant family and strong ties to others who identified and practiced similarly to me. However, at the same time, another experience of being Jewish was developing. This new sense of Jewishness was based on my early encounters with anti-Semitism and the resulting feelings of fear and shame. One morning the words "Go Home Jew Bastard" were scrawled on a mailbox. I recall

Catholic parochial school children, still dressed in their school uniforms, running after me screaming anti-Semitic slurs and I have vivid memories of the corner store clerk telling my mother to go back to where she came from. Despite the anti-Semitism I confronted in the Bronx, the proximity of my extended family provided a sense of security.

My mother did return to us after her visit to Israel, and soon after this my family left the Bronx and moved to Queens. Being separated from my extended family in the Bronx also further affected my feelings and perceptions about being Jewish. I lost an important buffer that my extended family provided. The Jewish people I met in Queens seemed unfamiliar to me. The synagogue was now a modern building. The beautiful stained glass windows of our temple in the Bronx and the closeness of the simple participatory celebrations of my grandfather's one room temple were gone. Some of my peers' parents were tatooed on their arms with the numbers assigned to them when they were in concentration camps, while others had nightmares about their horrifying experiences in the labor camps. In contrast to my Israeli immigrant community, the Queens communities seemed to be built on a culture of shared oppression, victimization, demoralization, and fear. They remained closed within their families and seemed to display strong prejudices toward other ethnic groups, including other Jews. Synagogue no longer felt like a place of safety and family and I began to feel like a foreigner among my own people. My inability to identify with these Jewish people was fostered by my early exposure to the proud, strong, assertive, and multiethnic "Israelis of New York." I am also sure that some of those differences were based on the shared sense of Israeli culture of having participated in the war and actively fighting back as opposed to being trapped in the death camps where fighting back was often a death sentence. The community I identified with was Jewish people who fled to Israel during their childhood and who were traumatized by their experiences of constant danger and profound losses. They were survivors who continued to experience threats of annihilation in Israel, but in Israel they had an army that fought back. Their grief and anger fueled their collective pride and commitment to their fellow Jews and their establishment of the State of Israel. They were descendants of a country and culture built on strong bonds of family, friendship, sharing, trust, and support. They grew up in an environment where their pasts were already too painful to talk about and they had no time to heal. Instead they danced the hora, joining hands and creating collective dances passed down from their diverse Jewish ancestries. Their dancing was an expression of joy but was also a way of managing the perpetual fear and threat that continued to plague their existence in their new home of Israel.

At 16, after feeling displaced and disconnected from the Jewish community in Queens, I visited Israel. I remember the profound emotions that surfaced as I gazed out the airplane window, crying as my country revealed itself from below. I had finally come home. I was overpowered by a familiar feeling that I hadn't experienced since leaving the Bronx, the strong feeling of belonging. After a month, I returned to New York focused on earning money so that I could go back to Israel, my homeland. My cousin, who was a director in a market research company in Manhattan, immediately helped me to secure a job as a telephone interviewer. I commuted to work every day after my classes. I gradually became consumed in my American life of work, school, and struggles of adolescence. It became increasingly more difficult to hold onto my positive feelings of Jewish connection. My strong Jewish identity gradually dissipated and was replaced by stereotypes of Jews created by anti-Semites. I felt conflicted when a coworker openly expressed her hatred for Jews after being treated in a demeaning manner by her boss who was a Jewish physician. I could understand her feelings of humiliation at the hands of a fellow Jew who treated her badly. In social situations, I noticed that people would politely move away from me when they discovered that I was Jewish. I learned how to dodge the question of my ethnicity. I consciously placed the "chi," a Jewish symbol connoting "life" that I wore on a chain around my neck, inside my shirt and eventually stopped wearing it altogether. I went to work on the Jewish holidays and stopped going to synagogue. At that time I concealed the fact that I was Jewish, an identity that had come to be associated with rejection and vulnerability. Childhood feelings of danger and differentness were rekindled and my goal was to assimilate. In contrast, my brother responded to the new environment by immersing himself more deeply in Jewish religion and customs. In the many places that he has lived he finds and regularly attends Saturday services at respective synagogues, finding the kinship and company of fellow Jews. My brother devoted most of his career to serving the Jewish community and is currently employed as an executive director for a Jewish organization that supports socially marginalized groups in Israel. It took many years for me to reclaim my Jewish identity. Gradually, it felt uncomfortable to go to work on the highest holy day, Yom Kippur, a day of fasting and atoning for your sins. I no longer choose to hide my identity as a Jew, yet I have never been able to find a synagogue where I could once again feel at home, surrounded by family as in the little Suhl in the Bronx.

In my family, the silence of my parent's experiences served as an artificial barrier for their ongoing suffering and left me feeling very confused. I thought that I could never truly understand the oppression and persecution they endured. The silence about what they suffered was profound. Even among their European friends and those who spoke their language it was understood that things were better left unsaid. My fluency with Hebrew dissipated, replaced by English for myself and my brother; my parents spoke German to one another. I thought that the American that I was becoming, the English speaker, would never be able to fully understand their hardship. The German of my parents seemed harsh and painful, so I came to be deafened to it. I believe this was a way of trying to protect myself from the anguish of their past. However, what I didn't realize was that I didn't have to be told the details of their experience or speak their language to absorb their pain. The pain of my parent's losses became my burden as well as theirs. Their survivor guilt became my legacy. Their depression became my responsibility. I learned that I couldn't protect myself from my parents' horrific experiences by deafening myself to their native language. Instead there seemed to be a shared unspoken language that we could all understand. Perhaps this is one of the reasons that I was initially attracted to sign language. American Sign Language (ASL) is an unspoken language, therefore it allowed me to keep my allegiance to my parent's "silence" around words but capture the underlying emotional experience. ASL is a very direct and richly expressive language that genuinely captures those underlying emotions. Given my background, it was a relief to me to be able to directly and fully communicate with people on an emotional level through a very expressive unspoken language, for there are many emotions and experiences that words are inadequate to capture.

American Sign Language encompasses the culture and experience of oppression for Deaf people as well as their suppression and discrimination. Their experiences seemed to resonate with me those experiences of my parents that were conveyed to me nonverbally. This clearly influenced my affinity for working with Deaf and hard of hearing clients. In my career as a psychologist, my work with Deaf individuals requires that I be able to openly acknowledge and support them in working through their emotional struggles and pain nonverbally, in silence. I am able to appreciate the nuances of nonverbal communication that can be so powerful and can appreciate how nonverbal communication in my family clearly affected me. I can understand the emotional conflicts of hearing children of Deaf parents who, unlike me, directly witness and experience the oppression and discrimination that confront their own parents who are living in a hearing culture that is often dismissive of that parent's competence. I can also understand what they must struggle with when coming to terms with their own bicultural identities. I believe that my work with the Deaf within their richly expressive silent language has helped me to become more in touch with my own and my family members' intense underlying emotional experiences. American Sign Language has given me a language that permits me to organize these powerful emotions that were unspoken yet passed on. These feelings that were festering inside of me could finally become symbolically realized without betraying my family's survivor cultural code of silence. Along with the unspoken pain and traumas of my family's persecution as Jews, my family gave me a strong sense of Israeli values that include the importance of community, sharing, and helping others. As survivors who lived by the principles of perseverance, integrity, commitment, and respect for others, they taught me both directly and by example how to persevere through challenges in my own life. Without an awareness of what compelled me to do so, I joined volunteer efforts to help people when I was very young. These traditions also find expression in my social activist and progressive political leanings.

In my mid 20s I started my own therapy to try and gain some understanding and sense of control of what felt like disconnected affects. In sessions, the silence was always difficult to endure as I struggled to keep the erupting emotions submerged and unspoken. These strong attempts to dissociate from my feelings gradually retreated and emotions began to emerge, were reexperienced, and were eventually understood within a context. Some were connected to my own experiences, but others were cut off affects belonging to my parents' that took refuge inside me. My Jewish heritage has very much influenced who I am as a therapist. I have a great capacity for compassion and am very committed to helping others. I am told that I have a capacity to create a climate of safety and acceptance that clients need if they are to explore feared aspects of themselves and/or revisit painful past experiences.

In my own therapy and supervision, I became aware of my need to fill my patient's silences and how doing so was connected to my family dynamic around silence. I consciously struggle to control this impulse so that my clients can have the space they need to establish their own pace. I listen to each persons' narrative respectfully understanding the importance of giving people the safety and time needed to tell their story and to have their struggles validated. I do this recalling how my mother was dismissed by those who didn't think her narrative and her pain was valid enough to be heard or supported, who used her survival against her and how harmful it was to her. I have come to understand that for people who develop in the midst of constant threats to their safety, from which there is often no escape, trauma from which there is no time to heal, only survive, that a very highly evolved and healthy family constellation would be needed to moderate the stressors and traumas of the social context of those times and experiences. Some people who survive trauma are fortunate enough to have an evolved family constellation to help them heal, and others are not so fortunate. So it is for my clients. In whatever way my client's choose to express their pain, I am there to listen, and in listening, I also learn.

A Process Without End: Seeking the Unrealized Yet Irrepressible Aspects of Self

JUDITH M. GLASSGOLD

INTRODUCTION

An exploration of the interaction between individual identity, family history, cultural meanings, and social context is always a work in progress. I do not believe that personal identity remains static, as it represents an individual's ongoing interaction with an evolving and dynamic context. The best metaphor is that of a tapestry that is being woven endlessly, with threads going back into the past but with new strands and fabrics always being incorporated. This article will highlight the significance of Judaism in my identity. However, I will also use Judaism as a lens to understand how social, historical, personal, and family issues interact within the self. This exploration is important to understand my own perspective and philosophy on psychotherapy and is a means of exploring the personal issues I bring to my therapeutic work.[1]

Meaning making through a self-aware personal narrative is a radical enterprise that undercuts the way our society addresses identity and difference (Rich, 1986a, 1986b; Martin & Mohanty, 1986). In our world, difference is managed—not embraced—through predefined categories. Most social categories are dichotomous: male/female, black/white, straight/gay, Christian/Jew, religious/atheist. The first term is privileged and superior to the second. Simultaneously, each category is predefined and thus the possibilities for each term are predetermined. Difference is defined as deviance, and then this label is used to justify oppression or exclusion from social power (Lorde, 1984). This definition of social categories limits the possibilities and the expression of alternate definitions of gender, race, sexuality, and

---

[1]I would like to acknowledge the influence of other members of the minyan project through the presentations we have given together: Beverly Greene, Andrea Bergman, Claire Holzman, Sophia Richman, Louise Bordeaux Silverstein, and Sara Zarem. I would like to thank K. M. Crosson for feedback and suggestions (for the title and the reference to Adrienne Rich's "Split at the Root") and Meg Harmsen for comments on an earlier version of this work.

religion. However, lived experience contains ambiguities, contradictions, and multiplicities that these categories cannot represent (Martin & Mohanty, 1986; see also Rich, 1986a, 1986b; Smith, 1991).

These social categories limit personal and group expression and also limit access to power. If these categories remain unquestioned, identity becomes a process of exclusion of realities and possibilities (Taylor, 2004). Rather, one is trapped in predefinitions of Whiteness, Blackness, femaleness, maleness, Jewishness, etc. These categories limit everyone through excluding aspects of what is possible, even those who are placed in the majority fear the aspects of themselves that do not fit, and then hide, conform, and at times attack those who represent difference.

For most individuals, adaptation to these categories creates internal divisions, generating fragmented selves and identities, producing internal oppositions and disconnections of silences and exclusions, so that one is "split at the root" (Rich, 1986b). For instance, in an essay by that very title: "Split at the Toot: An Essay on Jewish Identity," Rich confronts the family history, social context, personal meanings, silences, shame, and invisibility surrounding her Jewishness: "Split at the root/neither Gentile or Jew/Yankee nor rebel" (p. 101). This splitting process disempowers through both negative affects such as shame that stunt the imagination, making different realities and possibilities invisible. In order to rejoin our split parts and to regain our own personal agency we must become conscious of the inherited meanings from culture, community, and family and begin a process of integration, however tentative and incomplete that is (Rich, 1986b).

This type of exploration of identity, a process of deconstruction of existing meanings and of renaming the world, is a process of liberation— liberation from psychic and, at times, political oppression. In order to change and to resist any cycle of oppression, individuals must come to an understanding that oppression exists and acknowledge the complex way it has been incorporated into their being, through thoughts, meanings, perceptions, unconscious processes, and relations to others (Watts, Griffith, & Abdul-Adil, 1999). The ability to name the world as limiting, objectifying, and oppressive, immediately changes the world, as the individual perceives their place in the world differently and conceives of their social identity differently and can be a start to undo that oppression (Martin-Baro, 1994). Naming or renaming ourselves by changing existing meanings is changing the world: "To exist, humanly, is to *name* the world, to change it (Freire, 1970, p. 76).

At some point in order to resist inherited meanings and oppression, each person must embrace an active, conscious process of self-awareness that creates new possibilities through trying to discover that which is outside of consciousness, what is deeply felt and understood while being in the world. What I have learned through my own attempt to understand the past, create a present, and imagine a future, is that ultimately every person must create his or her own narrative through understanding these complexities of meaning.

PERSONAL HISTORY

In order to be effective as a therapist and to understand how history, culture, family, and other forces influence others, I need to understand how they have affected me. I was born in 1957 in the United States of parents also born here in the late 1920s, early 1930s. Three of my grandparents were born in Eastern Europe and emigrated here, one before WWI, the others before WWII; one set of great-grandparents emigrated in the 1870s, raising a family in the United States at the turn of the century.

Historical and social contexts frame much of my own and my families' possibilities. Persecution for being Jewish is the reason my family is now American and why so many are no longer alive. Forty years ago when my family was traveling in Eastern Europe behind the Iron Curtain my mother and I were told repeatedly, "You look European." That statement was meant in friendship and perhaps wonderment because they had never met Americans. However, a reality went unspoken by us: "We would have been European if my grandparents had not been driven out due to anti-Semitism." My paternal grandfather fled Russia in 1906 after terrible pogroms, when the young men who resisted had to leave to save their lives. My mother's family left growing anti-Semitism and the economic hardship that accompanied prejudice in Central Europe. Then there is that horrible truth that those who did not leave—brothers, sisters, cousins, aunts, uncles—are all dead; they were either shot in Poland or Russia or transported to Auschwitz at the end of the war with all the other Hungarian Jews, none in graves, many who remain unknown, erased from memory by the totality of loss.

Having been born and raised a Jew in the late twentieth century has meant my coming to terms with the history of anti-Semitism in Europe and the Holocaust. As Aharon Appelfeld, a Holocaust survivor describes, the definition of a Jew in the twentieth century evolved from being based on religious belief to being defined by blood ("The Nuremberg Laws," 1935). The Nuremberg Laws defined Jews as those linked by parentage, not those linked by religious practice or belief. Those killed in the Holocaust had many religious beliefs, but this did not matter; all that mattered to the Nazis was parentage or, more commonly, blood (Appelfeld, 2005). This imposed definition of who was a Jew was linked to some of the most oppressive and horrific events of the twentieth century and illustrates the power of oppressive categories to shape our lives: it directly controlled the fate of six million lives and of countless generations to come.

However, as part of the process that I see as essential to identity, I must reframe this situation to find sources of power; I can see my legacy of this tragedy and horror as presenting choices, as did Muriel Rukeyser (1944/1978), eminent woman and Jewish poet, writing during the war:

To be a Jew in the twentieth century
Is to be offered a gift. If you refuse,

Wishing to be invisible, you choose
Death of the spirit, the stone insanity.
Accepting, take full life.
The gift is a torment. . . .
But the accepting wish,
The whole and fertile spirit as guarantee
for every human freedom, suffering to be free,
Daring to live for the impossible. (p. 239)

In my mind, the personal challenge to forming a positive Jewish identity is to come to terms with the historic events and the personal impact of those events in order to embrace a Jewish identity while redefining what exactly that means. Does being a Jew mean accepting the definition in the Nuremberg Laws, blood versus belief? For those of us who have grown up after the Holocaust one must accept the gift of life, of not having endured the fate of so many others. For instance, in Appelfeld's (2005) view, to ignore or to deny a Jewish identity would be "immoral" and complicity with the attempts to exterminate the Jewish people. However, what it means to be a Jew is still in flux and open to definition.

For me, I cannot ignore the rest of the history of the twentieth century. Human history is a lesson in the existence of human evil. The genocide of the Jews was not the only example of genocide, and those who once were victims of injustice can become perpetrators of injustice. My lesson from this reality is that there must be a personal transformation from the powerlessness of a victim-of-history to agency, changing humiliation to compassion for the suffering of others and searching to develop personal and collective agency while understanding the force of historical events.

FAMILY[2]

My family's influence on me comes through tensions between individual, family, and community identities, primarily the interaction of gender (the roles of women in society) and sexual orientation. Much of the tension, pain, and suffering that resulted from these interactions were borne by individuals in silence, with some responding with indirect resistance and quiet opposition. At the core of these struggles are the lingering effects of my mother's Orthodox upbringing and her struggle with the restrictive aspects of her family's expression of that religious perspective. From looking at my family, it has become clearer that sexual repression is linked to the lack of social and economic opportunities for women. Many of these most powerful issues were hidden and denied for generations.

---

[2]This account of my family is solely my point of view, and some information has been changed to protect the identities of others.

My mother rejected her Orthodox upbringing, but never found another way of being religious or culturally Jewish. In that way she is loyal to her conservative Orthodox tradition, for in the mind of her father, a rabbi, and many of her religious relatives, religious belief defined Judaism, much as it had been in their towns of Eastern Europe. You are either Orthodox or you are not really Jewish. Her rejection of Orthodoxy and her older brother's rebellion through involvement with Reform Judaism separated them from their family of origin. Both my uncle and mother had complicated motives but were each in some way affected by the oppression of women that occurred in the Orthodoxy of that time and how it was practiced in my grandfather's house.

My grandfather had grown up in a small village in Eastern Europe and married into the extended family of the Chief Rebbe of the dominant city. He was Orthodox though more liberal than the Hasidic family he married into, yet far more conservative than what many these days define as Orthodox. He immigrated before WWII and became a rabbi in an eastern city. However, his inflexibility and intransigence on certain issues alienated my mother, despite her love for him. She, as the youngest, observed the lack of choices available to her sisters, who were blocked in their own lives due to my grandfather's religious views and his fear of what others would think. For instance, their choices for husbands were extremely limited, as they had to meet with the approval of their father, and career avenues other than motherhood were unlikely. Of course, it was not just Orthodox Judaism, what options were available in 1930s and 1940s for women?

My mother's anger was fueled by her own mother's frustrated wish for a little independence, even as slight as no longer having to cover her head with a wig as was required by my grandfather.[3] In addition, less consciously but even more intensely, the anger was deepened by my grandfather's refusal to address the presence of a man in his own congregation who had abused and was abusing young girls. Thus, it is not a mystery why my mother rejected the way of life of her father, for Orthodox Judaism is not just a set of religious beliefs; it is a way of life and a community. This community disappointed and betrayed its young women.

My mother's marriage was her first rebellion. My father was a scientist, not religious or observant. He had already separated himself from his family due to a refusal to submit to his father's will. Her marriage to him had was fraught with challenges. Thus, two rebels raised me, though they might not have seen it in that way initially: two individuals who had separated themselves from autocratic patriarchs. My brother and I were raised with no belief in a supreme deity and observed few cultural celebrations. When I asked at six, "Is there a God?" I was told, "Scientists haven't figured that

---

[3]Very observant married Jewish women cover their head in public, whether it is through wearing a wig or alternative covering. My grandfather requested that my grandmother always wear a wig, which was hot and unflattering.

out yet." However, it was clear we were Jewish, and Orthodoxy affected our lives in subtle ways, usually a rejection of any assimilation into the Christian mainstream rather than an embrace of Jewish religion or community.

As we never went to a synagogue except for weddings and bar mitzvahs, I did not realize how important Judaism was to my mother until I was 15. My mother's older brother was now a professor at Hebrew Union College, where he mentored and trained the first women rabbis. My mother was thrilled to go to the investment ceremony of the first woman rabbi ordained by Reform Judaism, a student of my uncle's. I went with her. Only in retrospect do I understand how important that was to her, as she was still searching for a place at the table of her people. Moreover, what if the life that was open to women in Judaism (and in the United States) in the mid-1970s had been open to her and her sisters? She has struggled over the years to come to terms with the internal and external barriers that her upbringing and family brought to her, sexism just being one. It feels more tragic and unjust, I believe, as she sees the changes that time has brought.

The form of rebellion authored by my mother was limited by the social context of larger society. She could disassociate from her family, but I am not sure she felt like she found an alternate path that satisfied her. She was then limited by the larger historical and social contexts. An identity focused simply on exclusion or disassociation has limited power and can be only the first step. My mother was "split at the root," her upbringing, loyalties, and yearnings dividing her and making alternatives seem impossible. Being unlike her mother and sisters took such tremendous energy, I am not sure there was enough left for the next step—creating her own narrative. That final step was left to my brother and me.

SOCIAL CONTEXT

Inherited meanings—from cultures and societies—shape our lives. Claude Steele in describing the theory of identity contingencies (Kersting, 2004) believes that every person's identity has aspects of possible social significance. What brings salience to any of these elements is how each is addressed by larger society: the labels, judgments, adversities, and privileges that come with each. Vulnerability, stigma, and a fear of attack can make one aspect of identity particularly important and dominate others.

My own identity is a mix of cultural messages and personal interpretation. Others' reaction to my name and my appearance is part of my experience of social categories and stereotyping and part of how I am defined as Jewish by others. My full name is Judith Miriam Glassgold. I was named for my grandmother Judith Miriam Kahane. Judith also can be interpreted as meaning "woman" in Hebrew, which makes it not simply a personal name but also the category. This word underscored for me my own sense of basic Jewishness.

My name is also one of the most "Jewish" things about me, as my own religious beliefs and cultural practices are not identifiably Jewish. Both my first, middle, and last names are commonly thought to be Jewish, which they are.

My names are important in not only how I name myself but also how I am perceived by others. Because of my name, people assume I am Jewish, which is true. However, they often then make additional assumptions about me based on how they define that word, usually without meeting me, without seeing me, and without speaking to me. Some clients (mostly Jews) pick my name out of the telephone book when looking for a Jewish therapist. This assumption becomes fodder for all sorts of projections and assumptions of what it means to be Jewish. This is often a source of initial identification and wish for understanding and mirroring but then can become an experience of difference. I also have to recognize that others define and experience Judaism in very different ways, perhaps based on faith, family heritage, and religious or cultural practices.

Then there is how I look, "The Glassgold's were always dark," says my aunt. My relative "darkness" and curly hair had great significance for me when I was growing up in an American society that idealized fairness and blondness, long before multiculturalism. Many people, especially those in New York, tell me I look Jewish, that very complex and troubling comment replete with stereotypes. Furthermore, geographical location is important. I have spent a great deal of my life in different countries. In those places, people usually consider me "something" or see me as different; however, I am not considered an American. I am often told that I do not look American because Americans (to those overseas) have light hair, light eyes, and light skin.

My appearance is important as it again influences the way people react to me, the assumptions they make that color our initial interaction as people try to fit me into familiar categories. In Latin America I was told, "you look Arab [like the many immigrants from Lebanon]." In suburban Connecticut a woman made a racist remark and then apologized as she thought I was Puerto Rican. Recently, when I went to Canada and went through the bilingual customs line the official spoke Spanish to me. One time as a teenager in New York City, I was particularly frustrated by being asked by a taxi driver, "What are you?" I had responded, "I am an American, my parents were born in America." He was not satisfied by this and went down every list of ethnic identities to figure out what I was. At that time, being American was not possible if one looked a certain way. And then what about ethnic favoritism, such as the behavior of counter men at a famous deli on the Lower East Side where I get free pastrami and my redhaired friend gets the cold shoulder. People make judgments based on appearances. Is that racism?

This sense of difference disappears when my appearance is unexceptional. For me this difference vanishes in sections of New York and New Jersey but also overseas in Israel, Mediterranean countries such as southern France and parts of Italy. The salience of these aspects vanish because I look like everyone else, and the impact can make what is foreign seem familiar. National boundaries disappear as well; it is indeed to disconcerting to feel more comfortable in Italy than in Boston. The awareness in Israel that being Jewish had a "taken-for-granted" quality gave me a sense of what it must feel like to be in the majority, a powerful but puzzling experience, highlighting its lack elsewhere.

Where I work, near New Brunswick, New Jersey, I am usually asked in Lebanese restaurants if I am Lebanese, and in one instance when I said, "I am Jewish," the owner replied, "Then we are cousins and neighbors" (children of Abraham and Israel/Lebanon). This was a positive experience between two people of nationalities described as different, as "others." That was because we chose to relabel ourselves—we defined our own relationship, ignoring the common objectifying categories in the United States where Jews and Arabs are enemies.

I could never deny my heritage, because my name and appearance mark me. Sometimes for me, because of the power of social labeling, Judaism feels like a race, imposed by appearance, color, and type of hair, eyes, skin, nose, as well as by name. Jewish identity can never be a choice. It is similar to what the writer Jean-Paul Sartre (1948) stated in his critique of anti-Semitism that appeared immediately following WWII: "The Jew is one whom other men consider a Jew" (p. 69). This is the terrible reality that some identities are not fully chosen and are imposed by others. The solution for those who believe in individual agency and the worth of the individual is to imagine how to reject and transform those imposed meanings and create personal significance, not to avoid or deny that identity or seek safety through impulsive and nonaware assimilation. Others may try to impose this identity, but it is mine to define.

For instance, my appearance does not have to represent an external, imposed identity. Rather, the ambiguities of my appearance help me see the flaws in our existing categories of race and ethnicity. To many I seem familiar. I confuse people; years ago in Boston I was told, "I have never seen a White person with hair like yours." More recently, I was told by an African American graduate student that I reminded her of her sister, who had my color skin, curly hair, and was a lesbian. A biracial (African-American/Caucasian) friend told me "I felt familiar" as her brother and sister look just like me. The range of color in her family and then the similarity between us has underscored how superficial preexisting assumptions and categories are, if people from such different backgrounds could look so much alike, perhaps we are just family.

INTEGRATION AND RESTORATION

I have been struggling with for many years—even without realizing it—with the labels and meanings that are imposed by others. Now I must ask, "What do those words mean to me?" Who am I in my own words? What is the identity that I am constantly creating?

A MINYAN OF WOMEN

When I came out to my parents as a lesbian over 25 years ago, all sorts of family secrets emerged. Finally, my parents began discussing other family members who could be considered gay or lesbian and who struggled with the historical and social limits of their life choices. The freedom to live outside of heterosexuality is recent. Heterosexuality has long been a form of social organization, not only a sexual/emotional orientation. For many women, with few economic or societal opportunities, heterosexual marriage was the only possible life.

One relative was encouraged by her father to become an engineer, but her parents also expected her to be tied to family and marriage. In the early 1950s she lived in Greenwich Village, which she describes as some of the best years of her life, but then left for Israel later to focus on the early socialist vision of Zionism, a classless and category-free society. She found a way to create a life in Israel, though not with regard to her sexuality but to live some of her ideals openly. Remaining in the United States and trying to be gay in the 1950s I think felt less possible to her without the sense of community and safety, which now exists for lesbian, gay, and bisexual individuals. The only identity that she felt was possible was as a Jew and as an independent woman. Her life was "split at the root" (Rich, 1986b) by social opportunities and homophobia.

Another female relative wished to become a classical vocalist and had talent—but who had ever heard of an Orthodox woman from a religious family singing opera on the stage? Instead, she was forced to marry a man she could not abide. Early in her 20s (60 years ago), she formed an enduring, deep friendship with a woman she now calls her partner. Now both widowed, they travel and share their most passionate life pursuits. Her life, though, at the beginning was "split at the root" (Rich, 1986b) has grown more unified over time. Of course, when I was growing up, all of this was invisible to me, as homosexuality has been invisible in Orthodox Judaism until very recently. In my limited genealogical research, I have found other potential gay and lesbian ancestors and family; this has left me wondering about all of the hidden stories and the erasure of same-sex attachments in our past.

For each of us the frame of the times shapes many of our possibilities and opportunities. Much resistance and rebellion are necessary to achieve a life in the face of stigma and adversity. For me, an important step was naming the efforts of the women in my family as resistance; this was empowering in itself, rather than only seeing their lives and hopes as frustrated. My family's history has also played a strong role in my ability to encourage others to redefine and resist. My hope is that although we cannot always define the frame of existence we can define what picture is in that frame. Identity can become an active creation that cannot rest on any given definitions for those predefinitions restrict. Finally, there is the influence of the social and historical milieu of my childhood: New York City during the late 1960s into the

1970s with feminism, Black Power, and the antiwar movement. These movements just encouraged the possibilities of choice and change.

Then there is the interaction between my Jewish, female, and lesbian identities that is so complex that it is impossible to separate the elements, as unraveling a tapestry would be destructive of the integrity of that effort. As this work focuses on Judaism, this perspective itself shapes the picture; another perspective would result in another view. How I am as a Jew is the basis of how I am a woman and a lesbian. Through figuring out how I am Jewish laid the way to address the stigma of being different, unwelcome, and excluded, a plight shared by all those defined as minorities in this society. Philip Roth in a recent essay describing his book (*The Plot Against America*) described how all groups who face stigma and exclusion must address feelings of humiliation and powerlessness (Roth, 2004). He asks, "How do you remain strong when you are not welcome?" (p. 11).

As a lesbian and as a woman, I must figure out how to stay strong and find the courage to create a life with meaning when faced with those who would label me as different and thus devalue and try to limit my very existence (Glassgold, 1995). I feel that being Jewish has made it easier for me to be a lesbian. The experience of overcoming the emotions of humiliation and powerlessness that came with the history and memories of the Holocaust, coupled with the pride and traditions of the Jewish people, made it easier for me to come to terms with and overcome the emotions that stem from the stigma prejudice regarding homosexuality.

However, as my identity as a lesbian has evolved, that identity in turn affected how I experienced being a Jew. It is perhaps why I appreciate now more of what Judaism can teach, in terms of history, survival, and its tradition of social justice. However, the feminist and lesbian movements present an alternative to the restrictions of Judaism around women's issues and sexuality. Judaism, in my family's history, has been at times a restrictive force, a limiting factor; feminism has been an alternative. In my life currently, my identity as lesbian seems more salient as it is more greatly stigmatized and presents more a greater demand for alternative meanings.

The lesbian and women's communities have made me aware and appreciative of a diverse community and diverse identities. When I sought role models, those who I found were lesbians, many women of color, like Audre Lorde, whose courage seemed large enough for the struggles ahead. As a White woman of privilege, the lesbian community has made me aware of difference, racism, and prejudice. This sense built on my experiences from childhood, growing up and visiting different parts of the United States and Europe where I grew to know many people who initially appeared different from me but with whom I developed close emotional ties. In college, when my Jewish friends and I were talking about what it meant to be a Jew and wondered where we could belong, I could not see limiting my "community of choice" or "family of choice" only to Jews, which is the isolation of

Orthodoxy. My lesbian identity, my identity as a woman, particularly an American woman and Jew born in the late twentieth century are all intertwined, and none can be separated. Many in my family have created community only among those like themselves. I cannot do that, for my identity will never be unitary. This in turn has influenced the sense of social justice that I bring from Judaism; justice must involve all people, not just one.

Emotional ties and relationships to others have had a powerful influence. My life partner and I share many values, though we are different in terms of those historical and social categories. Her parents are from German and Scottish backgrounds; she was raised going to a Lutheran church but can trace her family roots to Quakers. She grew up in a small town and I grew up in New York City. In a different historic moment, our relationship might have been very different.

Finally, as a therapist, I have worked with so many people very different from me. Their struggles, fears, hopes, and dreams are those I can feel. The emotional ties that are created between my clients and me make relationships based on artificial labels unimaginable. I gave up on the illusion that similarity brings safety or that similarity creates automatic loyalty a long time ago. My family is not to be found solely in those who seem similar, for home is not where you start from; home is a destination that you create with others.

IMPACT ON THERAPY: IDENTITIES

These issues have shaped my work as a psychologist and have led to my integrating different theoretical strands into my work: psychodynamic, constructivist and postmodern approaches, feminist, and liberation psychology (Glassgold, 1995, 2003, 2007). From my own experience of difference I have come to believe that identity is something that has to be actively created. One cannot deny social categories and labeling, but those categories must be transcended. Of course, the first step relies on models of psychodynamic psychology, understanding that many aspects of ourselves, especially those that contain shame, are sites of repression and fear and thus are split off from the psyche. These aspects of self must be recovered through introspection as well as relationships with others. From postmodernism, feminism, and constructivism, I have additional tools to understand the process of repression and alienation. Identity, itself, is a construction, a process, and often a struggle; the specifics are less important than the sense of movement. There is certainly a way I will always feel different: I am a Jew, but not as other people define it. I am an American, but not as other people see it. I am a lesbian, but not as society labels it.

Jewish life in America can provide a lens or a frame for understanding these issues. Rosen (2004), in an article on Jewish history in America, describes the process as one of a "struggle between ancient identity and modern belonging" (p. 19), framed by the process of immigration: "Immigration always involves making revisions—you either rewrite yourself or, if you are bold, try to revise the culture around you" (p. 19). Perhaps, even once having arrived physically in one location, we must constantly migrate to another place internally, making constant revisions, even if that other place is simply a place of new meanings.

In this historical moment, the open and diverse society found in the United States has permitted Jews to be free of the isolation and defensiveness that came with persecution that occurred for centuries. This openness has provided an unprecedented opportunity to define for ourselves what it means to be a Jew (Grossman, 2004, p. 5, as quoting S. R. Schwartz). As our society becomes more tolerant of even more aspects of human diversity, this potential becomes true of other aspects of identity as well. I have seen this in my lifetime to include the meaning of homosexuality, moving from deviance to difference.

The balancing of identities within historical context is the human condition representing both limits and potentials: "[I]dentity is not the goal but the point of departure of the process of self-consciousness, a process by which one begins to know that and how the personal is political, that and how the subject is specifically and materially en-gendered in its social conditions and possibilities of existence" (De Lauretis, 1986, p. 9). This process relates to all groups that must address losses of a homeland or ancient religious and cultural traditions, through immigration, colonization, and marginalization and oppression.

These issues became ever clearer as I worked with a young woman where my awareness of my own family history was particularly salient. It was a case of an immigrant Muslim family with a rebellious daughter. The irony was not lost on me, in this very polarized post–9/11 world, that here I was the granddaughter of Orthodox Jews trying to balance the feelings of observant Muslim parents with their daughter's attempt to integrate different sides of herself and create an identity as a modern American college student. Of course, there were some commonalities: code of dress, modesty, rules of gender, and sexuality, where at times I thought I was dealing with my maternal grandfather and heard the echo of my mother's childhood stories of resistance in my head. My awareness of the tension between traditional cultures and assimilation and integration into this culture informed my work with this young woman. As with many rebels, she was called bad and labeled as different and deviant. She did not see her struggle in wider terms. She experienced the conflict and was confused: was she being bad, as her parents told her, or was she like her friends? She identified as an American, a Muslim, and South Asian, and felt misunderstood by her parents and scapegoated for being strong-willed and independent, as she challenged their views of sexuality and gender. When I explained to her that this issue

was a result of the tensions involved with the clash of values and accultura-
tion, a common dilemma among children of immigrants, this interpretation
made these issues open for reflection and integration rather than a function
of a negative personality trait or moral failing. This nonblaming interpretation
opened up avenues for integration to her rather than dichotomous choices.

I also found myself being a translator between generations trying to
bridge the divide created by the conflict between her parents and herself,
while empathizing with both sides. I had to draw on my empathy for my
grandparents, who had watched their world be destroyed. The immensity
of that loss fueled their desire to re-create that world here. This woman's parents were faced with their fear of loss of their culture and fear of failing in
their quest to be successful while holding onto what was important in their
culture. Of course, paradoxically, as they became materially successful, their
children became more integrated into mainstream culture and incorporated
American values. This difference of cultures within generations in families
of immigrants is especially painful and creates separations and losses in families, a lesson I learned about from my mother's family and many other clients. The most powerful session for me was sitting with this client's
mother and mourning together her losses, in the present as an immigrant
who left her homeland, and as she perceived her future, with a daughter
so different from herself. In my own life, my work as a therapist has allowed
me to reunify my history, emotionally joining the loss and the rebellion,
healing another "split at the root" (Rich, 1986b).

As a therapist I strive to help others have the psychological freedom to
imagine their own choices and to create their own lives. The importance of
this process was illustrated to me when I started working with a woman who
was struggling to integrate her identity as an Orthodox Jew and a lesbian.[4]
My previous work to understand my own legacy permitted me to support
her process while understanding that it would be different from my own.
My own understanding of the women in my own family allowed me to be
open to a variety of outcomes, knowing that the ultimate goal would be this
women's satisfaction with her own life, not labels imposed by social movements or scripts imposed by religious beliefs. This woman's quest and many
others is a process of exploring how an individual can resist and rebel against
what is discovered to restrict and limit life. Then, more important, after that
recognition, and with the development of personal agency write his or her
script. No one has to receive passively what is given but can actively create
an identity, a life, and perhaps even change another's. I hope to overcome
the fear that because difference can make it difficult to belong, the only
option is to submit and conform. Rather, another possibility is to first face
the potential rejection that can occur when one resists and rebels—which

---

[4]This work is described in depth in Glassgold, J. M. (2008). Bridging the divide: Integrating lesbian identity and orthodox judaism. *Women & Therapy, 31*(1), 59–72.

is the only solution if one's life is to have integrity. Then, as a next step, find or create new communities of individuals who support new possibilities.

Perhaps, more simply, it is how to have faith and courage to create a life when it is outside the traditional definitions and limits. I try to help people to not only understand the choices that are presented but also to reject the exclusive dichotomies, whether it is the either/or mutually exclusive dichotomies of identity and gender or those external prejudices and labels that attempt to bind rather than liberate. There is also the assumption that these different identities must be completely congruent and not contain contradictory elements. Many of us have multiple identities, but we are told that these identities are not possible: you cannot be an Orthodox Jewish lesbian or feminist Muslim. One of my clients is female, Black, White, Christian, and lesbian. How can she make sense of the complexities of those contradictory elements? Perhaps the solution lies in realizing that it is only in those old dated definitions that these elements are contradictory. Alternatively, she can create new definitions where, though not completely harmonious, these identities can be woven into a personal melody.

Overcoming the belief that all identities have to be congruent and learning how to tolerate conflicts between identities is essential. At times that means rebelling, accepting one's differences, finding one's own path despite what the social messages are. This permits identities that are both more real and more complicated, enabling others to figure out how to be a republican, Catholic lesbian, or how to be a biracial lesbian, or how to be a feminist, assertive Muslim woman, or how to be an Orthodox Jewish lesbian. As one of my client's wrote:

> I feel that you constantly challenge me in the ways that I "make sense" of things . . . but truly—what you instill in me is a sense of impatience, [realizing] that I am living within a structure that is not an absolute . . . . That there are spaces within that structure and it is within those spaces that I can create my own identity—my own sense of agency.

RELIGION

We live in a time where religion has again sparked controversy. Due to the strange dynamics of our times, some of the fault lines of religious intolerance are around issues like same-sex marriage and homosexuality. This has even become an issue in psychology, where my professional life became intertwined with controversies that attempt to replace acceptance of lesbian, gay, and bisexual individuals with distortions of psychological science in the name of conservative religion. This controversy sparked for me a new interest in Judaism. The current political climate attempts to splice the connection of spirituality and homosexuality, attempting to split me at the root.

In the realm of politics, conservative voices try to define religion not only for themselves, but for others as well. To me, this has meant that those who differ, as I do, are made invisible, that my life is being shaped by laws determined by those of other religious beliefs who wish to force or compel me to live outside of my own beliefs. As a Jew, I am painfully reminded of the religious oppression that Jews have experienced historically, where others attempted to convert Jews by explicit force such as threats of violence or to oppress Jews by continuous disadvantage or hardship. These forces were not only religious but were found in the multiple laws that hindered Jewish participation in civil society, culminating in the abhorrent Nurenberg Laws of 1935, in which Jews were defined by others by their blood not by belief, discriminated against in civil law to the point of being told who they could or could not marry.

This context does affect me and has made me conscious of my spiritual beliefs and spiritual concerns, though my own beliefs are far more complex than those who wish to constrict religion would understand. This debate created by religious conservatives has made me more strongly aware of Judaism and more willing to reclaim that heritage. I have become involved in debates that I would have ignored years ago (Glassgold, Fitzgerald, & Haldeman, 2003; Glassgold, 2003; APA Task Force on Appropriate Therapeutic Responses to Sexual Orientation, 2009).

I have reconsidered what is faith and what gives inspiration. The inspiration I find is from a variety of beliefs—again multiplicity, not singularity: Thich Nhat Hahn's Buddhist (2004) understanding of the role of impermanence in understanding both suffering and social justice, the tradition of social responsibility and healing within Judaism, and the existentialist struggle to discover meaning despite chaos and oppression.

My spirituality is based on the constant struggle to act in spite of fear: for fear and faith, especially spiritual faith, are incompatible. Fear can never inspire true faith. True faith inspires courage in the face of fear. Faith allows the "courage to be" (Tillich, 1954). Those who resort to religious ideology to inspire fear of others in order to impose their faith or to bring unity to their faith do not truly inspire faith and only encourage compliance. The lesson of the persecution of the Jews and others in the twentieth century is that actions that arise from fear or hate are oppressive and can bring unjust and evil results. This lesson is true today, no matter who is labeled the scapegoat.

Human beings can cause such great suffering to each other. However, I cannot find the source of hope in a force outside of human beings, which is an evasion of the legacy of the genocides of the twentieth century and fundamentally an evasion of the problem of human evil. The only solution to that suffering must come from other human beings, not from hope for salvation from a divine being. Evil is a human trait, as are all those qualities we call Divine. The only solution must come from human commitment to humanity: Human beings must take responsibility for human actions, human evil, and human suffering.

Appelfeld (2005) recalls in his essay on the 60th anniversary of the liberation of Auschwitz a statement by a fellow survivor: "We didn't see God when we expected him, so we have no choice but to do what he was supposed to do: we will protect the weak, we will love, we will comfort. From now on, the responsibility is all ours." The solution lies in the ability of human beings to heal one another, to undo the harm and to show that despite hate, complacency, apathy, indifference, narcissism, selfishness—all those things—there is also hope, faith, love, compassion, nurturance, connection, and empathy. These positive human capacities must struggle with those deep flaws. The responsibility for that struggle is ours, the struggle against our own human limitations. I am proud, as a Jew, to be able call on the Jewish ethos represented by Pesach, the liberation of the slaves, and of *tikkun olam*, to heal the world through social action, as lessons for us all (Glassgold, 2007).

CONCLUSION: LIBERATION AND INTEGRATION

There are many personal meanings to these dynamics of resistance, rebellion, and loss. As many others of this minyan project have suggested, therapists are the keepers of secrets, and therapy is a place to address those terrible secrets of unexpressed pain and suffering. Therapy must be a place of healing and repairing the world—*tikkun olam*. When unexpressed emotions can be safely and truthfully spoken, therapy is a place we undo the fear and terror that created those secrets. As therapists, we create a place where those feelings of loss, shame, and humiliation can be resolved, and hopefully their negative impacts mitigated. Those things that cannot be named, as they put you in danger, can be expressed in therapy, and once resolved can be creatively articulated outside in the world. Many who I work with have borne pain, suffering, humiliation, and powerlessness alone and wordlessly. I hope to create a place for people to share their burden, finding the words to create new meanings for these feelings, and then discover a way to design a new life for themselves.

These feelings of pain and humiliation are essential to address if new identities are to be created. Social identities are not simply cognitive constructs; they contain emotional meanings and memories. These are the memories that must be uncovered, the feelings that are the consequences of these social categories and historical legacies. From my own family's experiences and through the eyes of my clients I see that the feelings and the memories of the events create generations of suffering (cf. Margalit, 2002) and become the roots of evil and injustice. The violence that comes from humiliation, the rage that springs from powerless anger only creates more of the same.

Exploring these feelings that result from oppression were therapeutic goals for me before I was completely conscious of their roots in my own background, but now that these roots are not split off from memory and now more fully conscious, these goals can be pursued with passion and energy and more fully integrated into my life. If as Eudora Welty (1983) writes, "all serious daring starts from within" (p. 104), then the continual exploration of my own life and the continual refinement of meanings are necessary for what I hope to achieve. My own identity as a Jew, a woman, a lesbian, and, most important, a therapist, must be where I start from, a continuous transformation that comes from weaving together all of the known and as yet unknown elements so that the phrase "Daring to live for the impossible" (Rukeyser, 1944/1978, p.239) becomes reality.

REFERENCES

APA Task Force on Appropriate Therapeutic Responses to Sexual Orientation. (2009). *Report of the task force on appropriate therapeutic responses to sexual orientation*. Washington, DC: American Psychological Association.

Appelfeld, A. (2005, January 27). Always, darkness visible. Op-ed Column. *Sunday New York Times*, Section A, p. 25, Column 2.

De Lauretis, T. (Ed.). (1986). Feminist studies/critical studies: Issues, terms and contexts. In T. De Lauretis (Ed.), *Feminist studies/critical studies* (pp. 1–19). Bloomington, IN: University of Indiana Press.

Freire, P. (1970). *Pedagogy of the oppressed*. New York: Seabury Press.

Glassgold, J. M. (1995). Psychoanalysis with lesbians: Agency and subjectivity. In J. M. Glassgold & S. Iasenza (Eds.), *Lesbians and psychoanalysis: Revolutions in theory and practice*, (pp. 203–228). New York: The Free Press.

Glassgold, J. M. (2003, August). Chair and discussant: Film: Trembling before g-d. Annual Conference of the American Psychological Association, Toronto, Canada.

Glassgold, J. M. (2007). In dreams begin responsibilities: Psychology, agency and activism. *Journal of Gay and Lesbian Psychotherapy*, *11*(3/4), 37–57.

Glassgold, J. M. (2008). Bridging the divide: Integrating lesbian identity and Orthodox Judaism. *Women & Therapy*, *31*(1), 59–72.

Glassgold, J. M., Fitzgerald, J., & Haldeman, D. (2003). Letter to the editor. *Psychotherapy*, *40*(1), 376–378.

Grossman, R. (2004, September 19). Finding freedom—350 years after its founders arrived as religious exiles, the Jewish community in America thrives. *Sunday Star Ledger*, *10*, 5.

Hahn, T. N. (2004). Impermanence. Retrieved July 19, 2009, from http://www.serve.com/cmtan/buddhism/Treasure/impermanence.html

Kersting, K. (2004, September). Social hurdles to true integration. *Monitor on Psychology*, *35*(8), 66.

Lorde, A. (1984). *Sister/Outsider: Essays and speeches*. Trumansburg, NY: The Crossing Press.

Margalit, A. (2002). *The Ethics of memory*. Cambridge, MA: Harvard University.

Martin, B., & Mohanty, C. T. (1986). Feminist politics: What's home got to do with it? In T. De Lauretis (Ed.), *Feminist studies/critical studies* (pp. 191–212). Bloomington, IN: University of Indiana Press.

Martin-Baro, I. (1994). Edited and translated by A. Aron & S. Corne, *Writings for a liberation psychology*. Cambridge, MA: Harvard University.

The Nuremberg laws on citizenship and race: September 15, 1935. Retrieved July 21, 2009, from http://www.mtsu.edu/~baustin/nurmlaw2.html

Rich, A. (1986a). If not with others how? In *Blood, bread, & Poetry: Selected prose 1979–1984* (pp. 202–209). New York: W. W. Norton and Company.

Rich, A. (1986b). Split at the root. Notes on Jewish identity. In *Blood, bread, & poetry: Selected prose 1979–1984* (pp. 100–123). New York: W. W. Norton and Company.

Rosen, J. (2004, September 12). The citizen stranger. Op-Ed Column. *The Sunday New York Times*, Section 4, p. 13, Column 1.

Roth, P. (2004, September 19). The story behind "The plot against America." *New York Times Book Review*, 10–12.

Rukeyser, M. (1944/1978). Excerpts from "Letter to the Front." In *Collected poems of Muriel Rukeyser* (pp. 235–243). New York: McGraw-Hill.

Sartre, J.-P. (1973). *Anti-Semite and Jew*. (George J. Becker, trans.). New York: Schocken Books. (Originally published in 1946 as *Reflexions sur la question Juive*.)

Smith, A. J. (1991). Reflections of a Jewish lesbian-feminist activist-therapist; Or, first of all I am Jewish, the rest is commentary. *Women & Therapy, 10*(4), 57–64.

Taylor, M. C. (2004, October 14). What Derrida really meant. Op-Ed Column. *New York Times*.

Tillich, P. (1954). *The courage to be*. New Haven: CT: Yale University.

Watts, R. J., Grifith, D. M., & Abdul-Adil, J. (1999). Sociopolitical development as an antidote for oppression—Theory and action. *American Journal of Community Psychology, 27*(2), 255–271.

Welty, E. (1983). *One writer's beginnings*. Cambridge, MA: Harvard University.

Elijah's Ghost: A Female Jewish Therapist Explores the Legacy of Love, Fear, Social Action and Faith

MARSHA PRAVDER MIRKIN

I could barely contain my five-year-old legs from galloping up the stairs rather than waiting by the elevator. I wanted to be on the sixth floor already, ringing and ringing the bell to Grandma Annie and Grandpa Joe's apartment and running in to see my cousins, aunts, uncles, and grandparents gathering for our family seder.[1] Instead, my parents insisted that we wait for the elevator, wait as it inched its way up the sixth floor, wait in front of the door with the wooden mezuzah. But the wait was rewarded. As soon as the door opened, I dashed in, winding my way through adult bodies to the tiny kitchen, checking to make sure the chicken soup, gefilte fish, and even the inedible chopped liver was all ready for us, checking that the huge table was set up in the small living room and that the silver cup of wine for Elijah stood regally beside the seder plate. Bursting with excitement, my cousins and I would scramble under the table, laughing, then heading for the refuge of my grandparents' tiny bedroom where we always met by the radiator, looking out over the cobblestone streets of the Lower East Side of New York City.

Yes, this night was different from all other nights. On this night, we celebrated the freedom of our people, but for me, the celebration was about my own freedom. No adults would chide me to sit quietly tonight. None would tell me to walk slowly or sing softly. I would even get patient half smiles from some unsuspecting adult who was unaware that a storm of cousins was about to practically push her over as we made our way through

---

This article is dedicated to the memory of my parents and grandparents. I am using stories told to me by my mother, as I remember them, while remembering the adage that "this is true, whether or not it really happened." I would also like to express my gratitude to Melissa Elliott, MSN, for her thoughtful review and editing recommendations.

[1]There are many traditions that make up a seder, but often a seder is the structured telling of the story of the Hebrew exodus from slavery. Often, families and friends gather to tell and discuss the story using a text called a *Haggadah*. The sages tell us to also invite people who would not otherwise attend a seder. A festive meal is generally served.

the remaining narrow area that was not taken up by the table. Then it would be time to sit down for the seder. On all other nights, my grandfather would pay most attention to my older cousin, a boy one year my senior. But this night was different. My grandfathers' proud eyes would rest on me because I, the only girl as yet in the family, had already learned Hebrew and was prepared to ask the ritual four questions in the tongue of our foreparents. Later, I would enthusiastically join in on the songs as my uncle banged the table while singing aloud in his gusty voice. I could almost keep up with him as he belted out the verses of the traditional seder song, Dayenu, which cited example after example of how we can live in the moment of the blessing without wanting more, even if there's more to be had. Then the entire family would join in the one word chorus, "Dayenu": it is enough for us. And it was. At those moments, I felt filled with the joy of family and ritual. It is enough. It is more than enough.

The night before we had celebrated the first seder with my grandma and grandpa Ehrlich, my mother's mother and stepfather. My feet moved more slowly toward their door. There would be no other children here. No aunts or uncles. Just me, my parents, and my grandparents. The love and gratitude that enveloped me there should have been enough. It should have been a "Dayenu" moment. My grandmother would be close to tears when I would read the sacred words in her sacred language. She would shake her head in both belief and disbelief, hug me, pride filling the room as much as the smells of chicken soup. It should have been Dayenu, but it wasn't. Grandma and Grandpa Ehrlich's house was somber. The seders were long; voices sang but didn't boom out with joy. I participated and I behaved. But I wanted to be at Grandma Annie's house.

Toward the end of the first seder, Grandma Ehrlich told me to open the door for Elijah. Every year, before the end of the seder, we opened the door so that the prophet could come in to each Jewish home and take a sip of the wine from his cup at the seder table. This is the prophet who Jews believe will usher in the Messiah, whose entrance would mark a time of peace. Elijah is also the prophet who according to Jewish lore unexpectedly shows up anyplace where there is someone in need, giving money to the poor, comfort to the grieving, hope to the hopeless. And, just when you think you know it's Elijah who visited, he suddenly disappears, only to show up on a road or at the home of someone else in need, only to keep showing up as an everlasting message that each of us has the responsibility to repair the world, even if it is one person at a time. Every seder, we have an opportunity to receive a visit from Elijah, who we are told takes a sip from the elaborate silver wine cup at the center of grandma's table and gives us the hope that he is still present and will be back again. The year before, I had yearned to see this prophet of kindness and miracles with my own two eyes, but each time I opened the door, he seemed to sneak in and out without my knowledge. My mother told me that he came and went in the blink of an eye, so this time, I had a plan. When Grandma told me to open the door, I went over, and as I opened it, my right fingers held my bottom eye lid open and my left fingers held my top eye lid opened, and I didn't blink. And there, quickly floating by me, was a thin ghostly figure with a long white beard, long white hair, and long white robe. Elijah! Right in front of my very eyes! I immediately left my post and ran back to the dining room screaming, "I saw him, I saw him!" The room was awash in excitement. My family joined in my joy and hugged me. Perhaps they even believed me. Even in retrospect, it is hard to know what my mother believed and what she did to play along with her precocious daughter. Here she was, an assimilated working woman who was a community leader and social justice advocate, and still, here she was, a Jew from Poland, carrying the profound faith, folk beliefs, and superstitions of her childhood.

But Mr. Ehrlichman was missing from our seder. A quiet man who loved my company, Mr. Ehrlichman was a boarder in Grandma and Grandpa Ehrlich's small two bedroom apartment. Always dressed in a suit and bow tie, he would sit in a high back chair in the living room and like a magnet, draw me to him. When I was turning eight, I began to wonder why Mr. Ehrlichman wasn't at our seders. I concluded that he must be with his wife and children. But then, why was he living with my grandma? I decided to check it out. "Mr. Ehrlichman," I asked, "Do you have seders with your wife and children?" Quietly, with profound sadness, he replied, "They died, Marshala, my wife and my children, everyone, they were killed in the camps." I didn't know what he meant. But I did know not to ask. Several months later, my mother showed me brochures for the summer camp she thought I should attend. I hesitated. Perhaps my mother picked up on my hesitation and thought I wasn't ready to go to away to camp at age eight, and that I should wait for the following summer. But I knew I was never going to any camp if that's where Mr. Ehrlichman's wife and children were killed. And why would my protective mother want to take that risk? I protested. I told her I wasn't going to any camp because children were killed there. And that's when I first was told the story of the Holocaust. And that's when it started to make sense to me when several months later, Grandma Ehrlich stroked my hair and once again sadly said, "You're the only one, Marshala, the only one left."

It would take time before I collected my family's story of the Holocaust, and as I did, I was both horrified by the tragedy and inspired by my mother's refusal to close her eyes to the pain that was happening so many miles away. In 1921, when she was four years old, my mother left Poland along with her parents and baby brother. It was a cruel leaving. Tormented by pogroms, they had spent many of my mother's early years hiding in their cellar, and my grandparents feared for their lives and the lives of their children. And yet, when they finally received clearance to leave, they were told that they could not take my grandmother's firstborn, a teenage son from an earlier marriage who was required to serve in the Polish army before being permitted to emigrate. Making a choice that no parent should ever have to make, my grandparents decided to leave Motl behind and bring him to the United States after he completed army service. But as the years passed, Motl fell in love and stayed in Poland to marry and raise a family. His second child was born in 1938, not long before his desperate letters started reaching my grandmother and her letters stopped reaching him. And, finally, his letters stopped coming. Forever.

So it is not surprising that when my headstrong, energetic mother started hearing about the Nazi oppression of Eastern European Jewry, she did what most others did not do in 1940—she believed what she heard, and she decided to take action. My mother had spent her adolescence longing to go to Barnard College, where she could get the education that she craved and that seemed so unavailable to her, the education that would make her in her own eyes a true American. My mother somehow found a way to take courses at Barnard and was thriving there when she went to a lecture by a representative of a group called "Vaad Hatzala" (translation: the helping community) whose goal was to save Jews during the war and resettle them after the war. She dropped out of college and joined the group, adamant that she could not continue with college under these circumstances and that it was her responsibility to help save European Jewry. My mother recalled to me with frustration and unspent anger that no matter how hard her committee tried, the U.S. government would not increase the quota of Jewish refugees allowed into this country during the Holocaust and knowingly turned boats of refugees away, boats that would have to return to Europe and concentration camps. Then, immediately after the war ended, my mother left for Europe to help identify and resettle refugees. She spent the next three years in Germany and France. I still have her papers, list after list of the names and information about refugees she helped to resettle, page after page of the forgotten whom she would not forget. She recalled a time when her organization gave her 25 boxes of Barton's candy to bring to France and Germany, candy that could be used as thank-you gifts or as bribes for cooperation with her mission. But underneath boxes 18 and 22 were hidden visas and cash. One time the police had been tipped off, and at the French-German border they boarded the train and went straight to my mother's compartment. She recalled keeping her cool, telling them she would cooperate if they only told her what they wanted. They started opening and dumping the boxes of candy, one after another, onto the floor of the train compartment. After rummaging through seventeen boxes, they stopped, sure that the tip was yet another false one. They left, and my mother got the candy, visas, and money to their destination.

During her time in Europe, my mother also told about being assigned to go to a French convent and orphanage where young Jewish children were hidden during the war. Years had passed since those children were secretly sent to the convents, and in the interim, many of the nuns who knew their identity were purposely transferred in an effort to protect the children and clergy. These young children survived the war out of touch with the Jewish identity that nobody could dare risk nurturing even if somebody wanted to. By the time my mother reached the convent and orphanage, it was unclear to everyone which children were Jewish and which weren't. And now the war was over, and the few surviving family members were looking for the few surviving children. But how do you figure out which of these children were Jewish, especially if they were girls or if parents chose not to circumcise a son because at that moment circumcision was a death sentence?

My mother, a young woman who could have been their mother, was told to gather the children and sing *Shma Yisrael Adonai Elohenu Adonai Echad, Hear O Israel, the Eternal is our God, the Eternal is Oneness.* When they were too young to know the words, many Jewish children heard their parents sing to them this statement of faith, the Shma, before bed each night. I myself had once thought of it as a lullaby to keep me safe through the night. And then, at dawn, the children would hear their parents sing the prayer again. These melodies were once as familiar as mother's milk, and just when both seemed lost, my mother sang the words once more. As she sang it, some children ran to her, hugged her, called her Mama. There were little children who had been scurried out of ghettos or passed through the underground or somehow had gotten out. Their mothers or fathers chose this path in desperation and had to let their children go to give them a chance to live. Some parents somewhere, alive or by this time dead, had to go to sleep every night, probably after saying the Shma, without knowing if their children were safe. And as my mother sang, the children's hugs or tears identified them as Jews. These words of prayer, hope, and commitment that graced my childhood and speak to me so profoundly in adulthood were powerful enough to cross the bridge of years and bring these children home. Some of the children were reunited with family members, and then there were the others, the orphans without ties to any home or country. My mother recalled a campaign to raise money to resettle these children, and her delight in meeting the actress Helen Hayes who agreed to financially support the least attractive of the children who would otherwise have the little opportunity to find a home. My mother's greatest gift to me as a therapist was her ability to bear witness to this overwhelming pain; to be fully present for the children and for the adults without distancing emotionally because of the intensity of their anguish. Although she paid a price for her commitment, she never gave up her voice and she never stopped speaking truth to power.

My father's experience was different. Born of Russian-Jewish immigrants into economic poverty on the Lower East Side of New York, my father profoundly understood the meaning of blessing. He found riches where others found poverty. He spoke often about family and neighborhood relationships and rarely about hunger, rats, and anti-Semitic taunts. If there was only one bathroom on his tenement floor, it was better than no bathrooms in the older tenements and shtetls. If the neighborhood was overcrowded, there were more children with whom to play stickball. If there was no money for special treats, he received more than enough from his violin lessons and social events at the Henry Street Settlement House and Educational Alliance. If there was a tragedy, then my father, while mourning, would talk about how this is a part of his otherwise blessed life. When I did something wrong, my father assumed I would learn from it, and that mistakes are also building blocks of life's wisdom. My dad understood "Dayenu," understood that each blessing is enough for us, and if our hearts our open, we will encounter more blessings on our journey. My dad's greatest gift to me as a therapist was that he could hold his strong sense of ethics and intervene gently while not judging others because he knew we are all wanderers on life's unmarked trails, bound to go off in wrong directions, and morally obligated to find a better path.

It is no wonder that after these experiences, my parents would have chosen to settle in a Jewish community and raise among Jews their only child, the one who would prove Hitler wrong by surviving and bringing a new generation of Jews into the world. I spent most of my elementary school years in a nurturant and supportive orthodox Jewish day school where I learned Hebrew at any early age. As much as my parents and grandparents loved the Hebrew language, I'm sure they also saw my knowledge of that tongue as a further rebellion against Hitler. For me, the ancient stories from Torah captured my imagination and I felt that the characters were people I knew personally. My school followed the Jewish tradition of encouraging multiple interpretations of holy texts and encouraged us to argue with and develop our own understanding of the holy words, so I was engaged from the start. Little would my teachers have predicted that their mandate to me to develop my own understanding of these stories would eventually lead me away from orthodoxy and toward more egalitarian forms of Judaism. A famous quote from "Pirkei Avot" ("Ethics of the Fathers" or "Ethics of the Parents") saying that "it is not our responsibility to complete the task, nor are we permitted to desist from starting it" would lead me to fight what I understood as sexism, heterosexism, and ethnocentrism practiced in some branches of Judaism and would fuel my dedication to social justice. In the struggle, I would also come to recognize some remarkably progressive ideas in Torah and Jewish tradition about women, people from communities who are not Jewish, and responsibility to humanity. But all that would come later. At this time, I was a young child learning beautiful stories about a beautiful people, taught to me by many who had been almost broken by the Holocaust.

So trust came hard to my community. After all, I was born just months before the Rosenbergs were executed more for being Jewish than for the charges against them, 8 years after the Holocaust killed much of my extended family and so many of my people, about 12 years after the United States turned away boats of desperate Jews whose only alternative was to return to concentration camps. While my people's history was largely ignored in public school textbooks, the texts of my childhood told me not only about the incredible contributions to society by Jews but also about a history of massacres of Ukrainian and Russian Jews, the murders and expulsions from Spain and England and later from Middle Eastern countries, the torture and killings of the Inquisition, the razing of Jerusalem and murder, enslavement, and expulsion of the Jewish population by the Romans who formally changed the name of Judea to Palaestina. And, of course, there is the more familiar, perhaps mythical but definitely central story of our people, the enslavement of the Hebrews in Egypt. "Whom should we trust?" was the mantra that surrounded me in my childhood. People had to earn trust. It wasn't taken for granted.

I'm suspicious of my trusting nature. I revisit that part of myself often. I still remember childhood neighbors saying, "Why would you have Christian friends? Would those so called friends have hidden you in the Holocaust?" What an incredibly high standard one must achieve to be trusted. Years later I realized how painful it was as I turned that question around on myself: If that's the standard, where would I fit? Would I risk my life and that of my entire family in order to hide someone in a different holocaust? I don't know the answer. It's humbling not to know the answer, but it does make me aware that even if I set the bar lower, trust needs to be earned. Nowadays, I understand and am not thrown by clients who come to me resentful and suspicious. After all, why should they trust me? Trust shouldn't be handed to me based on my past oppression, certainly not based on my current privilege, or on my belief in myself as a good person or even as a competent therapist. So I've learned to be patient with myself and with others and to give my clients time to decide if I'm trustworthy given the contexts of their past experiences as well as what I bring to the therapy. For example, several years ago I was seeing a couple, an African-American man and a Caucasian woman. At some point early on as we explored some of the dynamics in their relationship I asked a question about race. The man responded that race didn't matter in their relationship or in the therapy relationship. Two months later, with a playful "I got you" grin on his face, he shared (I don't remember the exact words), "You once asked whether race was an issue in our relationship. I said no. That's because I didn't trust you enough back then to say yes."

There is another critical message born from both the oppression and the privilege of Jews that became central to me as a woman and as a therapist. From the time I started Jewish day school at the age of four, I learned the Biblical passages stating that we are all made in God's image and commanding Jews to love the stranger, because we were once strangers in the land of Egypt. What an idea! Although we have a history of oppression, the Hebrew Bible also assumes that there will be times when we experience privilege, and during those times, we must remember what it was like to be brutalized and marginalized and we must resist making the unfamiliar person into "other." The tradition goes further than telling us to love the stranger. I was taught the words of Hillel, one of our most prominent sages, that "If I am only for myself, who am I? If not now, when?" Perhaps now is one of those times for the Jewish communities in the United States, a time of experiencing privilege and being responsible for recognizing it and acting for social justice.

So it is no surprise that I am a feminist and multicultural therapist. "Love the stranger." I feel that I have a radar screen tracking injustice, and I feel a responsibility to work hard to be on a journey that fights injustice. I am responsible for continuing to develop my own self-awareness and hold myself accountable for injustices in which I participate, knowingly or unknowingly. That I chose to be a psychologist who often fights injustice with my pen also comes from my parents and my tradition. After all, I was taught that I was from the "People of the Book," another name that Jews have for ourselves. Traditionally, when a Jewish child begins school for the first time or starts to learn the alef-bet (alphabet), he (in Eastern Europe, the "she" was often excluded) dips his finger in honey, writes with that finger, and licks it off. Learning is sweet. Writing is sweet. More than that, it is enticing. Thousands of years later, we are still reading and interpreting the stories written about our ancestors and we are still using them to commit ourselves to social justice. We are taught that our responsibility is tikkun olam, the repair of the world. Furthermore, our texts allow for argument and self-criticism; our prophets and sages call us on our actions if we are not making efforts to heal the world. For the past 20 years, the best way that I personally can challenge ideas that marginalize or devalue people is through writing.

I also do not want to romanticize my tradition, and while I have chosen this tradition, I do not think it is any better than religions chosen by others. Biblical writing can be interpreted in many ways and I know that Judaism has birthed some individuals who interpret the religion in ways that devalue others. I do believe that my parents, however, culled from Judaism many of its most progressive and humanistic values, and I'm grateful for that. But my parents also defined us as a separate community within the larger American community, one that is sometimes tolerated, rarely totally accepted, and often met with hostility. So, while they advocated for civil rights, added their voice to better conditions in the housing projects in our neighborhood, and worked closely and warmly with coworkers of color, they were insular in their private lives. My parents' friends were Jewish. Our neighborhood was primarily Jewish. Later when we moved to a less religiously observant neighborhood, I attended public schools where the student body was primarily Jewish and there was a generous representation of Jewish teachers. I was not supposed to date non-Jewish boys, and marriage to a non-Jew would have been met with fear that I was contributing to the destruction of our religion and culture. While over the years my parents came to embrace my Christian friends, they could not imagine why I would be interested in living in a predominantly Christian community and marveled that I could feel secure in that situation. As they began to soften their stance toward lesbian and gay couples, they still inquired whether my Jewish gay and lesbian friends chose Jewish partners.

I am in a different place now. The privileges denied my parents are not denied to me (at least not at the moment, although I do recognize the frightening growth of anti-Semitism and worry about the future security of the world's Jews). I am more curious about other groups and less insular in my choice of friendships, although I am deeply committed to progressive Judaism and I married a man who identifies strongly with Judaism. I don't experience my parents' fear or sense of betrayal when I enter a church or a mosque, and I can appreciate the spiritual strengths of traditions that aren't mine. Yet, at the same time, as Jews we are taught "zachar," remember. I remember that my mom was an immigrant and my dad the eldest son of poor immigrants. Their fears as well as their hopes are part of me. Their need to establish a familiar community in a strange and at times unaccepting land is both understandable and moving to me. So now, as a therapist, I love working with and consulting and teaching about immigrant families. I am curious about and interested in the beliefs that fuel their resilience as they struggle in their new and strange home. I have a visceral response to the woman who tells me about the papayas in her country of origin, and I can taste their sweetness and see their ripeness. I can feel her longing and her loss and see it reflected in the face of her little girl. I too was that little girl. I have a photograph in my mind's eye of the town square where my mother lived in Kladowa, Poland, the park in the square where she skipped with her friend during those brief better times; I see her leaving her home clutching both her doll and her fear. Even before I went back there four years ago and saw Klodowa for the first time, I missed the park of my mother's childhood and I knew that fear of loss can be transmitted across generations. Whenever I work with immigrant families, I try to understand the pre-, during, and postmigration experience, not only their own but also the experiences of the generations that preceded them and is part of their inheritance.

Both feminism and Judaism are influential in my life. When I was a child, my mother was by far the more assertive member of the couple within the home, but she was also constrained by societal injunctions. She worked, but it was part time and her office was in our apartment. My father did some child care and housework, but it was primarily my mother's responsibility. My parents sent me to a school that followed traditional gendered interpretations of Jewish law although they did not maintain their parents' strictly orthodox practices. My mother and my father communicated to me that I should pursue my education and enter a field of my choice and that it was important for me to earn an income on my own, but they expected me to marry and to marry a man. Although from the perspective of the American community in which I grew up, my mother's career was an anomaly, from my European Jewish heritage it was not. Women worked in the shtetls and towns. Often, women worked so their husbands could spend time studying Torah; often they worked just to make it possible for the families to survive. My mother worked in part because she needed the money. More than that, I believe, she worked for her intellectual survival and to feed the unrelenting responsibility she felt toward social activism.

But my mother paid a price for her awareness. The Holocaust took its toll on my mother, who helped the anti-Hitler effort but knew she was safely tucked away in America as her brother, sister-in-law, nieces, aunts, and uncles were murdered. I believe that the trauma of the Holocaust legacy stole my mother's joy, and gender roles kept her from usefully channeling her anger and leadership. As years passed and she no longer had a role in resettling refugees, she became depressed and easily angered. While the Judaism I know has permitted women (although not enough women) to be prophets, judges, leaders, and wisdom-bearers (the Hebrew word for wisdom is feminine), and while women in my family and in eastern Europe have worked for generations, the society into which my mother moved did not allow her to have that gender flexibility. My intelligent, energetic mother was asked by colleagues to move to Israel, to help form the Knesset (parliament) there, but she returned home after three years in Europe not only because she felt her mother needed her but because she internalized the unspoken rule that women had to marry and become mothers. She lost her enthusiasm for life in the process. As a therapist, I hope to question what is unspoken as well as what is spoken so that my client's decisions are made more consciously and with more awareness of the constraints that are being imposed. I've seen what can happen when trauma interacts with restrictions on ways of successfully channeling one's responses to trauma. I knew my mother as a victim of her history and her gender role, and I wish there had been a therapist in her young life who could have helped her develop her alternative stories, a therapist who saw herself or himself as a healer.

I also know that it was my mother's firm rootedness in the Jewish community and her community action projects and not just the love and devotion my father and I felt for her that helped her through her lifelong battle with depression. I therefore always understand mental health using an ecological framework. I cannot look at the individual without understanding the family, community, society, and contexts of race, class, gender, ethnicity, sexuality, religion, and more. It is through these contexts that we suffer, and it is from that same well that we draw our strengths. When an isolated, overwhelmed Latina widow came to me, part of our work was connecting her with a church and support group that felt familiar at a time when nothing felt like home. In another example, a first-generation Mexican-American lawyer, daughter of financially poor and traumatized immigrants, reported feeling a sense of well-being after years of struggling emotionally when she began to provide legal aid to Mexican-American immigrants.

It has been 52 years since Elijah's ghost floated by me, and it is only recently that I realized how much his ghost has been a part of me. After all, the mythical Elijah carries with him the hopes of our people: he speaks truth to power, he is there when we are at our lowest point, he takes personal responsibility to ensure that the poor and marginalized are given the sustenance they need and the hope that the order will change, he comes each year to our seders, he will always be with us. I hope to bring to therapy the feminist counterpart of Elijah. I want us as therapists to be there emotionally, relationally, spiritually, and cognitively with our clients; to understand their sorrows and their joys through the lens of the multiple contexts of their lives; to bear witness; to hold onto hope; and to experience the privilege of accompanying our clients on their journeys. I want my pen to keep writing and writing until the world we live in is transformed into a place of justice and compassion. Dayenu.

French, Catholic, Jewish. Outsider Within

LOUISE BORDEAUX SILVERSTEIN

As a Jew, one is automatically an outsider in many cultural contexts. However, my focus in this paper will be on how my Jewish identity has both reflected and constructed an ambiguous insider/outsider status within my own family. I will then turn to how this outsider status influences my professional work.

My mother was raised in an immigrant Jewish family. Her parents were born in Russia and Lithuania and were culturally Jewish. They emigrated to the United States in the early years of the twentieth century and settled in Cleveland, Ohio. My father's parents were French. They emigrated to New Orleans in 1874. My father was 30 years older than my mother. They met at the racetrack in Cleveland where my father was head of security and also owned and raced horses. They began living together after knowing each other for three months. Although my father had been separated from his first wife for 15 years, it took him another 12 years to obtain a divorce. Getting the divorce was a long and stressful process that broke his first wife's heart because of her religious beliefs and resulted in his excommunication from the Catholic church.

The first five years of my life I lived in New Orleans, in the city, and later running wild on a farm. My second language was French. I went to a French-speaking nursery school and to a very high French Catholic church. We said Hail Marys every day in front of a portrait of the Madonna and child in a room redolent with incense. I was very close to my father and felt loved and adored by him.

When I was five my father died, and my mother returned to her parents' home. In Cleveland, I was suddenly thrust into an urban, Eastern European Jewish lifestyle. My grandmother spoke Yiddish, kept kosher, lit candles every Friday evening, and observed the sabbath. Insofar as it was possible, she re-created the life of the shtetl where she had been born outside of Wilnius, Lithuania. Without a husband to support her, my mother was forced to seek paid employment, so my grandmother became my primary caretaker.

I cannot remember how difficult the transition to life in Cleveland must have been. However, I do remember getting off the train—the *City of New Orleans*—and greeting my grandmother, telling her that she was going to burn in hell because she didn't believe in Jesus Christ. *"Oy, Oy! Oy, gavolt!"* she cried, giving a *geshrei* (a scream). Somehow, we recovered from that shaky beginning and developed a very caring and loving relationship. Because my mother never again mentioned my father and our life in New Orleans, and because I spent the next 12 years living in the midst of my mother's Jewish family, I became identified as a Jew. I didn't repress my life as a French Catholic little girl, I just felt totally emotionally cut off from it.

Although I felt loved by my grandmother, I never felt like I belonged in my mother's family. My mother had a very competitive relationship with her two younger sisters, Emma and Pauline. They were blonde and light-skinned, like my grandmother, and had been her favorites. My mother had a darker complexion and dark hair and was allied with her father in the marital wars that my grandparents waged. My aunts had financially successful husbands and lived conventional, upper middle class lifestyles. My mother had a dead husband who had left her financially bereft. My name was Bordeaux, in a family of Goldsteins and Goodmans.

Despite my "otherness," my mother's family followed my grandmother's lead and was welcoming to me. Every Sunday one of the aunts would invite us to dinner. I felt embraced by the extended family as long as I was with my grandmother. However, I knew that I could never pass as one of them. I was too dark, too fat, too poorly dressed. I was my mother's daughter, and they were not fond of their older, disreputable sister.

I also had trouble fitting into the larger culture of Shaker Heights, Ohio. My last name, Bordeaux, was unpronounceable, and there was always a lot of snickering at school whenever the roll was called in class. I also did not have a father, which in the 1950s was like not having an arm. I always felt disabled, different.

There was also the question of money. In high school, friendships were defined, first by religion, then by class. I couldn't fit into the Jewish mainstream because my family didn't belong to either of the Jewish country clubs, my mother couldn't afford to send me to Mrs. Shapiro's for ballroom dancing lessons, and my clothing certainly did not attain the fashion standards required of the "popular" girls. Similarly, I couldn't fit into the non-Jewish mainstream because I was Jewish.

Ultimately, I developed three close Jewish girlfriends: two came from divorced families where their fathers had no relationship with them, and the third had a father who was chronically ill. The absence of male incomes in all of our families left us in more or less the lower middle class. The absence of a dominant male presence, and the fact that all of our mothers worked, allowed us more freedom than most middle class Jewish girls. Most of the time, our mothers had no idea what we were up to. We spent most of our time chasing boys, since this was the currency of self-worth in that era. Because none of us could fit into the upper middle class Jewish lifestyle of Shaker, we dated mostly non-Jewish boys and generally developed a "crossover" lifestyle.

My crossover lifestyle also led me to begin a flirtation with an African American boy in high school. We were young kids, 16 years old, studying American history together. We lived near each other and spent a few weeks walking home from school together. Although there was definitely a lot of sexual chemistry between us, we never got beyond a few kisses. After a couple of weeks, one of the "older" White Jewish boys, an 11th grader, began to call me "a nigger lover." Because of my vulnerability to my own outsider status in the Jewish community, I became very frightened by this epithet and began avoiding my Black friend. It took us 30 years to talk about this experience. At a high school reunion, I learned that the consequences of this crossover were much greater for him. He told me about how the football coach trumped up a reason to suspend him from the football team for a period of time. This suspension was very serious for him because he was going to college on a football scholarship. He got the message: Don't mess with a White girl. Learning about the differences in the consequences of our behavior was shocking to me, as was my complete lack of awareness of the implications of our friendship for him. This experience has generated a strong interest in confronting my own racism and insensitivity. Sensitizing the Yeshiva graduate students about racism and sexism has become a major focus of my academic work.

When it was time to apply to college, everyone smart [and White] at Shaker High was expected to apply to the Ivy Leagues. Instead, I applied to Sophie Newcomb, the women's college of Tulane University in New Orleans. I had no conscious awareness of wanting to return to my roots, wanting to return to a place where everyone knew how to pronounce Bordeaux. Yet, I stood up to the pressure from my friends and the guidance counselor and insisted on going to Newcomb.

When I got to New Orleans, I called my half-sister, Grace, my father's daughter from his first marriage. She refused to meet me. This experience was apparently so painful that I repressed it. I have no memory of that phone call. I didn't learn of it until Grace apologized for it many years later.

At Newcomb, I defined myself as part of the Jewish minority. This was somewhat problematic because I could not afford to go through sorority rush, which was the conventional pathway toward acceptance. Luckily, my roommate was a very cosmopolitan, Canadian Jewish woman who refused to go through rush because sororities were "too, too *passe.*" Her disdain provided a cover story that helped me avoid acknowledging my family's financial straits. We became notorious as the first two Jewish girls in the history of Newcomb who refused to rush. Thus she and I became part of the left-wing Jewish intellectual set, outsiders within the outsiders. Being a

Jew at Newcomb in the 1960s was interesting. One schoolmate from Dallas had never met a Jewish person before and asked to see my horns!

After graduation from college, I married a conventional, upper middle class Jewish man. Again, I had no conscious understanding that I hoped to become a Jewish insider. To my surprise, my husband turned out to be the "outlaw" in his family—of course, who else could marry someone like me? To his surprise, Louise Bordeaux turned out to be Jewish! So the hope that I would be welcomed into the bosom of a nice Jewish family didn't exactly work out. Still, as a "Silverstein," I came closer to joining the "Goldstein/Goodman" club.

This outsider/insider status has influenced my choice of profession, and my choice of a specialty within that profession. Becoming a family therapist has been part of my search for a family to belong to. Choosing to specialize in Bowen family systems therapy, which emphasizes reconnecting with one's extended family across many generations, has helped me find my own family. In retrospect, I think that I was hoping that doing family of origin work would give me the key to finding a way for my famil(ies) to accept me. Although I have not been accepted in the way that I had hoped (who ever is?), this work has helped me understand the emotional forces operating across the generations to overdetermine my outsider status.

Understanding these multigenerational roots, I have come to take my outsider position much less personally. I now realize that, because of the cultural/emotional clash between the two families, if I remain connected to both sides I will always be considered an outsider by each side. The only way that I could become an insider would be to deny or dissociate from one side of my family. This, of course, would be more damaging than absorbing the stress of being an outsider within.

Thus I remain very identified with both my Jewish and my French roots and have accepted that I will never feel fully at home in either community. I am close to both my Cleveland Jewish and Catholic New Orleans families. About 15 years ago, I hosted a large family dinner in which my mother and Grace (who is almost exactly my mother's age) met each other for the first time. Although this event was quite stressful, it also generated a new level of identity integration for me.

My insider/outsider status has had an impact on my academic life as well. When I decided to pursue an academic career after 10 years in private practice, it was very difficult to find a job in New York City. After being rejected in several places, I landed a job at the graduate school of psychology at Yeshiva University. Yeshiva is an interesting environment in that the graduate schools are all secular but the overall university and the undergraduate colleges (male and female) operate under the rubric of Modern Orthodox Judaism. As a secular Jew, I again find myself a Jewish outsider within an Orthodox Jewish institution.

However, with a name like Silverstein, I can pass for a member of the tribe, if not the family. That is, until I open my radical feminist mouth. Because I teach a course on the social construction of gender, I am "outed" early in each academic year. Although many of my views generate tension between me and some of my Orthodox Jewish students, I have learned a great deal from them. I have been privileged to have a window into a way of life that is much more complex and layered than a feminist outsider might imagine it to be. I have also been challenged to walk the walk of multi-culturalism in a way that is very personal. As a feminist, it has been difficult for me to embrace diversity to an extent that includes religious fundamental-ism, especially because this particular brand of fundamentalism represents my own cultural and religious origins.

My quest for insider status has helped me accept the ambiguity and complexity of life, and in this way has made me a better therapist. I now rea-lize that the forces generating the distance between me and both my father's and mother's families started many years prior to their marriage. For example, I now realize, that no matter how good I am to my Aunt Emma, my mother's sister, she will never love me as much as she loves Carol, her other sister's (my Aunt Pauline's) daughter. This is a continuing sadness for me. However, I now know that it has nothing to do with me and everything to do with the emotional triangle between my grandmother, my mother, and her two sisters. My mother was the outsider in that triangle, and as her daughter, I inherited that outsider status. It might as well be encoded within my genes.

Similarly, Grace would never forgive our father for the shame and humiliation that his divorce caused her mother. Because she could never completely separate her feelings for our father from her feelings for me, she would always maintain a wary emotional distance between us. In the early years after our reconciliation, Grace saw me as her ticket to heaven. She explained that she was worried about meeting St. Peter in heaven because she had not been able to stop hating our father. She was hoping that making peace with me would encourage St. Peter to overlook her hateful thoughts toward our father. Many years later, Grace ended her life in a nursing home, suffering from dementia. On my final visit, she was convinced that I was the devil standing next to her bed. And so I fell from the Gates of Heaven to the Gates of Hell, the ultimate insider/outsider experience.

Accepting the inevitability of these multigenerational emotional forces has helped me to stop blaming anyone in my family. Blocking blame may be one of the most important tasks of a therapist. As long as one is blam-ing others, one is not able completely to take responsibility for oneself. Focusing on the Other—on what our mother/father/husband/wife/any significant other—did or did not do, to or for us, is a way of giving up power, the power to change one's life for the better. Focusing on Self, in contrast, allows us to accept responsibility and mobilize our power to change.

The issues of sibling rivalry, emotional triangles, and conflicting family loyalties exist in every family. In my family many of these conflicts have been exacerbated by cultural and religious differences. Unbraiding the ethnic, religious, and emotional strands of my otherness has helped me to accept being an outsider within both sides of my family. On a good day, this has made it easier for me to help clients accept their sense of otherness. On a bad day, I tend to get too identified with that otherness and even to project it onto a client who may not be struggling with that issue at all.

To a great extent, my life has been organized around trying to become a cozy insider somewhere. However, when insider status is within my grasp, I "find" myself having climbed out onto a limb and in the process sawing it off behind me. When the in-group of the moment finishes off the amputation, I am (once again) surprised and hurt.

In the course of this lifelong struggle, I have made some progress recently. I am no longer compelled to be the outsider in every aspect of my life. In the past three years I have initiated a Holocaust research project at YU, studying the experiences of grandchildren of the Holocaust and exploring the possibility of creating a model teaching curriculum for high school students that teaches about the Holocaust and stresses the importance of protecting the rights of all minorities and marginalized groups. Focusing on this painful moment in Jewish history has brought me closer to many faculty members at YU and at universities in Israel as well.

Moreover, on a recent trip to Cleveland, I spent a lot of time with my cousin Carol, Aunt Emma's favorite. I am now beginning to have some appreciation for the burden of insider status. Still another surprise on the lifelong journey that is family of origin work.

From the Outside, Looking In

ANDREA J. BERGMAN

Thinking about and writing about my Jewish identity has been quite a challenging and rewarding process. My relationship with Judaism has changed and developed throughout my life, and I don't feel as if the journey is over yet. For me, one of the important themes that has remained consistent is one of affiliation and alienation, the feeling of being an "outsider" yet connected at the same time. That theme, more than any other, may have influenced my decision to become a clinical psychologist. As a therapist, I must always remain an outsider to my patients in some fundamental ways. But the connection between us is nevertheless extremely powerful.

Growing up, my mother and father were clearly ambivalent about any affiliation with institutional religion. I was born in the sixties and my parents were moderate hippies, rejecting many social conventions yet living a middle-class suburban lifestyle. They both came from a long line of ambivalent Jews, including my maternal grandmother who emigrated from Poland in 1939 when she was 16. Neither set of grandparents belonged to a synagogue, although my paternal grandparents kept kosher. I have no memory of setting foot in a synagogue until I attended a friend's bar mitzvah at age 13. We did celebrate the Jewish holidays with a festive family dinner, although I had no idea what these celebrations represented. During my early elementary school years, we lived in a relatively non-Jewish neighborhood, and I remember my parents commenting on how different the neighbors were because they were not Jewish. I didn't understand what that meant except that it made me feel different from everyone else and I learned not to advertise that I was a Jew.

There were other secrets as well, including those that I didn't even consciously understand. It seems that my parents were growing marijuana in our backyard, which they were keeping secret from everyone, including my sister and me. When I was in the fourth grade, my teacher was doing a lesson on debates and wanted the class to debate the legalization of marijuana (this was the early 1970s). None of the children in our rather rural, conservative suburb would volunteer to take the "pro" position so my teacher asked me to do it. I agreed and argued my case enthusiastically. After the debate was over, all of the other children gathered around my desk and started taunting me with statements such as "You are going to be a drug addict." I left school in tears and related the story to my parents when I came home, not consciously knowing about my parents' secret lives as pot smokers. This experience reinforced, on some level, my feelings of "other" but also illustrates my ability and willingness at a very young age to say things that others would not. This skill has allowed me, as a therapist, to facilitate the expression of uncomfortable and unpopular feelings, impulses, and thoughts of my patients. As a therapist, I am a keeper of secrets and I listen to things that other people don't want to hear, things that are underneath the surface and are perceived as unacceptable. As a therapist, I am able to listen, accept the unacceptable, and comment on things that other people hide or ignore.

Despite the great training I was receiving for my future career as a psychologist, my parents eventually tired of living in such an oppressive community. We moved to a more liberal, and predominantly Jewish, community, ostensibly for the highly regarded school system. I think that my parents wanted us to be surrounded by Jews without the need to join a synagogue. Unfortunately, given my complete lack of any Jewish education, I still felt like an outsider among my now mostly Jewish friends, especially since we were approaching the age for b'nai mitzvahs. As I entered adolescence, I felt awkward and shy regarding my body, mind, and soul. I dreaded attending the Saturday morning services during these coming-of-age ceremonies and felt like a complete foreigner, ignorant and ashamed. Luckily, I had few friends at this time so I didn't have many invitations to worry about.

Since I was clearly not having a bat mitzvah, my maternal grandmother decided to take me to Israel for my thirteenth birthday. For years, my grandmother had been telling us very vivid and scary stories of the Holocaust and her many relatives in Poland, some who had perished and some that had escaped to Israel. The relatives in Israel were my grandmother's first cousins and their descendants. This trip was instrumental in connecting me to both my family history and my Jewish identity. Throughout our stay in Israel, we were treated like royalty. This family that I had never met embraced me with such warmth and hospitality that I was astonished. The association I had felt between "family" and being Jewish was now strengthened. I felt that this was a missing piece of the puzzle of where I came from and who I was. I also felt a connection to these people and this country that had little if anything to do with religion. I was beginning to understand how I could be a Jew without believing in God.

Much to my father's horror, I decided that I would spend a summer in Israel when I turned 16. His greatest fear was that I would meet an Israeli boy, get married, and/or join the army. While in Israel, I lived and worked on a kibbutz where my cousins were residents. At the beginning of the summer, another cousin was getting married and my grandmother, mother, and sister had flown to Israel to attend the wedding. I was to attend the wedding with my cousins from the kibbutz since I had already started living there. While getting dressed for the wedding I noticed that my cousins were wearing very casual clothes (e.g., shorts) while I had brought a full-length gown to wear. I was feeling very self-conscious about my ostentatious dress and told my cousin that I didn't want to go to the wedding. She told me that I could also wear shorts since now I was a "kibbutznik." My head was now swimming with identities: American, Jew, Israeli, Kibbutznik! In the end, I wore my dress and, if my father had been there, he would have sighed in relief that I had chosen my American identity. Once again, I would belong but yet not belong.

In working through my issues with affiliation and alienation, it is not entirely surprising that I chose to do my graduate training in the South. On some level, I may have been stretching the limitations of how Jewish or non-Jewish I could be. Could I be accepted in a city where the Klan was marching just outside the city limits? After four years of graduate training in Atlanta, I decided to push the envelope even further and do my internship in Birmingham, Alabama. At this point, my father was wishing that I had married that nice Jewish boy in Israel.

By beginning my professional training in a place where I continued to maintain my "outsider" status, I began to explore how these factors might affect my therapeutic work. Initially, I tended to focus on similarities rather than differences between my patients and myself. Historically, this was my way of dealing with the feeling of being an outsider, so I was pretty good at it. This skill has served me well in making connections with patients and developing a therapeutic alliance. On the other hand, I have learned that my status as an "outsider" may also facilitate the therapeutic relationship. For example, when I was on internship in Alabama I sometimes treated patients with little education or economic resources. During my treatment of one such family who was living in a trailer park on the outskirts of the city, it was disclosed that a grandfather had molested several of the girls in the extended family. Despite the religious, social, and cultural gap that separated me from this family, we were able to work together with the entire extended family in uncovering their secret and getting help for all of the girls. I believe that my comfort in discussing unacceptable and distasteful material, as well as my status as an "outsider," may have provided some safety for the family in disclosing their secret.

When I lived in the South, being from New York was synonymous with being Jewish. Both patients and other (non-Jewish) professionals made certain assumptions about me based on the way I talked and dressed, since these factors usually gave away my Yankee background. I felt awkward being lumped into a category that I did not fit into. How could I explain that, while I was Jewish, I did not observe religious holidays or attend synagogue?

Ironically, after moving to Alabama I decided that, for the first time in my life, I wanted to attend services for the high holidays. I felt a need to affiliate with other Jews and explore further what my Jewish identity meant. It was not difficult to locate the other Jews in the hospital, and I was welcomed into the small Jewish community where I felt a curious comfort, although I understood nothing of the Hebrew services.

Moving back to New York after internship, the significance of being a Jewish psychologist had greatly changed. I was neither special nor unusual, and my religious background seemed irrelevant to most of my patients. What has become much more salient, to both patients and colleagues, is my theoretical orientation. It has been my experience, in the New York metropolitan area, that psychodynamic psychotherapy is akin to a religion; adherents often believe based on intellectual faith and their own experiences rather than on empirical evidence that either confirms or disconfirms its principles. This is not necessarily a criticism. Since psychotherapy is based on a relationship, which is difficult to quantify and measure, it is not surprising to have a viable theoretical orientation that is not based on empirical evidence.

I have always identified myself as eclectic, being trained in both cognitive-behavioral and psychodynamic approaches. Now I find myself feeling like an outsider in both "circles" because I do not affiliate exclusively with one or the other. Luckily, I am comfortable in this position given the practice that I have had throughout my life. This dual identity allows me access to the benefits of both approaches, where I can pick and choose that which makes sense for me and for my patients/clients. I am often surprised by the ease in which I can navigate both professional realms. For instance, while seeing a particularly difficult borderline patient, I sought supervision from an accomplished psychoanalyst. The support and insight that she provided were priceless, and she provided an anchor for me during the unpredictable and violent storms of a borderline therapeutic relationship.

Just as I am struggling to find a "home" for my professional identity, I am in the process of finding a "home" for my Jewish identity. I am married to a man who was raised in a Conservative Jewish home and we are both very active in our Conservative Synagogue, despite the fact that I cannot understand much of the religious services. I feel a sense of community in my shul and I am proud that I am providing my daughters with the sense of spiritual community that I did not have as a child. Despite my active involvement in my synagogue, however, I still often find myself sitting in meetings and services feeling like an outsider looking in. This realization brings a smile to face, with the knowledge that my lifelong experiences feeling like an outsider have contributed to my unique abilities and strengths as a therapist.

As my children get older, the questions are becoming more complex and less easily answered. Since I had never participated in religious school, I was not quite prepared for the indoctrination into the religion that they are now experiencing. This has made for some interesting dinner conversation regarding my belief in God and whether a lack of such belief means that I cannot be Jewish. The complexities of culture, religion, and belief are difficult concepts to explain to elementary aged children who are more comfortable with concrete categories of right and wrong. Hopefully, through my outsider status in my current nuclear family, I can now teach my children tolerance and the subtler shades of gray that they will encounter all around them.

Unexpectedly, there is also something that my experiences as a therapist have contributed to the development of my relationship with Judaism, and that is faith. I have learned the necessity of faith in every aspect of life through the privilege of having access to the intimate details of the most painful sorrows and joyful triumphs of people's lives. I know that sometimes there are forces operating beyond explanation, beyond science, and certainly beyond my comprehension, and I have come to appreciate that force. As a psychologist, I have a yearning to quantify, measure, and analyze everything, but I am also learning that there might be some elements to the healing process that we will never uncover, and that this just might not be a bad thing.

Culture as Both a Lens and a Veil

CAROL R. HEFFER

Like the wise men describing an elephant, we all see the world through our own unique perspective. What we perceive when we encounter the elephant depends on where we're standing in the room, who we're standing with, and where the room itself is located. We see through the eyes of our ancestors, our culture, our race, religion, economic status, families, and teachers. And we, in turn, are seen by others through their unique lenses. The depth and complexity of our development—who we are, how we think, our perceptions of the world and one another—make each encounter with another person a unique and singular journey. The more we can understand our own personal journey, the more we can begin to appreciate and grasp the depth of another's experience. This seems intrinsic to the work of a therapist.

My own journey has been enhanced and enriched by my being born a Jewish woman. There are endless arguments about whether Judaism is a religion, a race, or a culture. Discussing Judaism as a race is always disturbing to me, as it was used as a rationale for the extermination of Jews during the Holocaust. For me, Judaism has always been both a culture and religion. It represents a unique way of life, customs passed down through the ages, affected by the way our ancestors saw the world and how, via the Jewish Laws, we impacted one another. I believe Judaism is underrepresented in the broader considerations of cultural diversity and in the multicultural discourse. It is sometimes difficult for non-Jews to appreciate how profound the effect of being Jewish can be. It is hard for some to see Jews as a minority, a group of approximately 14 million people, because of our powerful and enduring impact on our communities, society and the world.

For me, the essence of psychotherapy is inextricably bound to my upbringing, which includes my understanding of Judaism and the world. One of my earliest memories about being Jewish was when I was young and attending youth services at my temple. It was a conservative temple, with some orthodox families. We were learning about our connection to G-d and our responsibility to that connection and our connections to our society and the world. In this connection, I felt as though I had both ultimate freedom and ultimate responsibility. Whatever I did to prove myself in this world was between G-d and me; there was no other intermediary. This meant that I was responsible for my actions, for how I cared about the people and the world around me. I took this responsibility very seriously. It made me feel very free, very alive, and very powerful. This became a core value for me, a value that motivated me to both engage in my own psychotherapy and to become a psychotherapist myself. My own psychotherapy has helped me to practice being the best person I can be, and I try in my work as a psychotherapist to help others experience the thrill and the responsibility of their freedom. These are my highest ideals and aspirations. Yet, the struggle of being human means that I must also embrace my imperfections, my shadow side. That is part of my individual journey as well as my therapeutic goal for my own clients. Everything does not need to be healed immediately. My personal work in psychotherapy has taught me to embrace patience and process instead of perfection.

Personally, what I have always loved most about my culture, are the stories. Our history as a people and my own individual history within my family of origin is rich in joy, pain, and struggle. My family was not short on tales going back to experiences in Russia, Austria, Germany, and the Ukraine. My mother's name was Ricca, her mother's name was Sarah. Sarah's mother was Sophie and her mother was Chavah. Chavah's mother was Devorah. My sister is Jessica, her daughter, Dara, and now Harlie, Dara's daughter, has recently joined us. All these women! I have heard stories all of my life, sitting around the dining room table, the kitchen table, cooking, laughing, crying, and laughing until I cried. My great-grandmother, Sophie, came from a *shtetl*[1] outside of Kiev. Her parents ran an inn and her father was a teacher. He taught my grandmother to read and write, which was uncommon for women of her generation. She came to America with my great grandfather, Charles, who was my namesake. Sophie and Charles ran away together to Latviah because she was betrothed to another and they loved each other. There they lived and worked until they saved enough money to journey to America. When they left Latviah, my great-grandmother was pregnant with my grandmother, Sarah, who was born on the Fourth of July, 1898, in America. The voyage here was difficult. The passengers were packed in, living in close, hot quarters. My pregnant great-grandmother was exhausted and nauseous from the pregnancy and the rough trip. As the story goes, she was feisty and beautiful. Apparently,

---

[1]A *shtetl* (Yiddish: שטעטל diminutive form of Yiddish shtot שטאָט "town") was typically a small town with a large Jewish population forced to live there by Germans in pre-Holocaust Central and Eastern Europe. Shtetls (Yiddish plural: shtetlekh) were mainly found in the areas that constituted the 19th century Pale of Settlement in the Russian Empire, the Congress Kingdom of Poland, Galicia, and Romania. *Wikipedia, the free encyclopedia.*

the ship's captain took pity on her and permitted her to come up top to the deck for fresh air, and a cup of tea—a memorable story that I loved hearing again and again.

On my father's side there were also strong women and men. My last name, Heffer, is from my father's maternal lineage, not his father's. My grandmother was already here when she met my grandfather. She had already started a business on the Lower East Side when they married, so Grandpa went to work for/with her. The customers would call him Mr. Heffer, my grandmother's name. He and Grandma decided he should change his name to hers so not to confuse the customers, He and Grandma and my father's oldest brother, Milton, all had their names changed to Heffer, my grandmother's family name. And so I carry the maternal name. It was a powerful, radical act. It added fuel to my fire of independence and pride as a woman and a devotion to my name and roots. I think of how confident my grandpa John must have been to take his wife's name. The story is that he was completely devoted to her. In the 1970s, when feminism was reignited, this story inspired and validated me. This story validated my pride in my feminine strength and inspired me to challenge the patriarchal values that the feminist movement then explored and challenged.

Grandpa John came to the United States at the age of 11. He won a lottery in the Ukraine, and came all by himself across the ocean. He made a good life here; he met his wife, and had four sons, all good husbands and fathers, four daughters-in-law, and eight grandchildren. How brave he must have been to make such a trip alone and to know no one when he arrived. How brave all these immigrants must have been. When I went to Ellis Island to honor where they landed, it was such a powerful experience that I cried. I thought about my great-grandmother's cousin. He was sent back because he was ill. I cannot imagine what it was like to have traveled so far, at such expense—physically, emotionally, and economically—and then to have to return. This happened to many people who have made that journey and happens still. I tried to imagine what those immigrant returned to: pain, persecution, poverty, possible death. Looking at the photographs on display at Ellis Island, I was struck with their rich ethnicity, with faces alive with hope, joy, pain, and mischief. These stories encouraged my adventurous spirit. They opened my eyes to the struggles people have taken on to find safety in their worlds and peace in their hearts.

Sophie and Charles settled on the Lower East Side of New York City and they worked hard making clothing. My great grandfather would go to work all day in a sweatshop. My great-grandmother stayed home because she was pregnant and, so I was told, modesty dictated that she remain home. They saved pennies until they could afford a sewing machine of their own. Then great grandpa would bring work home and they would both sew into the night to make enough to start their own little business. With the money they made they sent for the rest of the family. The cruelty of the czar and the continual *pogroms*[2] made them resentful of Russia and worried for their kin. As a result, they rejected their Russian background while embracing their Judaism and America. They went to school immediately to learn English and to lose their Russian accents. They gave up speaking Yiddish. Yiddish was the international language of Ashkenazi Jews from Central and Eastern Europe. It was derived from a combination of German and Hebrew. For them, Yiddish was the language of their oppression and they spoke it only to keep secrets from their Americanized children. They did not want to use a language that they were forced to use by their oppressor. They did very well for themselves and their family but left behind their Russian culture and part of their pain. Jews in Germany were not allowed to speak German, which is where Yiddish originated. Jews in Russsia and Poland were not allowed to speak those languages, so they too spoke Yiddish. While there were many Jews who gave up speaking Yiddish to make it easier to assimilate in America, this was not the case with my family. I was always told that Yiddish for them represented their oppression. They spoke Yiddish in Russia because they were not permitted to speak anything else, not because it was their choice. There was no ambivalence in my grandparents as with many Jews, regarding being Jewish. They often talked about how disturbing it was to them that many Jews changed their names or felt compelled to hide their identity out of fears for their safety.

I was born in New York City in 1948, the same year Israel was born. I always felt a kinship to Israel. I grew up in a region that approximately half of the world's Jewish population calls home, yet I was raised in a predominantly Catholic neighborhood. Steeped in Jewish culture, my family was part of a small enclave of Jews who had chosen to leave the safety of a larger Jewish community and make their homes in a Catholic neighborhood. I believe this was the beginning of my understanding of feeling like an outsider. That sense of outsiderness was a mentality that would help me to understand the struggles of people who fall outside of the mainstream expectations and common wisdom of their communities. Our neighborhood was made up of post–World War II families, of soldiers who were returning from the war. For these families, marrying and having children necessitated more space, prompting the move from the city to the suburbs. The ethos was to be "American." There was no sense of what I was to do with my identification with my Russia roots, as being Russian was a conflicted identity for my grandparents and Russia was then the Cold War "enemy" of the United States. My family didn't have much that was positive to say about the country from

---

[2]*Pogrom* is a Russian word meaning "to wreak havoc, to demolish violently." Historically, the term refers to violent attacks by local non-Jewish populations on Jews in the Russian Empire and in other countries. The first such incident to be labeled a pogrom is believed to be anti-Jewish rioting in Odessa in 1821. Copyright©United States Holocaust Memorial Museum, Washington, D.C. Encyclopedia Last Updated: May 4, 2009.

which they barely escaped with their lives. Hence, my connection to and understanding of what it meant to be Russian was largely colored by negative memories.

The stories I was told of my ancestors' time in Russia had a powerful impact on my sense of safety and security. They spoke of how the soldiers would eat and drink with my family at their inn, befriend them, and then viciously turn against them. On Christian holidays, as well as at other times, the soldiers and people from the surrounding towns would ride their horses through the *shtetl* murdering Jews and wreaking havoc. I am told that they once pitchforked my great-granduncle. The story was that my great-grandmother could only watch breathlessly as her brother was suspended in the air. However, despite the danger involved, my great-great-grandmother, Chavah, took action. She called to the soldier by name. Through his drunken frenzy, he recognized her and he released my great-granduncle alive.

These stories reverberated in my mind and have left an imprint of fear, worry, and suspicion. The question that arises from this is who can be trusted, for what, and for how long. When will they turn? Even now, when I meet new people, these are questions that flash through my mind. Clearly issues of trust come up in my work with clients, and knowing my sensitivity to issues around trust, I have to pay special attention to my countransference in this area.

I was in first grade when I realized there was something different about us. A classmate commented about my praying differently than the others and suggested that I was not holding my hands in the "right" way during school prayer. At the time I was not putting my hands together in the way that people of some faiths do when praying. I asked my mother why we did this "wrong." She responded that we weren't wrong, but we were not like everyone else. We were different. It took me a while to understand the difference between "doing it wrong" and doing it "differently." How easy it is to label differences in a perjorative way. How difficult it is to assimilate when one is different. Can one assimilate? Is assimilation possible? Is it desirable? What are the psychic costs of not assimilating? How does one build a bridge across difference? How do we hold on to the reality that we are different while striving for the ideal that we are all one in our humanity is the challenge? Our conversations at the dinner table and with friends often questioned whether we could trust assimilation. Clearly assimilation hadn't worked for the German Jews who saw themselves as very assimilated into German society yet perished horrifically in the Holocaust. My father would remind us that although we were Jewish and proud of Israel, we were Americans first. Not only is this a continuing dialectic in my own life but also in my work as a therapist. I use my spiritual understanding that we are all human beings who are learning to live together, who have more things in common than are different, in my work with clients. I believe that if we focus on our similarities rather than our differences it will counteract the isolation that many people experience that keeps them stuck in their pain. When stuck in their pain they can be unable to see resources and solutions outside of themselves.

Facing anti-Semitism as a child was difficult. Growing up, balancing the pride in my culture and yet wanting to fit in was challenging. It was difficult then and still raises conflict between defending myself and remaining engaged with people who devalue Jews and therefore devalue me. I am aware in my work with clients how pride can give rise to emotional conflict. Sometimes pride is their greatest hold on self-respect, particularly in untenable situations. It is a defense that is delicate and powerful. It is delicate because it is built on hurt. It is powerful because it gives the person a sense of strength; however, the sense of strength is illusory. The sense of strength is really a pretense because it is not based on a healthy decision about the person's best long-term interests, it represents fear, defiance, and self-protectiveness.

The fact, idea, or feeling of being the outsider made me endlessly curious about what the lives of other people were like. I was frequently reminded that I was different. I was the "Jewish" friend when introduced to friend's families, or when I went to friend's country clubs and told not to let anyone know that I was Jewish. I recall driving to Brooklyn for Passover when I was very young. I would sit in the back seat of the car, looking into other cars, other worlds, wondering what they were doing, where they were going, what their lives were like. I was aware that my reality was probably very different from theirs. My curiosity led me to want to experience other ways of being and to know lives that were very different from mine. I have deliberately chosen jobs and career paths that would let me experience life with people who were different. During my most overtly radical feminist years I was as a carpenter working with men. I wondered, despite my frustration with their misogyny, how men were hurt by the sexism in our society and how they maintain their humanity. My encounters with people who were different has challenged my acceptance and my understanding of people from other cultures as well as those from similar cultures and their different choices. It is not surprising that I chose a career as a therapist, where my work requires—demands—that I step into the shoes of others and experience life from their vantage point. This is something I have been doing in some way or other since I was a child who felt different from others.

Part of my Jewishness is the constant desire to learn. It is not that other cultural groups do not want or do not encourage learning among their members. It is that learning is an explicit part of Jewish law. Studying the Torah and Talmud, questioning, participating in your community and society, challenging and reevaluating its laws are cultural and religious expectations of Judaism. It is what has led us to success and what has also left us open to attack. Reading and writing were and are essential to religious study and participation in the world, and it has historically led to a higher level of literacy among poor and peasant classes of Jews than their non-Jewish counterparts.

Keeping records for the landholders, collecting taxes, and lending money were the jobs that Jews were permitted to hold. We did the dirty work of the owning class such that they could maintain greater distance between themselves and the people they exploited. The fact that Jews were dispro-portionately literate made them overdetermined candidates for such jobs. These kinds of jobs made us intermediaries between the land-owning classes and the workers. Although we were not landowners or part of the ruling elite, as we were usually not permitted to own land, we became the face of the landowner and the target of resentment of working people that the landowners were exploiting. This has been the underlying impetus that drives anti-Semitism. However, we survived through knowledge.

Because Jews were targets of resentment we were often scapegoated and made targets of violence in most of the countries we inhabited. Hence, Jews were often forced to flee their homes with little notice to find safety, even when it was only temporary. Having to flee with little notice usually meant that there was no time to gather possessions. You had to leave taking only what you could carry. You could always carry your knowledge to some other place and start over again. Knowledge was one of our most important survival tools.

Being Jewish meant being socialized to always ask, "Why?" Studying the Torah and Talmud has always involved endless questioning, analyzing, reflecting, thinking, and seeking new understandings of ancient teachings. Hence it became infused into Jewish culture and the very way that Jews inter-act with one another and the world. In religion, work, school, and in our relationships there is endless questioning. In one of my intimate relationships there was a constant struggle between my partner and I with my constantly asking *why*. After our relationship ended and I attempted to process what happened with other Jewish friends they pointed out that it was normative for me to raise questions because it was a part of my cultural reality that I had been unaware of in my interactions with my partner. What I came to realize was that it was this cultural aspect of myself that my partner could not understand or accept and that at the time one I was not fully aware of. This aspect of being a Jew means asking why of ourselves, society, the Bible, the world. Among Jews it is the first step to gaining wisdom.

One important guide I have had in building bridges to the experience of others and in valuing connection with difference is embedded in another story from my childhood. When my family came to New Hyde Park they wanted to belong to a temple. They went to the only temple in the area, a small schul near the border of Queens. When they entered the schul they were greeted by the shamus.[3] My parents realized they were in an orthodox temple when the shamus started to seat my parents in two separate sections,

---

[3]sha·mas (shä'məs) noun *pl.* shamosim sha·mo'·sim (-môs'im) a synagogue official who pro-vides various services, often one who manages day-to-day affairs.

one for men, one for women. My parents did not wish to be separated. The shamus, sensing their discomfort and wanting these two young Jews to feel at home allowed them to sit together at the back of the temple. They stayed for the service and joined the congregration. The shamas captured the spirit of the rabbi and Jewish community who decided to open the doors to the rest of the congregation. Eventually, a compromise was made: the enclave of orthodox Jewish men, dressed in their black hats and beards could doven[4] at a table in the front right side of the temple near the altar and the other congregants could be integrated, men and women, in the body of the schul. These orthodox men were loving and gentle to me. My memory of the wise shamas smiling at me with sparkling eyes always brings joy to my heart.

As I reflect on the importance of the shamas and the schul to me, I am reminded of how I have been critically shaped by my desire to learn. I will attempt to summarize my understanding of how my being Jewish has affected my work as a therapist. A client recently read a quote to me from an unknown source: "Most of my great discoveries have been flashes of deep insight into the obvious." What is obvious to me is that people are always more than what they appear to be on the surface. Most situations and human dilemmas have a personal/internal aspect and a social/external component. People are harmed most when they feel responsible for their devaluation when it is really social or systemic forces that are culpable. However, if we attribute all problems and all pain to external or socially systemic causes, you take no responsibility for your own contribution to those problems. Since your contribution to your own dilemma is something that you do control, failing to recognize what that contribution is means that you lose the opportunity for growth. People cannot control nor are they responsible for everything that happens to them. What they do control is how they respond and what they learn from painful situations. The challenge is to discern the difference between your own contribution and that of systemic forces. The process of making those distinctions is where psychotherapy can be most helpful.

My work as a therapist comes from the core of what I have learned as a Jew. I deeply respect people and feel people have a responsibility to themselves and their community, which if not fulfilled can leave them feeling empty and isolated from others and themselves. I also respect people and their struggles, and when I lose sight of this I know I must examine myself and my countertransference. I believe that life is a gift that we are given to use to the best of our ability, in balance with others. And in this way, my Jewishness and my identity as a therapist come together and embrace each other.

---

[4]to daven (*third-person singular simple present* **davens**, *present participle* **davening**, *simple past and past participle* **davened**) (intransitive) to recite the Jewish liturgy; to pray.

Am I Jewish?

BARBARA LEVINE RODRIGUEZ
(PSEUDONYM)

When others ask me what I am, I say I am Jewish. I cannot categorize myself in any other way. Both of my parents were Jewish; all four of my grand-parents were part of the large Russian Jewish migration at the turn of the last century. However, apparently, like others who were requested to write for this volume, I also responded to Beverly that I was not representative and could not speak for other Jewish people. In fact, as the years have passed, I have come to feel more and more different and alienated from Jewishness as I experience it in America today. This was not always so for me, and it is a source of considerable pain.

I always knew I was Jewish. I was named for my deceased paternal grandmother, a deeply held tradition among Ashkenazi Jews. Up until the age of 5, I lived with my parents and my maternal grandparents. My grand-parents spoke English to me and my parents but Yiddish to each other. When I was about 4, my grandmother began to teach me to read letters in the Yiddish alphabet. My grandparents remained a major and significant presence in my life until my grandmother's death when I was not quite 8 and my grandfather's death when I was 15.

As I was growing up, I had little contact with my father's family. Both of my paternal grandparents died before my birth. My father's mother had died when he was a young child, and his father had left him and his sister, separately, with various relatives. The sister eventually married a German-American Protestant man from the Midwest, and she hid her Jewishness from the community in which they lived. As a result, she wanted no contact with my father, who bore a very easily recognizable Jewish name and appearance. Therefore, I never met my aunt. My father's father remarried and had two other children but never took my father to live with him in his second marriage. Despite this, my father maintained some contact with these two half-siblings, and I knew both of them. We saw them once or twice a year. My father's identity as a Jew was an ethnic one, not based in religion. It was connected to his sense of himself as a "mensch"—someone who despite the poverty and chaos and losses with which he had been raised was honorable and decent in his interactions with others. In addition to the terrible hurt he suffered from his sister's rejection, my father carried other experiences associated with being Jewish that he shared with me. He remembered ethnic gangs of kids on the Lower East Side who staked out turfs and how dangerous it was for him as a youngster to be in the Irish sections of town. My father was a big baseball fan and played on local teams as a young man; he told of a time that he played on a team sponsored by a local parish and gave a Irish version of his name so he could play (although all his teammates knew the truth). In his younger years, he worked in offices that were dominated by Irish people. He was friends with many, but he also experienced "jokes" that were not so funny. The main message that my father left me regarding being Jewish was the importance of not denying who you are.

My father also had a significant positive impact on me as a woman. Despite his lack of education, he expected that I would go on to college and become a professional. He would identify careers for me, like international journalist or criminal defense attorney, as being great careers for a woman, and it never occurred to me as a child that this was a peculiar distortion of the reality of assigned women's roles in the world. He never emphasized to me the importance of finding a marriage partner, and, in fact, derided people we knew who placed such an emphasis on it for their daughters. I think that his strong opinion about not denying who you are and his lack of tolerance for relegating women to the role of sex object/meat on the marriage marketplace resulted in my confusion about why so many Jewish women I knew were preoccupied with straightening their noses or lightening their hair. In this way, I don't think I have some of the internalized self-hatred that many Jewish women seem to have.

In contrast to my lack of interaction with my father's family, we lived with my mother's parents until I was five, and my maternal grandmother was probably my primary attachment figure. It is she whose face and hands are in my earliest memories. Each of my maternal grandparents had come from a large family, with many siblings, almost all of whom had migrated to the United States in the early part of the twentieth century. There were many great-aunts and great-uncles as well as their children and grandchildren who were part of my life as a child. All of the people in my grandparents' generation were heavily identified as Jews, but as secular and progressive in their orientation. My memory is of conversations among them at family gatherings that took place in both Yiddish and heavily accented English. As a very young child, I thought that the aging process involved developing both gray hair and a Russian Jewish accent.

There were major family gatherings of my grandfather's family at the home of my great-aunt twice each year—at Thanksgiving and at Passover. While my great-grandfather (my maternal grandfather's father) has been a very religious man, who spent his life at the synagogue studying and teaching children Hebrew, none of his eight children followed his religious observance.

This was very apparent at our Passover seders, where neither my grandfather nor his siblings would have anything to do with reading the Haggadah or any religious practice. The wonderfully gracious and giving hostess, my great-aunt, had married a man who came from a more traditional family. In deference to them, she would have her brother-in-law (her husband's sister's husband) read the Haggadah at one end of the table, while everyone else carried on a conversation about the events of the day, as though this was just any family gathering, with an outsider who happened to be present and who had an agenda that was different from everyone else's. These events also included my only exposure to any kind of kosher food restrictions. Again, in deference to her in-laws, my great-aunt had a separate set of plates for Passover and did not serve dairy with meat. However, despite the lack of real religious observance, the story of Passover was never lost on me, in that it clearly identified Jewish people to me as those who had been oppressed and should never oppress others.

My maternal grandparents were extremely political people. My grandfather and one of his brothers had been very active in the underground in Russia before the revolution. There were stories of time spent hiding in the woods and activities involving distribution of underground newspapers and leaflets. He and all of his brothers left Russia (actually Belarus) one by one to escape the draft. While his family had been poor, they were a tight-knit group, evidenced by the continuing family gatherings described. After five brothers had come, they paid the way for their parents and two younger sisters to join them in America. My grandfather and his siblings all learned to read and write Hebrew, Yiddish, and Russian, and all of the sons had skilled trades before coming to the United States. In contrast, my grandmother's mother had died in childbirth when my grandmother was five, leaving the father, who was an itinerant peddler, with a slew of children. The children, including my grandmother, were "apprenticed" out to wealthy families or shopkeepers. My grandmother, at age five, was essentially a servant in a wealthy family's home, where, according to her stories, she had to stand on a stool to make the bed because she was so little. Unlike my grandfather's childhood, my grandmother's girlhood was one of loss and lack of protection; siblings died, were raped, and were exploited. Needless to say, none of them were educated, and they were barely literate in their native languages when they came to America.

My maternal grandparents met in Russia, in the underground revolutionary movement, and fell in love. My grandfather came here first and sent for my grandmother. They considered themselves "freethinkers" and they never formally married, either in the synagogue or in city hall, because they felt that neither the state nor religion should govern what people do in their private lives. They were together from the time they were in their late teens until my grandmother's death, and they were proud of their unmarried status, as they felt their being together was a continuous choice. When they came to this country, my grandfather worked as a cabinet maker in construction, and my grandmother worked as a superintendent of an apartment building in which they lived. They both learned to read and write English, and they quickly became active in the same political movements in which they had been active while in Russia. These were Jewish, left-wing, secular movements. After the revolution in Russia, my grandmother wanted to return to Russia to help build the country, but my grandfather refused, saying he had grown accustomed to in-door plumbing. However, both my grandparents, and especially my grandmother, became active in the Communist Party in the United States. My grandmother's active involvement continued from the founding of the Communist Party in 1919 until her death in 1953.

For my grandfather, his involvement was more talk than action, although he did talk a lot. At those family gatherings at his sister's home, the discussion was often political, and the arguments were between those who considered themselves socialists (and read the *Jewish Daily Forward*) versus those who considered themselves communists (and read the *Freiheit*, the Jewish communist paper). My grandfather was often in the midst of those heated arguments, although I understand that it was my grandmother who always managed to get everybody there to give some financial contribution to a cause she was espousing. These arguments were vigorous, but loving, and, for me as a child, had the same quality as the arguments that the same group of people engaged in about whether the Brooklyn Dodgers or the New York Giants or the Yankees were the better team. My grandfather also liked to flaunt his nonobservance by going to work on Jewish holidays (e.g., Rosh Hashanah) in his work clothes. My grandparents routinely argued about this because they lived in Jewish neighborhoods, and my grandmother did not want to offend the neighbors needlessly.

In contrast to my grandfather, my grandmother was the real doer. During the Depression, she was part of regular brigades that would scour the Bronx for families on the street who had recently been evicted and move their furniture back into their apartments. She regularly made street-corner speeches, mostly in Yiddish, about causes in which the party was involved. During the course of such speeches, money was always collected. There is one family story that involves the arrest of my grandmother during one of those speeches. She had a tin can with some money she had collected. As the police were carting her off, she saw a man she didn't know and he motioned for her to give him the can. She gave it to him, because she thought it would be better for some man on the street to have the money rather than the police. When she arrived at the police station, a lawyer arrived, and the charges of begging could not be sustained because there was no can and no money. Later, my grandmother found out that the man had brought the money to the Communist Party office and alerted them to my grandmother's arrest.

My grandmother also was the more powerful of the two within the family. My grandfather turned over his paycheck to her and she paid the bills. She made all major decisions within the family. She was extremely protective of her children to the point of being overcontrolling so that both my mother and her brother had significant difficulty standing on their own throughout their lives. However, because I only knew her until I was eight, I did not experience her as limiting my freedom. In those days before television, I did not attend preschool but spent most of my waking time with my grandmother, who played with me, taught me card games, let me drink a little bit of coffee in a big glass of milk, and protected me from my parents' admonishments. To me, she was a very involved, supportive, proud, and encouraging grandmother, who cherished me and delighted, particularly, in my intellectual ability. One clear message I had from her was that I was smart, that I had opportunities she never had, and therefore I had an obligation to do something meaningful and productive with my talents.

My grandmother's death was profound for me. I didn't yet know the details of her political life, but I knew the nurturing role she had played for me, the power she held in the family, and the high esteem in which she was held by everyone who knew her. Her death had an additional consequence; my mother had always been extremely dependent on her and essentially parentified me subsequent to my grandmother's death. Thus, with the loss of my grandmother, I also gained a huge responsibility as my mother's confidante and emotional parent. My internalization of my grandmother as a lost primary attachment figure has dominated my life. She had two other grandchildren (the daughters of my mother's older brother), but I was the only one who lived with her, and I was the only one for whom she left a letter to be read after her death. The letter instructed me to work hard in school and be a productive person who contributed to others. It has been the cornerstone of my life and I think of that message as quintessentially Jewish, in the way I understood Jewishness. I learned more about her life and what she believed after her death than I could have known as a young child. That knowledge continued to contribute to my sense of self long after she was gone.

My grandmother involved my mother in Communist Party activities from the time my mother was a small child. My mother was a Pioneer and then a member of the Young Communist League. However, my mother was a much more timid person than was her mother, and, although she remained left-wing in her thinking throughout her life, she dropped out of all activities upon her marriage to my father. My father, who was a very bright man despite not finishing the eighth grade, was also rather left-wing in his politics. However, both my parents became very frightened of the Communist Party connection in the context of the McCarthy era.

I was a young child during the early 1950s. Once of my earliest memories of television is of my father watching the Army-McCarthy hearings and my realization that this was a significant event that I didn't understand at all. I did not understand my family's connection to the Communist Party until I was an early adolescent, when my mother communicated this history to me in hushed, whispered tones, letting me know that this was a very secretive and dangerous affiliation. This, much more than my Jewishness, was my secret identity, although, in reality, it was *my* Jewish identity. The political values my family held were strongly imbued in me from as far back as I can remember, before I understood them to be dangerous and secretive, and they are very connected for me with my Jewishness. The belief in the dignity of all people, the anger associated with exploitation of others, the conviction that we all have a duty and obligation to utilize whatever gifts and skills we have in the service of others and the betterment of humankind and the respect for learning were values that I associated with being Jewish.

My parents were working class and very working class identified. I grew up with a very clear sense of being a child of the working class economically and politically but with aspirations for higher education and professional level work. Much of that working class identification also had a Jewish quality. My mother, who had left college after a semester, returned to work as a secretary when I was nine. My father was a semiskilled factory worker who was unemployed four months of the year during the industry's "slack season." He worked as an "underpresser" (pressing the lining of completed garments) in a "ladies' coats and suits" business. While there were people of several other ethnic groups who also worked in his factory (specifically, I remember mostly Italians and one Cuban woman), the people I heard about from him were mostly Jewish. My father was a member of the ILGWU (International Ladies Garment Workers Union), a union dominated by Jews at that time; I marched in Labor Day parades with him. Money was an ever present issue in my childhood in that I was aware that my parents worried about it. However, I always had food, a roof over my head, and clothes to wear. My parents saw to it that I was exposed to everything they could manage that was free or available at reduced rates: museums, children's plays and concerts, the library. I took piano and music theory lessons from a teacher from Julliard who was part of a low-cost music school sponsored by the local "Y" (Young Men's–Young Women's Hebrew Association).

My parents wished for me to become a college graduate and a professional but they also clearly communicated to me that, whatever your station in life, there was pride to be had in being a hard worker who provided in a steady and responsible way for one's family. In addition, they communicated that no matter how successful you might be, that was never justification for thinking you were better than others whose circumstances had not allowed that success. A story often repeated with disdain in my home was about a male family member who had married into an assimilated and economically well-off German-Jewish family; the mother of the bride stood at the door at the ceremony and directed the "Americans" (her family and business associates) to one side of the aisle and my family to the other. Members of my family were enraged and the arrogance and insensitivity of the bride's mother was held up to me as an example of horrible behavior never to be engaged in by any decent person.

The local "Y" was my entry into another major socializing factor in my life: my summer camp experiences. For most of my childhood and adolescence, I attended a Jewish camp that came out of a settlement house model. The fees were very minimal and based on a sliding scale. I would guess that my parents paid near the bottom of that scale. Those who ran the camp were social workers. The overarching philosophy was one of cooperation and noncompetition. We never had "color wars" at this camp. Most of the campers and counselors were Jewish; however, I would say that most were secular Jews for whom religious observance occurred minimally if at all. The food was "Kosher style" in that meat and dairy were not served in the same meal, but the kitchen was clearly not kosher. A routine prayer was said in Hebrew at the start of every evening meal, and, because I came from a totally nonobservant family, I heard and learned that prayer in camp for the first time. Another Jewish tradition observed in the camp was "Oneg Shabbat." On Friday nights, we had an all-camp special program of some sort, but the programs often focused on significant social issues. My experience of the camp was that the mission was to develop in the children a sense of social consciousness, and I believe that many of the campers must have been, like me, "red diaper babies," although this was not fully discussed. For example, one of the Meeropol brothers, a few years my senior, was a camper and eventually a counselor at the camp. "Meeropol" is the adopted name of the children of the Rosenbergs, who were executed as Communist spies in the early 1950s. After their parents' death, the Meeropol brothers were adopted by a family friend, who changed their last names to protect them as they were growing up. Other counselors had been in the South and active in the civil rights movement. At the camp, we sang many more songs that came out of the civil rights movement than songs coming out of the Jewish tradition. The camp leaders were extremely concerned about the arms race with the Soviet Union, and I remember there being a major celebration at the camp in 1963 when the nuclear arms proliferation treaty was signed. At the same time, there was also support for Israel and celebration of its successes. I remember a big 10th birthday party for Israel in 1958. Israeli folk dancing was a major activity that I took part in and enjoyed. The backdrop for all of these experiences was the Nazi Holocaust and the experience of Jews as an oppressed group who identified and allied themselves with other disenfranchised, exploited groups to fight injustice worldwide.

I attended public elementary school in the South Bronx. At the time I was there, the neighborhood was a White ethnic neighborhood (Jews, Italians, Irish, and smatterings of many other more recent European refugees from World War II). My friends were primarily Jewish and Catholic, and I do not recall any tension or difficulty associated with this. I was more aware of religious education and the role of religion among my Catholic friends, who typically left school one or two afternoons a week to attend religious instruction. After sixth grade, I experienced very academically competitive junior high school and high school settings, where the great majority of the other students were Jewish. Being Jewish in that setting meant being part of the dominant group and not having to think about it any further.

I was in for a rude awakening upon entry into college. I attended one of the "seven sister schools" at a time when they were all White and all women. The school was dominated by graduates of elite private preparatory schools who were bluebloods (Protestant, old money and connections, coming out parties, segregated country clubs). Immediately, for the first time in my life, as a Jewish, working class, scholarship student from a public high school, I personally felt like an outsider. Several specific painful events left me feeling targeted and humiliated. I began to try to connect with others along dimensions with which I identified, and I recall attending a few meetings of the Hillel group on campus. For the first time, I felt really different from other Jews. Many of these students came from economically privileged backgrounds and were also more religiously observant than I was. They spent a lot of time talking about and planning weekend mixers with Hillel groups on equivalent men's campuses, and I did not have the money to take even these small trips. I found a home in the small left-wing movements on campus, in the form of the civil rights group and the fledgling Students for a Democratic Society (SDS), and "came out" politically at that time. My closest friends through college and through graduate school were other students involved in civil rights, antiwar activities, and eventually feminist groups. This is where I spent my energy and got my support. I did note in that period that Jewish people were overrepresented among the White people in these groups. I did take pride in this overrepresentation, believing that my experience of what it meant to be Jewish mirrored theirs and that the reason for the overrepresentation reflected Jewish progressive values.

I completed my graduate training in psychology, but the program I attended had a heavy emphasis on understanding normal development in its social and cultural context. I entered the work world in the early 1970s with a commitment to serving the underserved, with a wish to give back to those who struggle to make it but who may not have had all the advantages I had. I became heavily involved in left-wing political activity in my own right for a good part of that decade and began working professionally in underserved communities of color. During that decade, as part of both my political and professional work activity, I discussed, studied, and considered racism in the United States. I became much more aware of both the intrapsychic toll it takes as well as the role it plays in the larger society, by keeping apart exploited people who should be natural allies. I began to see racism as a primary issue in the United States and throughout the world. My perspective has been that racism results in the particular oppression of people of color but also functions to give some small privileges to poor White people who contribute to distrust and tension among working class people of different races. I saw and continue to see myself as maintaining the Marxist values with which I was raised, even though I believe that all of the countries that have called themselves communist have fallen short or actively betrayed those principles.

While I initially considered my perspectives on racism to be highly consistent with my identification as a Jew, I became increasingly aware that my Jewish identity was unlike the identity of most other Jews I knew and met. In the 1950s and 1960s, most young Jews I knew considered themselves allies of Blacks in the struggle for civil rights. However, over time, I became aware that my reactions to national events was different from other Jews. Unlike many, I embraced affirmative action programs seeing that the barriers broken by them helped all disempowered groups. Perhaps, of more significance, unlike many other Jews, I was never distanced or frightened or turned off by the "anti-Semitism" many Jews perceived in some of the Black community. The response of many Jews to both militancy and to the Black power movement that evolved out of the civil rights movement was fear; they saw the removal of Whites (who were primarily Jews) from civil rights groups as anti-Semitic, and they saw the conflict between Jewish teachers and community groups in urban areas as anti-Semitic. I distinguished Black militancy and the need for a sense of self-sufficiency and potency from Black nationalism. I understood the need on the part of the Black community to gather without the presence of people who had been dominant in the past and develop a sense of selfhood separate from Whites, just as women needed time without men. On a political level, ultimately, I think that alliances must be forged among working class and exploited people across racial, religious, gender, and ethnic lines, and that primary identification on any basis other than class ultimately leads to more oppression. It is clear to me that dictators in Africa can create regimes as stratified and brutal as any that can be created by Europeans, and I do not believe that a Black ruling class would ultimately be any more benign than a White ruling class. However, Black nationalism in the United States does not feel threatening to me because racism against Blacks is so central to the way the United States functions that I do not perceive any realistic threat of a Black ruling class emerging at this time from Black nationalism and oppressing other Blacks or Whites. As I thought about these issues, I adopted a more internationalist perspective in which I viewed all forms of nationalism as ultimately reactionary, recognizing that they might seem somewhat progressive in a particular moment in history; to me the concern about any form of nationalism was that it had the potential to mobilize masses of people to achieve ends that would not serve the majority of that particular group but would serve only an elite few. However, I did not and do not personalize that concern or see it as a danger to me.

Another major issue defining the gulf I feel from the Jewish community is my concerns about the State of Israel. As I became more aware of both Israel's domestic and international policies, I began to see Zionism in its current form as more clearly reactionary with each passing year and as a much greater threat in the current world than Black nationalism in the United States. Once nationalistic, reactionary forces have control of a government, their power to damage others is much greater. When Zionism emerged as an answer and response to the persecution and extermination of European Jewry, it had a progressive face. However, ultimately the need to establish safety along ethnic, religious, or racial lines creates enemies of people who should be allies, literal and figurative walls between Palestinians and Israelis, and interminable pain. I see the policies of the State of Israel as morally and politically wrong and cannot defend its positions in the world any more than I can defend the positions of the United States as represented by its ruling class. My feelings about the State of Israel have led to my increasing sense of distance and alienation from the Jewish community. It has become virtually impossible to go to any event at which significant numbers of Jewish people are present without what seems to be to be unthinking support of Israel becoming a dominant theme.

The other factor that has contributed to my alienation from the Jewish community is the family I created. In the mid-1970s, I married my husband, a man of color, and we have two children. Increasingly, I have begun to see the world through their experiences and their eyes. I see the small daily humiliations that are the experience of people of color in America, and I am increasingly put off by White people who cannot acknowledge that this exists. It is particularly difficult for me to face this denial in Jews, many of whom immediately want to turn any discussion of racism in the United States into a discussion of anti-Semitism, sexism, or anything else except racism. As a Jewish woman (and especially given my experience in college), I am acutely aware that there are multiple issues at play in this society. However, I am also aware that, as a White woman, I stand somewhere in the middle of the privilege structure and I feel a sense of responsibility and connectedness to those lower on this structure not to deny the centrality and potency of their experience.

My choice to become a psychologist was largely determined by the parentified role I had toward my mother as well as my grandmother's injunction to use my intellectual ability to contribute to the well-being of others. My professional work as a psychologist has been almost entirely focused on providing services to oppressed and underserved communities and to individuals who have been victimized. This comes from my identification and respect for the struggles they face and my wish to give back. I do not equate education with intellect, nor status in life with morality. Some of the smartest and most moral people (including clients) I know have histories filled with experiences of adversity and humiliation. I don't see myself as a spiritual person, but I do have a deep sense of history, historical movement, connections between peoples and across time, and of being a link in a chain of human progress. This belief led to my interest in being trained as a family therapist.

I believe deeply that multiple layers of experience (personal, familial, social, historical) impact people's behavior, and my choice of a graduate program was influenced by that. My attraction to systems thinking reflects my belief that I have gotten to where I am in because I have stood on the shoulders of others whose struggles enabled me to grow. I am enormously grateful to the efforts of those who have gone before me, both my relatives and all people who have fought to make the world a better place, and I have tried to give that sense of continuity of struggle over generations to my children.

I have not and would never deny that I am Jewish; I am truly my father's daughter in that sense. I think I look Jewish. My maiden name is easily recognizable as a Jewish name and I use it routinely as my middle name. However, it has become harder for me to say I am Jewish and explain what this means to me, because its definition for me is so tied to the political values espoused in my family. The difficulty feels related to two issues. First, it is connected to the secrecy associated with my grandmother's political affiliation, as interpreted to me by my parents and reinforced by years of living in America, where even "liberal" has become a dirty word. Of even greater significance to me, however, is the internal conflict I feel about where most of the American Jewish community seems to be politically, socially, and morally. I cringe at all of the Jewish intellectuals who have become neocons, like Paul Wolfowitz. My friends and relatives from years past suddenly do not seem to be the people I knew as a child. I feel very "other" from them and hidden in my beliefs and perspectives. I am mortified by the massive and ostentatious bar mitzvahs and weddings that seem to have become the norm in suburban Jewish communities. I am astounded at the sense of entitlement that underlies moving into land that others dwell on and then by the condemnation of dehumanized people who react violently. I am angry at the rejection of affirmative action as discriminatory against them by members of the Jewish community, given the success the Jewish community experienced in response to what was essentially an affirmative action plan for European Americans after World War II (this is the thesis of an excellent and well-documented book by Karen Brodkin titled *How Jews Became White Folks and What That Says About Race in America* that was recommended to me by one of my children). In short, I am confused about what happened to the secular, progressive, Jewish community that I felt a part of as a child. I experience a sense of betrayal by a Jewish community that seems to have become increasingly right-wing and something other than the one with which I identified as I grew up. Therefore, I often find that I feel more connected to people of color and their struggles than to the concerns of most of my Jewish contemporaries. I am also aware that, as a White woman, I have been privileged in American society and continue to enjoy a variety of comforts that come with that status, so I know that, much as I might feel a connection, I don't share experiences and I am an "other" to people of color as well, including my own husband and children.

In my therapeutic, teaching, and supervisory work, I find that I have an easier time with people from almost any ethnic background. Because my name identifies me, Jewish people with whom I come into contact immediately recognize me as Jewish. Internally, I struggle particularly with these interactions if it is assumed that we share a religious background, or that we share support for the policies of the State of Israel, or that we share feelings of distrust about Black–Jewish relationships in the United States. Any assumption of a shared identity that is not based on respect for human dignity and struggle leaves me with discomfort. To confront this in any real way, to be "out" with other Jews about who I really am and how this defines my Jewishness leaves me feeling further alienated. In contrast, I have a much easier time exploring issues of difference and its meaning with non-Jewish clients, particularly people from working class backgrounds or people of color. I can listen with interest and empathy to their experiences, including their experiences of Whites and of Jews, without any sense of personal discomfort. The interest and ability to do this comes from my connections to my grandparents, my secular, progressive, very Jewish identified grandparents, connections that form the bedrock of my existence but leave me feeling estranged from the Jewish community today.

Reflections on a Carpathian Legacy

KORNELIA HARARI

My parents and I are Russian immigrants from a small city called Munkacs in the Carpathian Mountains. Munkacs has one of those convoluted and confusing European histories, particularly over the past century. It's been, in turn, part of the Austro-Hungarian Empire, democratic Czechoslovakia, Nazi Hungary, communist Soviet Union, and, currently, the Ukraine. Through my grandparents' childhoods, the Carpathian Mountains region was filled with an ethnic mix of Hungarians, Ukrainians, Germans, Slovaks, Czechs, gypsies, and Jews. After World War II, the Russians took over and were added to the Carpathian ethnic fabric, taking the place of most of the Jews who had been exterminated in Auschwitz and other death camps.

The earliest Jews in Munkacs were recorded in the mid-seventeenth century. Before World War II, Munkacs contained a vibrant community of 11,000 Jews (over 40% of Munkacs was Jewish), including a large and famous Hasidic sect, some members of which survived the Holocaust and transplanted themselves to Boro Park in Brooklyn. My maternal grandfather, Yankl, grew up as part of this sect, and he often showed me with pride his copy of the *Minchas Eliezer*, a well-known book of Hasidic thought written by the original Munkacher Rebbe. He often boasted about having been circumcised by the rebbe and beamed about my brother's circumcision by the rebbe's grandson, his successor. While my maternal grandmother, Rozsie, was raised in a home that was not Hasidic or particularly religious, her family was still very connected to their community and observed the basics of Orthodoxy. My paternal grandmother, Feige, was born to religiously devout and Hasidic parents, but photos of a wedding shortly before Munkacs was plunged into the Holocaust reveal that the younger the family member in the picture, the more assimilated and modern he or she appeared to be. My paternal grandfather, Hershy, was the least observant of the bunch. He was orphaned by his Hasidic parents by the time he was 10 years old and rebelliously left his extended relatives in Munkacs to support himself through the streets of Central Europe. If not for Hitler's mad goal of murdering all of the Jews of Europe, I think Hershy might have assimilated in Vienna where he lived before the Nazi rise to power, soon losing his Jewish identity. In fact, his life was saved by an SS officer whose daughter he had dated years before. The officer recognized Hershy in the selection line at a concentration camp and picked him out to be his personal slave, offering him extra food and incongruous protection until the end of the war. Before the war broke out, however, Hitler's rise sent Hershy back to his extended family and the relative safety of Munkacs.

I always imagined pre-Holocaust Munkacs as a utopian Jewish shtetl, a varied but strongly identified Jewish community filled with a mix of Hasidim and "enlightened" secularists, socialists and Zionists, minus the Cossacks and pogroms. In this environment, there was no escaping the integral Jewish aspect of their lives and identities, even for those who were not particularly religious or observant. This strong Jewish identity was passed on to my parents after the war, even as they were inculcated with communist messages of the uselessness of religion. They have pointed out that, despite a lack of formal Jewish education as they grew up, the rate of intermarriage in Munkacs among their generation was quite low, and nearly everyone they know sent their own children to Jewish day schools when they eventually arrived in the United States. Of course, communism devalued religion while highlighting differences between religious groups, particularly between Jews and non-Jews, paradoxically reinforcing and strengthening a sense of Jewish identity among many.

All of my grandparents were Holocaust survivors. The relative safety of what was then a democratic Czechoslovakia quite suddenly and drastically morphed into the restrictions and dangers of ghetto life for one year, then the unthinkable transports to extermination and concentration camps for just short of a year before their liberation from the Nazis. Despite the now-infamous rumors and warnings from relatives and friends in other parts of Europe and Palestine, the Jews of Munkacs could not believe the stories about what Hitler was doing. One of Feige's sisters came back to Munkacs from Palestine in 1940, on a mission to get as many Jews out of Europe as possible. No one believed this gun-toting, pants-wearing woman's stories of mass murder, and she returned to Palestine alone. By the time the Jews of Munkacs understood the danger they were in, it was too late for them to escape. My grandparents never knew when their respective parents, siblings, and other relatives were killed. May 7 was the first day of transports to the death camps and marks the observed Yerzheit of all the Munkacs Jews whose actual date of death is unknown.

My mother knows almost nothing of her parents' Holocaust experience, or, for that matter, of their early lives at all. This was simply not spoken of.

She says that children never even thought to ask their parents such personal questions. She knew the bare facts—that her parents had been through a horrible war and most of their families were killed—and did not dare to ask anything more. When I ask her how she imagines the war might have affected her parents and the way they raised their children, she denies that it might have had any effect at all. Her conscious version of the events is that the war was horrible, people suffered and died, but then it was over and everyone went back to their regular lives. Yet she admits that as a child she never wanted to cause her parents any more suffering than she knew they had already experienced. My mother did all she could to make life easier for her parents, having internalized a sense that her parents, particularly her mother, could not handle any more pain. She was constantly striving to be the perfect child, never causing trouble, always at the top of her class, always reliably caring for others, including, from a young age, her parents. Like other children of Holocaust survivors, she has always felt responsible for being unable to ease her parents' lives in some way, often blaming herself for any mishap or discomfort in their lives as well as in the lives of others close to her. Her survivor guilt has driven her to limitless attempts at perfection in terms of dedication to her parents and other family members, at times confusing self-sacrifice with being "nice" and "good." She could never do enough to erase the pain and anguish my grandmother continued to experience in the forms of anxiety, severe depression, various real and imagined physical ailments and diseases, and repeated entreaties to God to spare her from the hospital and imminent death. I will never forget what must have been the first words I learned in Hungarian: *Oy, Ishtenem, shegesh megeck!* (Oh, God, help me!) I've wondered if, in some essential way, this has made my mother feel like she was not good enough in all of her relationships. She seems to always believe there is something more that she could have or should have done, even when her actions are objectively more selfless than most people would be willing to bear.

Even after losing nearly all of his family in the war, my mother's father was as religiously devout as one could be in Russia at the time. Risking a sure prison sentence, he prayed in clandestine prayer groups in Munkacs on the Sabbath and holidays, often leading the service as cantor. My mother was raised in a home environment that respected and valued religion, but, since she was a girl, her Jewish education was scant and superficial. Being a product of his time and place, when I went through my own stage of strict Orthodox observance and prayed three times a day, Yankl tried to discourage me, saying I was doing too much for a woman. I think that, for a long time, my mother's associations with practicing Judaism were of warmth and familiarity, mixed with feelings about it being irrelevant and backward. This became even more complicated when my brother and I became observant in our teens, and with my brother's continuing movement toward ultra-Orthodoxy.

Whereas my mother was aware of her parents' war-torn past but denying of its impact as she was growing up, my father's parents' past suffering
was less salient to him than was their concern about their present and future
while in Russia. The messages he got about the war were less about the pain
and losses that had been inflicted and more about surviving other peoples'
hatred toward him as a Jew. From early on, his father proclaimed Zionism
as the only guarantee of safety for Jews, and, starting in the 1950s, repeatedly
attempted to get a visa out of Russia. (He was finally allowed to emigrate to
Israel in 1974.) My father was stamped with a sense of being different from
and hated by the goyim, and he was brought up on the need to prove himself
better than them. The only way to survive hatred and discrimination, apart
from leaving Europe, was to be better—smarter, stronger, and more successful. This was constantly reinforced by the communist policy of discrimination, imposing quotas on the number of Jews allowed into schools of
higher education and various professions. To get into college, Jews had to
work harder and perform better than the non-Jews in their class. My father's
Jewish identity became cumbersome but also a source of pride when he saw
that despite the discrimination around them, and through the centuries, Jews
could and did succeed. He was motivated and driven in large part by the
force of others' hatred and the barriers they placed in his way.

My father's trademark perfectionism arose in the context of attempting
to prove to others that he was deserving of his place at school, at work,
indeed in the world. Even his immaculate home and factory, with spotless
broom closets containing measured and evenly spaced hooks specially
installed for cleaning implements, prove that he meets the highest standards.
Sometimes it seems that those Jews who don't meet such standards are seen
by him as deficient in some way, because they do not prove the important
rule of being better than the goyim. If others don't meet his standards of
perfection, his association with their tribe leaves him vulnerable to character-
ization as less than perfect, compelling him to distance and separate himself
from them. Thus, the need to be better than the goyim has a corollary—
disliking Jewish subgroups who are not perceived by him as better. This is
about a different kind of other, Jews who are different from him and threaten
his position in the goyish world in which he tries to prove himself.

My father's relationship with Judaism has always been deeply ambivalent. His parents fostered a strong Jewish identity in their children by observing some of the Jewish traditions (they hosted an annual secret Yom Kippur
service) and by their embrace of Zionism, but they often spoke negatively
about rabbis and other religious figures from their past. They often blamed
rabbis for the murder of their families because they had discouraged community members from emigrating to Palestine or the United States before
the war. Palestine and the United States did not have the religious infrastruc-
ture that Munkacs did at the time, and the rabbis were concerned about
losing their community members to secularism. When my father speaks of

this, I am sure he echoes his own parents' sentiments when he says these rabbis' true concern was only for their own livelihoods.

Despite my father's hostility toward religious Judaism and anger at those who have sustained it, he also feels a deep pride in being Jewish. His ambivalence extends to other aspects of his Jewish identity and personal history. He has expressed pride in coming from a nation that produced Einstein but resents feeling that one needs to live up to that to be considered worthy in society. There was the pride of his mother's resistance during World War II by putting sand in the German bombs she was forced to manufacture in Birkenau but shame and pain in the mere fact that Birkenau existed. His ambivalence is stark because he grew up knowing he could never escape being Jewish, being reminded in Russia time and again of his vulnerability as a Jew. At the same time, both of his children are Orthodox. My brother is in fact quite the paradigm of right-wing ultra-Orthodoxy. Can you just imagine the conversations over Sabbath dinners? More recently, my parents have also come to take on some of the trappings and traditions of Orthodoxy and are now peripherally part of a modern Orthodox community.

Though my parents were not particularly observant while I was growing up, my brother and I were always imbued with a strong sense of being Jewish. Being "Jewish" meant being different from most others, both hated and better in some way. I always had trouble understanding why they sent me and my brother to Jewish Day School. I remember the hostility toward religion my parents, particularly my father, often expressed growing up. He tried to teach us what he had learned in school as a child: religion is the opium of the masses and that it is for people who are unsophisticated and old-fashioned. I suppose he would have been happy for us to be identified as Jews who are knowledgeable of our history, proud of Jewish accomplishments and a bit wary of those who were other, but certainly not practicing. I am sure he did not expect that my brother and I would become Orthodox. For some time my parents must have been confused about how, in the land of opportunities and assimilation, their children had become even more strongly identified as Jews than they ever were.

My own journey to Orthodoxy was part a search for spirituality, part obedient Hebrew Day School student, and part differentiation from my parents. Exposure to Orthodox practice and lifestyle got me interested, and even as a child I felt spiritual fulfillment from various aspects of my religion. I loved going to synagogue where my grandfather was the cantor, and I was often stirred by his prayers. Many of my classmates came from Orthodox homes, and there was something about being part of the Orthodox community that seemed beautiful and appealing to me. I had also internalized the authority of God and the Torah through my Hebrew Day School education and earnestly decided when I became bat-mitzvah that it was time for me to follow through on what I had learned. In parallel to my mother's guilty obedience to authority I quickly learned to feel guilty when I ate the slightest questionably kosher food or accidentally ripped toilet paper on the Sabbath, an act that is forbidden on the holy day. As I learned more in school, I felt I had to follow all the halacha (Jewish laws) to a T, even those most of my peers were not observing. I modeled my father's perfectionism in the way I practiced Orthodox Judaism. I thought I would be even more perfect than my parents if I only followed the rules that were so clearly laid out for me. Sorotzkin (1998) wrote that strict adherence to Jewish law lends itself to perfectionist attitudes, something I clearly experienced as an adolescent.

At one level, religion fulfilled in me a yearning for spirituality, perhaps a legacy of my deeply religious ancestors. At another level, becoming religious acted out the strains of survivor guilt and perfectionism that I had adopted from my parents. At still another level, it had allowed me to separate from my parents, while surpassing them in terms of perfection. The separation was the key. The more they resisted my attempts to be religious, the more zealously I held my position. I remember one fight about my emerging religiosity ending with my father saying that he was ashamed to have me as a daughter because of my refusal to travel by car with him to visit his friends on a Saturday (travel by car is forbidden on the Sabbath). I knew then that I would never give up on my new religious identity, both because of how meaningful it was to me but also because my parents were so set against it. Religion also helped me to deal with some of my adolescent crises. Forging an identity was simpler, because so much of it could be determined by religion. The structure and restrictions of Orthodox Judaism also made it easier for me to negotiate a discomfort with my adolescent sexuality. As I became more comfortable with myself postadolescence, I allowed my identity to become less rigidly tied to religion and more authentic. I still identify myself as modern Orthodox, but am now less strictly religious and more critical and cynical of Orthodox Judaism, often struggling with its meaning in my everyday life. I have given myself permission to feel confusion and express doubts about religion, and I have learned to accept living in a world of ambiguities.

One of the interesting and exciting things about writing this chapter is the opportunity to think about the points at which some of my identities have collided and influenced one another. I've never before considered the ways in which being raised through my family's particular experience of Jewishness might influence my identity as a beginning therapist. One influence that now seems clear is that my mother trained me to have the same sensitivity to others' emotional states as she had to those of her parents', particularly emotional pain. I have always felt a pull to be there with others in emotional distress, and even at times when my own interests conflicted with theirs I have found myself compelled to help. While I'm sure my tendency to do this was, to some degree, lack of assertiveness and a need to feel needed, there was also a need to alleviate the pain of those around me and a sense of responsibility to do so. There was never any question in my mind that I would choose a helping profession. In examining my choice, it seems, at least in part, a sort of repetition compulsion. I am mastering the art of helping others and easing their pain and suffering, something my mother has spent much of her life trying to do for her parents.

Both my parents live with an insecurity that is based on not feeling good enough. My mother's inability to meet her impossible expectations of relieving her parents' pain has left her feeling overwhelmingly guilty and responsible for everyone around her. My father's (not entirely unreasonable) paranoia about his safety in the world has made his pursuit of perfection paramount in the hopes that it could offer him both a sense of self-worth and some protection against discrimination. My mother's guilt and father's paranoid perfectionism have found some form of expression in me, affecting me both personally and professionally.

Particularly as a beginning therapist, I have often felt not good enough, despite rationally knowing that I am a novice and receiving positive feedback from supervisors. From the start of my training, I thought I had to be the perfect therapist. Any mistake I made felt earth shattering and I was guiltily certain that I had ruined the therapeutic relationship, or worse, the client. When clients dropped out of therapy, I was always quick to blame myself—there must have been something I should have known to do differently, something I said or did must have turned the patient off of therapy forever. While I know all therapists-in-training understandably feel insecure about their abilities, my early insecurities and worries felt somehow more acute than those of my peers and friends. My exaggerated fear of making mistakes resulted in the paradox of wanting to tell all to my supervisors in an effort to abrogate responsibility for my imperfections versus wanting to hide my mistakes so as not to appear incompetent. Fortunately or not, my guilt most often led me to tell all.

With increased training and practice I am now more confident in my abilities as a therapist and spend less time second-guessing myself. Though I am still somewhat uncomfortable knowing I will never be a perfect therapist, I am now striving for competence rather than perfection. I've also achieved a finer understanding of clients' responses to therapy, keeping me from feeling too personally responsible for their reactions. It seems I may be living a pattern of hypervigilant perfectionism and guilt when embarking on something new; becoming Orthodox in adolescence and a therapist in early adulthood are only two examples of this. With time, I work on adjusting my unrealistic expectations and allowing myself to be comfortable with a more authentic space within a new aspect of my identity.

Another way in which my family and personal experience with Judaism affected my early work as a therapist was in my admittedly irrational experience of a slight but nagging feeling of being judged at work through a prism of being Jewish rather than simply for my work. I felt that in some way my performance represented something greater about the Jewish people and our collective competencies. My experience has been that this attitude is reinforced in the greater Jewish community. Whenever we went on school trips in Hebrew Day School, there was a serious talk between the teachers and students about how we represented the entire Jewish community to the museum curators, security guards, and random others we were about to encounter. The boys' yarmulkes and girls' long skirts would surely mark us as Jews, and they wanted to be sure we were aware, even hypervigilant, of our behavior. There was always an emphasis on the responsibility of individuals to favorably represent the group in public, thereby serving as a *kiddush Hashem*, sanctification of God's name, rather than a *chilul Hashem*, desecration of God's name. This is understandable considering a Jewish history filled with persecution, but in the safer context of New York City in the 1980s contributed to a continuing sense of cultural paranoia. In some way this has stayed with me, and in various work environments I have had to consciously remind myself that I represent only myself. At first, it further complicated issues of self-disclosure to my patients. I was extremely ambivalent about revealing my Jewish identity; for example, by revealing that I was rescheduling an appointment because of a Jewish holiday. On the one hand, I did not want to hide the strong identity of which I am proud. On the other hand, I found myself feeling anxious about how patients, particularly those who were not Jewish, would respond to even the subtle self-disclosure that would ensue by wearing a Jewish star on my necklace. In my internalized version of cultural paranoia I felt pressured to be an even better therapist to my non-Jewish clients if at some point it was revealed that I was Jewish. In my mind, being the better therapist would ensure that my clients (or supervisors and administration for that matter) wouldn't leave their work with me with a bad impression of the Jewish people.

My clinical internship placement at Maimonides Medical Center some years ago helped to relieve some of this pressure, presumably because the hospital is so institutionally and culturally Jewish (the hospital serves Boro Park, a neighborhood with one of the greatest concentration of Hasidic and other ultra-Orthodox Jews in the world). In the relatively protective cocoon of my internship I was able to refine my therapeutic skills and more clearly define myself professionally. By the end of the year I found myself feeling more comfortable with and confident about my abilities, allowing me to put my cultural paranoia in perspective.

The greater awareness and clearer perspective of my internalized paranoia has helped me to stem my feelings of professional insecurity at my postdoctoral internship and beyond. Yet even in writing this chapter I have struggled with how honestly to portray my family and experiences of Judaism, worrying that this brief sketch might be perceived both as negative and representative of Orthodox Jews rather than of my personal experience.

It has been difficult to end this essay, perhaps because so many questions about the meeting of my various identities continue tug at my mind.

I wonder about what aspects of my Jewish and family experience I have not yet accessed in formulating an understanding of myself as a person and as a therapist. And I wonder about what I have more consciously chosen to exclude here, and why. I continue to struggle at the intersection of maintaining a paranoid privacy in the interest of personal safety and publicly exposing myself in the interest of openness and honesty. I end with what I hope is a satisfying enough compromise.

REFERENCE

Sorotzkin, B. (1998). Understanding and treating perfectionism in religious adolescents. *Psychotherapy, 35*(1), 87–95.

I've Always Known I'm Jewish, but *How* Am I Jewish?

CLARE G. HOLZMAN

There's an old maxim that says that there are as many definitions of a Jew as there are Jews. My own experience tells me that even one Jew may have many different definitions of herself as a Jew over the course of a lifetime. In this article I will trace a narrative of my identity as a Jew growing up in a particular family, in a particular geographical location, at a particular time in history. I will highlight the ways in which various facets of my Jewish identity have shifted in content and in salience over time. Finally, I will describe some of the ways in which my identity as a Jew impacts my work as a therapist.

FAMILY HISTORY AND JEWISH IDENTITY

Recent theory and research on identity development support viewing identity as complex, contextual, and fluid (Barrett, 1998; Bhavnani & Haraway, 1994; Goldberg & Krausz, 1993a; Rathzel, 1994; Steinberg-Oren, 1997). There were particular circumstances in my life that I believe made my sense of my identity as a Jew especially ambiguous and changing. One is that not only my parents but all four of my grandparents had rejected the Jewish religion (although not Jewish identity) long before I was born. Thus Jewish religious beliefs and rituals were never a routine, taken-for-granted part of my daily experience. Another is that my parents were highly ambivalent about ethnic and cultural identities. In their political belief system, the only divisions that mattered had to do with class. Racial or ethnic loyalties were viewed as undermining working class solidarity.

At the same time, my parents' life experience had been such that being Jewish was a major organizer of their lives. This was particularly true of my mother, who had been born in 1907 in Chudnov, a *shtetl* in the Ukraine.[1] My mother's parents, in their youth, had rebelled against the norms of this

---

[1] A *shtetl* was a village inhabited entirely by Jews. It was a close-knit, culturally and religiously homogeneous community surrounded by non-Jews who were intensely anti-Semitic.

community. My grandmother had left home to attend a pioneering program that trained midwives in modern obstetrical techniques. My grandfather, whose parents had wanted him to become a rabbi, wanted to study engineering in Zhitomir, the large city closest to Chudnov. When he was denied admission to engineering school because he was a Jew, he stayed on in Zhitomir and became a political activist. However, both he and my grandmother returned to Chudnov to earn a living and start a family. Thus my mother grew up immersed in the culture of the shtetl, particularly as embodied in the person of her paternal grandmother, while simultaneously hearing her parents' biting critique of that culture.

By the time she was 13, my mother had experienced World War I (1914–1918), the Russian Revolution (1917), the Polish-Ukrainian War (1918–1919), the Polish-Soviet War (1919–1920), and the civil war between the Red Army of the Communists and various White Armies that wanted restoration of the old regime (1919–1920). Each of these events had included *pogroms*[2] instigated by the armies that advanced and retreated through Chudnov like opposing teams moving up and down a football field.[3]

My father, born in New York City in 1914, had grown up in a neighborhood where various ethnic groups lived side by side but kept their distance from one another. The anti-Semitic violence he had encountered as a boy in the streets of Washington Heights was far less lethal than the anti-Semitic violence my mother had witnessed in Chudnov. It had, however, provided frequent reminders that being Jewish was a significant part of his identity.

I am aware of four distinct aspects of Jewishness that are relevant to my identity as a Jew: (a) Jews as targets of persecution, (b) Jewishness as ethnicity, (c) Jewishness as religion, and (d) Jewishness as race. I will discuss each of these in turn.

JEWS AS TARGETS OF PERSECUTION

The earliest and most intense messages I got about being Jewish were (a) that being a Jew was not optional and (b) that to be a Jew was to be in danger. I was born in 1942. I was not yet three years old when the concentration camps in Europe were liberated and the full horror of the Holocaust became

---

[2]The *American Heritage Dictionary* defines a *pogrom* as "an organized, often officially encouraged massacre or persecution of a minority group, especially one conducted against Jews."

[3]Armies that were active in the region between 1914 and 1920 included the Imperial Russian Army, the German Army, the Polish Army, the Ukrainian Army, the Communist Red Army, various counterrevolutionary White Armies, and the Cossack Army. There were also deserters and demobilized soldiers from the various armies who were making their way home as well as bands of brigands taking advantage of the breakdown of authority (Channon & Hudson, 1995; Polish–Soviet War, 2009; Polish–Ukrainian War, 2009; Prior, Wilson, & Keegan, 1999; Russian Civil War, 2009; Ukrainian People's Republic, 2009).

widely known to the American public. For my mother, the Holocaust confirmed and amplified the lessons of her childhood about the peril inherent simply in being a Jew. She was scornful of people who thought they could assimilate and disappear into the general population. There had been people in Germany, she told me, whose ancestors had converted to Christianity, people who did not even know that they had Jewish ancestry. The Nazis had tracked them down through public records and had sent them to the concentration camps. When the state of Israel was created in 1948, the Law of Return defined a Jew as anyone who said he or she was a Jew, allowing individual self-definition (and encouraging rapid expansion of the Jewish population of the new state). My mother defined a Jew as anyone *other* people, the people in power, said was a Jew. In retrospect, I realize that my mother was not as thorough-going a social constructionist as this implies. If I had asked her, I think she would have said that her definition applied for all practical purposes but that the descendants of Jews remained Jews even if no one on the face of the earth knew it or had any way of finding out. At an intuitive level, I agree with her.

From my earliest years my mother tried to prepare me for life in what she perceived as a hostile, dangerous world. She did her best to negate any notion I might have about the United States being a place of safety for Jews. "Don't ever get the idea that it can't happen here," she would tell me. "It almost did." Among other things, she told me about a pro-Nazi rally that had filled Madison Square Garden before the United States entered the war. Since I had been to Madison Square Garden to see the circus, the image of thousands of seats, all of them filled with screaming people who hated me, was very powerful.

My mother firmly believed that all non-Jews were anti-Semitic, no matter how enlightened they seemed to be. I don't know how old I was when she first warned me to watch out for people who say, "Some of my best friends are Jews." I do know it was before I was nine, because I have a visual image of the conversation taking place in the living room of our apartment in the Bronx, before we moved to Queens. Nor do I remember what, if anything, she said about why such people were dangerous. Thinking about it now, what occurs to me is that the statement is usually made when the person has just been confronted about her or his anti-Semitic attitudes or behavior. If no one can escape internalizing the oppressive belief systems that are prevalent in their culture, the people who deny their anti-Semitism are the ones who haven't taken responsibility for recognizing and changing it.

My first direct encounter with anti-Semitism occurred in the playground when I was seven. A group of children trapped me on the monkey bars and told me that I was going to go to hell because I had killed Christ. They cited the nuns at the local parochial school as the source of this information.[4]

---

[4] It wasn't until the Second Vatican Council in the early 1960s that the Catholic Church decreed that Jews were no longer to be held personally responsible for the Crucifixion.

They continued to taunt me for what felt like a very long time. I had no idea how I was going to get away from them or what they would do to me next. I think they eventually got bored and left. I went home in tears.

Later experiences with anti-Semitism were much less frightening but still unsettling. A few examples out of many:

- A girl in my class in high school, who was of German descent, told me with utter conviction that Hitler had done a lot of good things in Germany and that it was a myth that he had murdered six million Jews. The story had been made up, she said, by Jews who wanted Germany to pay them undeserved reparations. I was stunned. I had no idea how to begin to formulate a reply.
- A coworker shared with me his alleged observation that whenever a Jew and a non-Jew owned competing stores in the same neighborhood, the Jew always prospered and the non-Jew went broke. I was not convinced by his claim that he was simply expressing admiration for Jewish business acumen. This time, after the initial shock at what I was hearing, I recovered enough to point out that his statement was a thinly veiled version of an age-old, ugly stereotype. I added that if Jews had some kind of insider knowledge about how to succeed in business, it had somehow bypassed my family. Shortly after arriving in the United States, my grandfather had been swindled into investing in a candy store. Within two years he had filed for bankruptcy because he couldn't bring himself to swindle someone else to get his investment back. I doubt that my words changed my coworker's thinking, but I did feel less like a helpless victim.
- I have witnessed Jews in progressive and/or feminist settings being inter-rogated about their views with regard to the State of Israel in order to establish their credibility and right to be heard on issues of racism and anti-Semitism. Members of other racial/ethnic groups were not subjected to this litmus test.

When *The Diary of Anne Frank* first appeared in English, I was about the age Anne had been when she went into hiding. It was easy for me to imagine myself in her circumstances and sharing her fate. My mother and her parents had fled the Ukraine when the Communists overthrew the democratic socialist regime my grandfather supported. After two years in Poland waiting for visas they had made it into the United States by the slimmest possible margin. The immigration laws of the 1920s, drastically restricting immigration from Eastern Europe, took effect after they had received their visas and paid for their passage, but before they had entered the United States. They had been held at Ellis Island while Congress debated a bill allowing entry to people in these circumstances. It was chilling to think that if their departure had been delayed by even a few more months, or if the bill had failed instead of passing, they would have been returned to Europe and would have been in Hitler's path 15 years later.

The stories I was told at home, the books I found on our bookshelves, the movies I saw had a lasting impact. I still have nightmares about being hunted by Nazis. Something inside tells me not to make myself conspicuous, not to talk too much or too loudly in public settings, not to express my opinions too forcefully, not to be too quick to step into a leadership role. If I do any of these things, I experience a wave of anxiety afterward. This response is partly the result of gender and class socialization. But it also reflects an unconscious conviction that someone, somewhere, is thinking, "That pushy Jew needs to be taken down a peg" and is getting ready to do the job.

Avoiding appearing boastful, self-confident, or optimistic has another source in Jewish culture: fear of attracting the attention of the "evil eye."[5] My parents would have vehemently denied being influenced by such a superstitious notion. Nevertheless, I think that at some level they felt that not only anti-Semites but some mysterious, malevolent force would strike them down if it noticed their good fortune.

Another legacy of this transgenerational or intergenerational transmission of trauma (Root, 1992; Schlosser, 2006) was a lot of early training in being constantly on the alert, scanning the horizon for danger, anticipating everything that could possibly go wrong, and finding a way to either prevent it or fix it. I don't think my parents had ever heard of Murphy's Law, but their own version of it was implicit in their interactions with me: "If something can go wrong, it will, and when it does it will be your fault." Even small slip-ups—an overdue library book, getting caught in the rain without an umbrella—brought stern admonitions: "How could you have allowed that to happen? You should have known better. You have to pay more attention to what's going on around you." No matter how trivial the real-world consequences of my lapse, it was evidence that I was being careless, and carelessness could be fatal.

I was also expected to be constantly attuned to my mother, who bore the unhealed wounds of layer upon layer of trauma, and to adapt my behavior to what she could tolerate. These expectations were enforced by my father, whose first priority was protecting my mother. Increasing the difficulty of the task were family secrets I was forbidden to inquire about or figure out for myself, even when numerous clues were lying around in plain sight. I was not to know what my parents' political affiliations had been in the 1930s. I was not to know that my mother was seven years older than my father and had been married to someone else for 11 years. I was not to know that the breast surgery she had undergone when I was seven was a radical mastectomy, not the removal of a benign cyst. I was not to see anything

---

[5]*Evil eye* is a look that is believed by many cultures to be able to cause injury or bad luck on the person at whom it is directed. The term also refers to the power, superstitiously attributed to certain persons, of inflicting injury or bad luck by such a look" ("Evil Eye," 2009).

unusual or inappropriate in her intrusiveness, her need to control every aspect of my life, her intolerance of any expression of anger or even difference of opinion. As an only child, I had no allies in my family who could provide a reality check. Nor did my mother permit close relationships with relatives outside our nuclear family. I became a very obedient, if emotionally inhibited and chronically anxious, child, teenager, and young adult.

JEWISHNESS AS ETHNICITY[6]

When I started writing this chapter, it took me a while to identify the specific content of my family's Jewishness. There was actually quite a lot. My mother used to entertain me with stories about the lighter, more picturesque side of childhood in the *shtetl*. Her first language was Yiddish, and her English was sprinkled with Yiddish words and phrases. We often ate traditional Jewish foods, either cooked by my mother or brought in from the deli and the bakery. There were folk tales, and jokes that celebrated Jewish *chutzpah* (gall, brazenness, impudence) and a particular kind of wacky logic carried to an utterly illogical conclusion. ("In the first place, I never borrowed your pot. In the second place, it was already cracked when you gave it to me. And in the third place, I returned it to you in perfect condition.") We felt a kinship with elements of popular culture that were by and about Jews. We listened on the radio to Jewish entertainers like Eddie Cantor, Jack Benny, and Milton Berle. We read best-sellers by Jewish authors about Jewish life, like *Marjorie Morningstar* and *Exodus*. We went to see "Fiddler on the Roof" and my mother pronounced it authentic, except that the characters' clothing was too clean and there wasn't enough mud in the streets. We were proud when a Jew made the news because of a special achievement, and cringed when a Jew disgraced himself or herself publicly.

There were also values that I learned from my parents that they didn't explicitly label as Jewish. One was a reverence for books as physical objects. It was so ingrained in me that it was a long time before I could underline or make marginal notes in my college textbooks. I realized later that the origin of this reverence was probably reverence for the sacred scrolls of the Torah, which are so precious that the text is never touched. I also believe that my parents' commitment to social justice ultimately derived from Jewish teachings dating back to the Biblical prophets.

Often, when my parents heard about a new development on the local, national, or international scene, they asked each other, "Is this good or bad for the Jews?" At one level, this was a metaphor for "What are the practical implications of this? Is it a good thing or a bad thing?" At another, they were

---

[6]The Jewish culture described in this section is, more specifically, Eastern European Jewish culture, which is one among many Jewish cultures worldwide.

quoting the punch line of an old joke about the tendency of (Jewish) human beings to evaluate all information in reference to themselves. Fundamentally, however, I believe that, consciously or unconsciously, the question was an ever-present filter through which they viewed the world.

Eventually I encountered a term for Jews who don't practice Judaism but do identify as Jews: secular Jews. But being a secular Jew is an active process. Secular Jews value the culture and work to preserve it and pass it on to the next generation. As I said earlier, I think my parents' political views were in conflict with what they called ethnic chauvinism. I was taught that there was nothing to be ashamed of about being a Jew, but nothing to be particularly proud of either. There was a *schule* (a school, not to be confused with *shul*, or synagogue) in my neighborhood to which some of my parents' secular Jewish friends sent their children to learn Jewish culture and the Yiddish language. When I wanted to go too, my mother said she could teach me Yiddish at home for free. She borrowed an elementary textbook and went over the first article with me. I don't remember what happened next, but we never got past that first lesson.

Thus many of the things that were culturally Jewish about us remained unlabeled fragments with no organizing framework to hold them together. Some were so much a part of generic New York culture that I didn't realize that they were Jewish in origin. Others I thought were my family's idiosyncrasies. I've learned more about what is Jewish about me in anthropology and sociology classes and through my own reading as an adult than I learned growing up. Culturally, I don't feel qualified to claim the title "secular Jew," but I do feel Jewish enough to reject the pejorative label "bagel and lox Jew," applied by some to people whose sole expression of their Jewishness is what they eat for brunch on Sunday.

JEWISHNESS AS RELIGION

To most people, one of the defining characteristics of a Jew is observance of the Jewish religion, and in that respect my family definitely didn't fit in. My mother regarded religion as a deliberate hoax designed to pacify the oppressed. She said she didn't believe in God, but she got so angry when she talked about Him that I think she was furious with Him because of the horrors He had allowed to happen in the world. Refusing to believe in Him was how she expressed her rage and pain.

My father was more of an agnostic than an atheist. I asked him, when I was 5 or 6, if there was a God. His answer was that many people believed there was, but that nobody knew for sure. As a boy, he had decided shortly before his 13th birthday that he wanted to have a bar mitzvah (in those days a simple religious ceremony followed by modest refreshments, not the lavish social event it has become). He had arranged, completely on his own, to take a crash course in Hebrew to prepare for it. I no longer remember what it was that disillusioned him shortly afterward; it involved something the rabbi did that he perceived as hypocritical. He stopped attending services, but he didn't become bitter, as my mother had. In college he took an elective course in the history of religion, an unusual choice for an engineering student.[7] He kept his textbooks and encouraged me to read them and discuss them with him when I was old enough to understand them. He believed that there was a rational basis for religious practices. For example, the dietary laws had probably been sound public health measures in a hot climate with no refrigeration.

Some time before the age of nine, I discovered that other children believed you couldn't be a good person unless you believed in God. For a few years I succeeded in believing, or at least considering it possible, that there might be a God. I prayed nightly for things like world peace and my grandfather's recovery from a crippling stroke. (I also wished for those things on the evening star. I had learned well my parents' lessons about taking multiple precautions.) Then I learned from my Jewish peers that believing in God might help you to be a good person, but it wasn't enough to make you a good Jew. There were 613 commandments you were supposed to obey. My parents explained that we didn't do all those things because what mattered was being fair and honest and kind. That made sense to me, but I also wanted to belong and to be approved of by my friends. I asked for and was given a Star of David to wear on a chain around my neck, and a menorah to light at Chanukah. My parents, for reasons that had nothing to do with religion, sent me to Jewish summer camps for five years. I enjoyed the Friday night and Saturday morning services and memorized some of the prayers and songs. Even after I stopped believing at age 15,[8] I still enjoyed the rituals and the sense of community, although I wasn't motivated enough to attend services other than weddings and bar mitzvahs.

As soon as I started attending elementary school, the Jewish holidays became an issue that I would wrestle with for the next 40 years. The majority of my classmates were Jewish, so on most Jewish holidays our classroom was typically occupied by four Christian classmates and me, trying to explain what I was doing there.

"I thought you were Jewish."
"We are, but we're not religious."
"Then what makes you Jewish?"
"We just are, okay?"

---

[7]Rereading this, it occurs to me for the first time that my mother married the engineer her father had wanted to become. Interesting.

[8]The death of a family friend in a loft fire, along with 25 other victims, was something I couldn't reconcile with the existence of an omnipotent and benevolent God.

Meanwhile my Jewish friends regarded me as a traitor who caused our (non-Jewish) teachers to question the legitimacy of the numerous Jewish holidays they observed by staying home from school.

My parents did, however, keep me home on the High Holy Days, Rosh Hashanah and Yom Kippur. My mother's reason for doing so, and for staying home from work herself, came straight out of her childhood in the *shtetl*: There was no reason for us to flaunt our unbelief. It would be offensive to our religious neighbors to see us so flagrantly violating community standards. People would talk about us.

My father said he stayed home from work because he didn't want a repetition of an experience he had had years earlier in which a coworker had said to him, "The city is so much nicer when the Jews aren't around." I didn't understand until decades later that he was doing more than avoiding an unpleasant experience of anti-Semitism. He was coming out as a Jew, refusing to pass.

But just taking the day off wasn't enough to avoid causing a scandal. If I left the house I had to wear a skirt, not jeans. I couldn't ride my bike. I couldn't be seen carrying shopping bags home from the supermarket. It all started to feel hypocritical. Instead of passing as a gentile, I was passing as a Jew, in the sense of "person of the Jewish faith."

Over the years I've tried various ways of handling the High Holy Days issue. For a while I went to work on the holidays, but there was something alienating and unsatisfying about doing so. Then I stayed home in solidarity with Jews who did observe the holidays and were sometimes penalized for doing so. Later I adopted my father's rationale, staying home as an assertion of my identity as a Jew. Currently I regard the holidays as part of my cultural heritage.

I've recognized for a long time that all religions can have very real benefits for those who participate in them. Belief, ritual, prayer, and community can have powerful and positive psychological and physical effects. I experienced those effects as a child at camp, and again when my son, unwittingly following in his grandfather's footsteps, decided that he wanted to have a bar mitzvah. We accompanied him to services every Friday night and drove him to Sunday school every Sunday morning for three years. It helped that the rabbi was one of the first women to have full charge of a congregation. She was gradually introducing nonhierarchical and gender-neutral elements into the service, and her sermons emphasized ethical and humanistic interpretations of the Scriptures and the Law. She called it *tikkun olam*, the mending of the world. For me, it resonated with my parents' teachings about social justice. I even went to some adult education classes, which I found fascinating, and considered continuing to attend services after my son's bar mitzvah.

Unfortunately, shortly after the bar mitzvah the rabbi decided to move back home to California. Her replacement was a retired army chaplain. He conducted the services in a manner that suggested that they were an annoying obligation to be disposed of as quickly as possible. Needless to say, he had no problem with the hierarchical and sexist elements in the prayers.

Thus ended my brief stint as a Jew in the sense of "member of a Jewish congregation."[9] It hadn't lasted long enough to be internalized as an enduring part of my identity. It did, however, contribute a lot to my understanding of my heritage. It also increased my receptiveness to spirituality, which to me means experiences of transcendence and community.

JEWISHNESS AS RACE

One more aspect of my identity as a Jew has to do with race, specifically with the question, "Are Jews White?" I think it's useful to break that down into two separate questions, one easily answered and the other more complicated. The easy question is "Are all Jews White?" The answer, of course, is no. There are communities of Jews all over the world who are physically indistinguishable from their non-Jewish neighbors.

The more complicated question is, "Are *any* Jews White?" In my mother's classification system, Jews were not White, and it was dangerous to delude themselves that they were. The KKK targeted Jews as well as Negroes, as I was taught to call them, and the Klan was still a force to be reckoned with in the 1940s and 1950s. It followed that Jews should ally themselves with Negroes, because we had a common enemy and similar aspirations.

I think that even for my mother this was more of a political stance than a core identity. She wouldn't have had to warn me if it hadn't been easier to think of ourselves as White than as non-White. When I'm with White Christians, I'm more aware of not being Christian than of being or not being White.

Among my family and friends, myself included, there was a certain moral smugness about being a Jew and therefore not White. It allowed us to think we weren't racist. It came as a shock to me in the 1980s when I encountered the concepts of White skin privilege, passive racism, and unconscious racism. Acknowledging and taking responsibility for my Whiteness was a painful process.

I have come to recognize that in this country, at this time in history, Jews who look like me are functionally White. I think it's important to keep in mind, however, that this is a fairly recent development (Brodkin, 1998; Jacobson, 1998) and that there are some highly organized and vocal groups, such as neo-Nazis and White militia organizations, who still disseminate the old rhetoric. Today if I'm asked if I think Jews are White, I respond with

---

[9]My son's participation also ended. He later encountered neopaganism and became a Wiccan high priest. But that's another story.

another question (also a Jewish cultural characteristic): Compared to who? I think Melanie Kaye/Kantrowitz (1992) got it right when she wrote that Jews are either "the closest of the coloreds to White or the closest of the Whites to colored" (p. 145).

CONTEXTUALITY OF JEWISH IDENTITY

As I move from one social context to another, the salience of my identity as a Jew and the relative importance of its different aspects vary. In New York City I move through my days as a White person with the White person's privilege of not having to think about my race very often. Although only about 25% of New Yorkers are Jewish, Jewish culture is very much a part of the cultural fabric of the city, so I feel that I'm on home ground. New Yorkers are also less likely than other Americans to assume that everyone is a Christian, so I don't feel that I have to keep coming out as a Jew. When I leave New York, things shift.

I lived in Baltimore for two years while my husband finished medical school. The large Jewish community there lived for the most part in the sub-urbs. We lived in student housing, an all-White enclave in the midst of a poor and working class African-American community. The medical school community was not only almost entirely White and mostly Christian, it was also largely Southern, which to me was synonymous with virulent anti-Semitism. Those were the only two years in my adult life when I lit a menorah during Chanukah and put it in the window. I did so in a spirit of defiance toward my White, Christian, Southern neighbors. My intended message was, "Whether you like it or not, I'm here and I'm not going to be invisible."

I also spent two years as a graduate student at the University of Cincinnati, which had an almost entirely White, Christian student body and faculty. We lived near the campus in a very White, Christian neighborhood. Everyone seemed to have blond hair and blue eyes. This was the only time in my life when I was self-conscious about my "darkness" (black hair, brown eyes).

Comparing my experience in Baltimore with that in Cincinnati, it seems to me now that in Baltimore the presence of the surrounding African-American community positioned me as one more White person in the medical school community. What differentiated me from the other White people was my Jewishness. In Cincinnati, the marginality of my Whiteness was more salient.

FAMILY DYNAMICS, JEWISHNESS AND PSYCHOTHERAPY

David Bakan (Bakan, 1958), among others, has written about the parallels between Freudian psychoanalysis and the Jewish mystical tradition. Both regard the surface of what is communicated as concealing a deeper, hidden meaning that must be painstakingly unearthed in order to release its power. Both regard multiple, even contradictory interpretations of a single text or behavior as the norm. The Jewishness of psychoanalytic thinking may have contributed to my receptiveness to it. Although my thinking has moved away from some of the content of classical psychoanalytic theory, I remain fascinated by the process of collaborating with my patients to unravel the meanings implicit in the stories they tell about their lives.

I knew in junior high school that I wanted to study psychology. A gifted science teacher gave my class an assignment that sent me to the encyclopedia to look up "mind" and "brain." I followed the cross-references for hours. The same teacher helped us to understand the disturbing behavior of a teacher who, in retrospect, I would diagnose as having a narcissistic personality disorder with borderline features. The prospect of learning to understand the behavior of the important people in my life was a lifeline I grabbed with both hands. A year or two later, when I read about the career options for someone with a degree in psychology, I knew that I wanted to be a therapist.

It's hard to imagine a career choice for which years of attempting to meet my parents' needs could have better prepared me. As a therapist I'm rewarded for using the skills I learned as a child: I help people to heal emotionally by engaging with them empathically, striving to see the world from their point of view and disclosing my own thoughts and feelings only when it's in the patient's best interests. At the same time, I'm not only permitted but required to do what was once taboo: I get to ask all the forbidden questions, bring up unmentionable subjects, point out inconsistencies, and piece together the answers to the mysteries. Professional ethics mandate that I maintain the boundaries appropriate to the relationship even if the patient wants us to overstep them. Thus I have firm backing for meeting with the patient only at the designated time and for the designated duration, limiting telephone contact between sessions and declining offers to enter into a dual relationship. Professional ethics also require me to give a high priority to my own self-care in order to preserve my ability to be an effective therapist. This provides a dramatic and welcome contrast with the self-abnegation demanded of me by my parents. When I am working with a patient who persistently tries to shift the boundaries, I sometimes feel an internal pull to go to excessive lengths to accommodate what she has persuaded me she needs. At those times, I find it useful to discuss my work with colleagues. I count on them to ask, "Why on earth would you be willing to do that?"

Family dynamics have influenced my therapeutic style in both positive and negative ways. Sensitized by my mother's controlling and intrusive behavior, I am wary of replicating it. Thus I lean toward a nondirective approach. Based on the patient's responses to my interventions, I intuitively adjust my activity level. I want her to experience my presence as supportive without distracting her from her focus on herself. I also tend to be reserved in my expression of emotion. This meets the needs of some patients, matching their own preferred level of emotional intensity. For others it provides a calm and reassuring stability within which they can give free expression to their own emotional storms. On the other hand, some patients need more expressiveness from me than I can currently provide and experience me as cold or aloof. When verbally attacked, I still sometimes fall back on my old response of doing my best to disappear (a strategy that worked well with my parents, less well elsewhere). When this happens, some patients feel abandoned, while others seem not to notice. Bringing myself back into connection with the patient involves remembering that I am not in danger in the present. Often this takes the form of silently reassuring and comforting my own inner child.

Jews have historically been perpetual outsiders, and this is a role I find very familiar. For most of my life I have perceived myself as marginal to whatever group I found myself in, including groups of Jews. Throughout my childhood I consistently chose adult approval over that of my peers and assumed that conforming to the adults' expectations was the way to get that approval. As a result, I remained on the fringe of every peer group, from my neighborhood to school to summer camp. As a psychotherapist, I am paradoxically both inside and outside the patient's life. My patients tell me their most private thoughts and feelings, their life stories, and their hopes for the future. Over time, if the therapy goes well, we come to deeply appreciate and care about one another. On the other hand, we do not participate in each other's lives outside of my office. I hear a lot about the people in the patient's life, but I rarely meet them. Thus being a therapist allows me to experience some of the rewards of an intimate relationship while remaining within my comfort zone at the periphery.

When I'm working with a Jewish patient who is religiously observant, has had an extensive secular Jewish education, or is an ardent Zionist, I am vulnerable to feeling that she perceives me as not enough of a Jew or the wrong kind of Jew. There is a temptation, which I try to resist, to display what knowledge I have acquired about things Jewish in a fruitless effort to win the approval I longed for as a child.

Remnants of my mother's indoctrination about the ubiquitousness of anti-Semitism influence my emotional response when a non-Jewish patient expresses a stereotypical belief about Jews. There's an internal lurch that I feel when a non-Jew says that Jews are rich, or smart, or clannish, or greedy, or that Jewish men make good husbands. (Jewish patients may also express anti-Semitism, but I am less hypervigilant in that situation.) The first challenge for me is to notice my emotional response and then set it aside for later self-exploration. I remind myself that the fact that I hear a statement as anti-Semitic does not mean it actually is, in the present context. If the comment is tangential to the issue the patient is working on, I may say nothing about it. If the time is right for exploring the basis for her beliefs about Jews, I look for an intervention that will encourage her to do so but will not induce shame. This is particularly delicate when the patient hasn't thought about whether I'm Jewish and suddenly realizes, after the fact, that I may be.

As a therapist, I am frequently faced with deciding whether and how to come out as a Jew, with all of the concerns that accompany any act of coming out. My intent is to handle self-disclosure as a Jew the same way I handle other aspects of self-disclosure, such as my sexual orientation or whether I have children. I don't routinely identify myself as a Jew to new patients, nor do I mention it in my handout about myself and my practice; it feels intrusive to provide the information before it's requested. I do, however, give a direct answer to a direct question, as part of the process of informed consent to treatment.

I don't remember a non-Jewish patient ever asking at intake whether I'm Jewish; most Jewish patients don't ask at intake either. Jewish patients who do ask usually put it in a context of wanting a therapist who will understand their experience as a Jew. Of course, as this article and the other articles in this collection amply demonstrate, there are many different ways of being a Jew, and being Jewish has different meanings and different consequences for different people. There may be things it is easier for me to understand than it would be for a non-Jewish therapist, but that may not always be the case. There may even be times when we both assume that I do understand and it may be some time before we realize that we're talking about two different things. Furthermore, even when our experience coincides, it will be important for the patient to put her experience into her own words and to connect with her own emotions about it. It's the telling and retelling in the presence of an empathic other that opens up possibilities for change.

Some Jewish patients may seek out a Jewish therapist in order to ensure that the therapist isn't anti-Semitic, although I don't remember any of my patients ever stating that explicitly. It is worth noting here that Jewish therapists, myself included, may harbor some degree of conscious or unconscious anti-Semitism. There may also be a difference of opinion between therapist and patient about whether a particular belief or attitude is anti-Semitic.

If an orthodox Jewish patient asks if I'm Jewish, I will volunteer the information that I'm not religious because I think that has direct and legitimate relevance to her decision whether or not to work with me. Similarly, if I know a patient was referred to me because I'm Jewish, I'll ask if it's important to her to work with someone who's religious, and decide together whether to immediately refer her to another therapist or explore the issue further.

Even if the question doesn't come up in the initial interview, I think most Jewish patients quickly recognize that I'm Jewish, whether from my last name, from how I talk, or from my familiarity with aspects of Jewish culture or religious practices. Non-Jewish patients may pick up the same cues. If our usual appointment time coincides with one of the High Holy Days, I will say explicitly that I need to reschedule because of the Jewish holiday. If the question is asked later in the therapy, I will answer it concisely and then explore what prompted them to ask and what it means to them that I am.

CONCLUSION

I started writing the paper that evolved into this article in 2001. Not surprisingly, given the conceptualization of identity that I set forth at the beginning of this article, my relationship with my Jewishness has not remained static over the past decade. The writing process itself has involved summoning up memories, thoughts, and emotions going back 50 years and more and trying to put them into words that will make sense to others. Hearing the narratives of other contributors to this volume has shaped my own account by showing me where my experience has been similar to theirs and where it has been different. Reading published accounts of Jewish identity and experience have furthered the process (Goldberg & Krausz, 1993b; Siegel & Cole, 1991, 1997).

My writing process has coincided with and interacted with my participation in an ongoing series of dialogues with diverse groups of people. We share a commitment to expanding our own self-knowledge, listening deeply to one another, and building a network of long-term, heartfelt relationships to support sustainable leadership for social justice at the individual, the interpersonal, and the institutional level. These dialogues have taken place within Be Present, Inc., a national, nonprofit organization founded by Black women, then opened to women of all races, and then to men of all races.[10] I have had numerous opportunities to talk in an emotionally connected way, and in the presence of both Jews and non-Jews, about the role my Jewishness has played in my life. I have heard other Jews talk about their experience of being Jewish and have heard non-Jews talk about their experiences with and perceptions of Jews. Be Present has become my home community, a community in which my way of being a Jew is a valued contribution to the collective process that furthers our shared goals. It is in this setting, more often than in any other, that I participate in Jewish religious rituals. I am able to do so without feeling inauthentic because part of my contribution to the ritual is speaking about my relationship to it as a nonbelieving, nonpracticing Jew.

In writing this article and in my work in Be Present I have been gathering up the unlabeled fragments of my identity as a Jew and giving them

---

[10]More information about Be Present Inc. can be found at www.bepresent.org

greater coherence, clarity, and specificity. I now have a more solid sense of my location in the vast, multidimensional array of ways of being a Jew. I have a better understanding of how I got here, why it makes sense that I am here rather than somewhere else, and why here can feel very different depending on what is going on around me. I am no longer perplexed by the question, *"How* am I Jewish?"

REFERENCES

Bakan, D. (1958). *Sigmund Freud and the Jewish mystical tradition.* New York: Schocken.

Barrett, S. (1998). Contextual identity: A model for therapy and social change. *Women & Therapy, 21,* 51–64.

Bhavnani, K.-K., & Haraway, D. (1994). Shifting the subject: A conversation between Kum-Kum Bhavnani and Donna Haraway, 12 April 1993, Santa Cruz, California. *Feminism & Psychology, 4,* 19–39.

Brodkin, K. (1998). *How Jews became White folks and what that says about race in America.* New Brunswick, NJ: Rutgers University Press.

Channon, J. W., & Hudson, R. (1995). *The Penguin historical atlas of Russia.* London, England: Penguin Books.

Evil Eye. (2009). *Wikipedia, the free encyclopedia.* Retrieved July 21, 2009, from http://en.wikipedia.org/wiki/Evil_eye

Goldberg, D. T., & Krausz, M. (1993a). Introduction: The culture of Identity. In D. T. Goldberg, & M. Krausz (Eds.), *Jewish identity* (pp. 1–12). Philadelphia: Temple University Press.

Goldberg, D. T., & Krausz, M. (Eds.). (1993b). *Jewish identity.* Philadelphia: Temple University Press.

Jacobson, M. F. (1998). *Whiteness of a different color: European immigrants and the alchemy of race.* Cambridge, MA: Harvard University Press.

Kaye/Kantrowitz, M. (1992). *The issue is power: Essays on women, Jews, violence, and resistance* (1st ed.). San Francisco: Aunt Lute Books.

Polish–Soviet War. (2009). *Wikipedia, the free encyclopedia.* Retrieved July 22, 2009, from http://en.wikipedia.org/wiki/Polish-soviet_war

Polish–Ukrainian War. (2009). *Wikipedia, the free encyclopedia.* Retrieved July 22, 2009, from http://en.wikipedia.org/wiki/Polish%E2%80%93Ukrainian_War

Prior, R., Wilson, T., & Keegan, J. (1999). *The First World War.* London: Cassell.

Räthzel, N. (1994). Harmonious "heimat" and disturbing "auslander." *Feminism & Psychology, 4,* 81–98.

Root, M. P. P. (1992). Reconstructing the impact of trauma on personality. In L. S. Brown, & M. Ballou (Eds.), *Personality and psychopathology: Feminist reappraisals* (pp. 229–265). New York: Guilford Press.

Russian Civil War. (2009). *Wikipedia, the free encyclopedia.* Retrieved July 22, 2009, from http://en.wikipedia.org/wiki/Russian_Civil_War

Schlosser, L. Z. (2006). Affirmative psychotherapy for American Jews. *Psychotherapy: Theory, Research, Practice, Training, 43,* 424–435.

Siegel, R. J., & Cole, E. (Eds.). (1991). *Jewish women in therapy: Seen but not heard.* Binghamton, NY: The Haworth Press.

Siegel, R. J., & Cole, E. (Eds.). (1997). *Celebrating the lives of Jewish women: Patterns in a feminist sampler.* Binghamton, NY: The Haworth Press.

Steinberg-Oren, S. (1997). Bris, Britah: Parents' first lessons in balancing gender, culture, tradition, and religion. In R. J. Siegel, & E. Cole (Eds.), *Celebrating the lives of Jewish women: Patterns in a feminist sampler* (pp. 9–17). Binghamton, NY: The Haworth Press.

Ukrainian People's Republic. (2009). *Wikipedia, the free encyclopedia.* Retrieved July 22, 2009, from http://en.wikipedia.org/wiki/Ukrainian_People%27s_Republic

I Am the Rabbi's Daughter

BETH A. FIRESTEIN

I am the rabbi's daughter. This simple fact has shaped and colored every aspect of my childhood and adult existence. I loved being the rabbi's daughter, and this positionality separated me from everyone except my sisters, who were also Rabbi's daughters. It separated me from those I wanted to be like and from those I never wanted to be like. It connected me to my Judaism and separated me from my Judaism. This fact shaped my choice of profession and denied me access to certain professions. It complicated every other facet of my identity formation, adding to my internal conflict as I came to terms with discovering myself as the bisexual, feminist, polyamorous, Jewish psychologist that I am today. And I am still the rabbi's daughter.

SHAME, PRIDE, AND IDENTITY

My entire life has been a dance between shame and pride, and this dance has played out through the discovery and exploration of every aspect of my identity. I remember being the only Jewish child in virtually every one of my elementary, junior high, and high school classrooms. Due to differences between my family's socioeconomic standing and the socioeconomic position of the majority of our temple's congregants, I rarely attended the same public schools attended by other Jewish children. My father made a much lower salary than most of his congregants. He raised a family of six on $11,000 a year and the charity of temple members who were doctors and dentists, while many of his congregants owned successful businesses, belonged to country clubs and wore fashionable clothing and jewelry to Sisterhood events.

My mother never felt she fit in, and she really never did. She was the rabbi's wife, and she struggled with the conflict I was to inherit from her: that disturbing tension between shame and pride in having a status that was esteemed yet alienating, honorable yet disadvantaging, special yet in some respects inferior to the positions held by other temple "wives." I came to feel conflicted about my mother's conflict. I would admire her beauty and relished the scent of the Shalimar perfume she would don when getting dressed up to attend a special event at the temple. I would feel the tension of the painful discussions and arguments she had with my father every five years when the board of directors discussed renewing my father's contract. Although this was never discussed with the children, we were nonetheless affected by the ugly political struggles between my father's allies and his enemies over issues such as our family's salary for the next five years and whether he would be retained in his position. The net effect was to tarnish my experience of Judaism in the context of organized religion by connecting me emotionally with the least spiritual elements of temple life.

Elsewhere I have written that my experience as a rabbi's daughter was similar to that of a child involved in the life of the theater with a family whose father is a lead actor. The experience in front of the curtain differs significantly from the experience of growing up and seeing the drama of the theater played out from behind the curtain. My father was a lead actor on the stage of the "theater" of organized religion. The beautiful, moving, and mystical quality of the show was different for members of the temple than it appeared to members of our family as we grew up behind the stage.

GROWING UP JEWISH AND BISEXUAL

As I moved into my teenage years, my mother rejected her role as rabbi's wife, and although I didn't realize it at the time, this influenced both my own relationship to my Judaism and the emergence of my feminist identity. As my childhood innocence passed into the early years of my adolescent yearning, I watched as my mother spent more and more Friday nights at home in front of the television, venturing out only to the most important Jewish services and events, and our (the children's) attendance at services waned as well. Once I left the house, I felt uncertain whether to be proud of my mother for her feminist rebellion against the expectations associated with being a rabbi's wife or angry at her for her failure to support my father in his profession. He sacrificed so much of his time and his personal life to his rabbinical work, it is hard to imagine the embarrassment he probably suffered in not having my mother at his side through many years of his career. This further complicated my relationship to my Judaism, and I became increasingly confused about Judaism's role in my life.

By the time I left for college in the mid-1970s, I was definitely a secular Jew, and my Judaism took a back burner to other emerging facets of my identity. I fell in love with a woman who was my college roommate and my best friend and discovered the joys of sex in many of its diverse forms. Ironically, I attended Southern Methodist University, a private university in Dallas, Texas, known for its very Christian School of Theology (a part of campus we termed "the God Quad"), yet I could only afford to attend this private undergraduate institution of higher education because my father was clergy and, therefore, we were offered a partial scholarship on tuition reserved only for children of clergy. Such paradoxes riddled my existence.

My college roommate and I formed a support system of two. We were the only two "girls" on our campus who did *not* go through Rush Week to join sororities, and I am convinced that we were probably the only two bisexual women in our dormitory—at least the only two I knew existed at SMU. As we wound our way through the joys and tribulations of first same-sex love within the conservative bastion of a religiously affiliated Bible belt educational institution, I identified strongly with my emerging status as a sexual minority. First, I was a woman who loved sex and was not ashamed of loving it, and second, I was a woman who felt love, sexual attraction, and desire for both women and men, and this made me neither straight nor lesbian. When I was introduced to the term "bisexual," I felt it completed my understanding of myself in a very important way.

For reasons I do not fully understand, I always rejected the shame projected onto me by the culture around my sexuality. Perhaps my years of experience in transforming the injury of stigma related to being Jewish in a predominantly Christian, Southern culture somehow prepared me for transforming the adversity of another stigmatized identity into a source of personal pride and celebration of difference. I know for certain that the mastery of this mystery of transformation set the stage for the development of my positive self-esteem and further, for my ongoing and lifelong commitment to making the world a diversity affirmative and sexually safer place for others, both like and unlike myself. I came to believe deeply that being different can be a good thing and that it is possible to take pride in our differences rather than feeling ashamed of them. These experiences also affected my personal relationship choices.

Looking back, it is perhaps not a surprise that one of my closest friendships originating in the SMU days turned out to be with an African-American man involved in a polyamorous relationship with an older White woman. He had been recruited to SMU as a football player and by the time I met Tim Seibles, he had given up his football scholarship and was pursuing his true passion—writing poetry. He is now a highly regarded, nationally recognized professional poet and professor of creative literature at Old Dominion University in Norfolk, Virginia. Our incredible and spiritual friendship has continued and grown for over 30 years.

EVERYTHING I HAVE BECOME, I HAVE ALWAYS BEEN

My interest in psychology began early in my educational life. From the first time I took a high school class in the subject, I was entranced with this body of knowledge. I couldn't get enough. Natural curiosity and my ever-present and continuous desire to learn eventually led me to an undergraduate degree in psychology and my decision to enroll in an American Psychological Association approved PhD program in counseling psychology at the University of Texas at Austin. Thus began the long journey that led to the eventual integration of my sexuality, my feminism, my spirituality, and my career as a psychologist. Apparently divergent streams of interest periodically intersected and the convergence of these streams of passion resulted in the progressive integration of more and more facets of my being.

At the time of this writing, I am celebrating 24 years as a practicing psychologist—half of this time spent as a staff psychologist and the director of a campus-based Office of Women's Services and half of this time spent in an increasingly diverse and eclectic private practice, specializing in women's issues, LGBTQ issues, and support for those engaged in the meaningful explorations of alternative lifestyles. My Judaism remained on the back burner throughout much of this period of my professional development, though I felt periodically called to explore my Jewish identity in personally relevant and professional important ways.

The Jewish Women's Caucus of the Association for Women in Psychology certainly provided the most stimulating call to reapproach and explore my Jewish identity. The Jewish Women's Caucus posed for the first time in my life the possibility of integrating two critically important facets of my identity—my feminism and my Judaism. My ambivalence about my Jewish identity was the primary limiter in my exploration of that nexus of the personal and the professional. Furthermore, I now understand that I had always felt a need to choose between being Jewish and being myself. Given the choice to be Jewish or be myself, a sexually empowered, feminist, bisexual, queer-identified woman, I had always chosen to be myself. Yet, it has become increasingly important over the years to reconcile my inner conflicts about my Judaism with the rest of my identity and this search for spiritual integration comprises a substantial part of my current life journey.

SO AM I A JEWISH THERAPIST?

For many years it has been easier to say that I am a therapist than it has been to say that I am Jewish. My Jewish identity has certainly been invisible at times, even to myself. The most accurate measure of my conflict about my Jewish identity has been the degree of my denial of the impact and importance of Judaism on my life and my identity, which is exactly why I so welcomed this opportunity to write about it.

For many years my Jewish identity was such a source of emotional pain to me that I simply ignored my Judaism. Although I occasionally participated in services or observed Jewish holidays, for the most part

I simply disengaged from my identity as a Jew and went about my life finding spiritual fulfillment through quasi-Jewish, quasi-Buddhist, and nature-based approaches to spirituality. I found my spiritual nourishment through personal growth, the exploration of my nighttime and daytime dreams, and by closely watching and learning from others who seemed to emanate a sense of serenity and spiritual wholeness. My resistance to organizational religion persisted and I could no more join a dojo or follow a guru (spiritual teacher) than I could see my way to joining a temple or synagogue. Yet, my Judaism remained important to me in some profound, immeasurable way. I began to realize that I couldn't feel complete about my healing or fully integrated in my identities until I addressed this important omission in my life—my Jewish self.

COMING OUT, COMING TO TERMS

I have spent my entire life in communities in which I was a minority by virtue of my gender, my Jewishness, or my sexuality. I truly have no idea what it would be like to live among other Jewish people. My attendance at National Association for Women in Psychology (AWP) conferences is probably the closest I have come to experiencing Jewish community in over 30 years away from my Jewish childhood home. For whatever reasons, there seem to be a disproportionate number of Jewish women psychologists who join feminist psychology organizations. I think it reflects the intellectual values and curiosities characteristic of many Jewish women. We want to understand how things work, who we are, and how others experience their lives. And then there is the Jewish value of *tikkun olam*, the Judaic concept of "repair of the world" that we can participate in through our work as therapists, educators, and researchers.

In the last 14 years, I have begun to more actively address the question of my Jewish identity: what it means to me and how I live that identity in the world. I notice that it has become more important to me to allow the fact that I am Jewish to be a visible, acknowledged aspect of my identity, both inside and outside of the therapy room. Within the consulting room I find that the vast majority of my clients are not Jewish. Among the Jewish clients with whom I have worked, some are secular or cultural Jews, some have interfaith religious lives, and a few have been observant Jews.

I notice that I usually "come out" as Jewish to my clients who are Jewish, just as I frequently come out as bisexual to my nonheterosexual and LGBTQ clients much more frequently than I come out to my straight clients. In the context of a client's exploration of their own spirituality or religious practice, I sometimes feel it is important to allow them the benefit of understanding my frame of reference and the context that influences my responses to them on religious or spiritual matters.

Occasionally, I disclose my religious upbringing to very religious (usually Christian) clients so that they can make an informed decision about whether they wish to work with a non-Christian therapist. I have become increasingly comfortable with my own ability to work effectively and nonjudgmentally with very religious clients, even some fundamentalist-aligned religious clients; rarely has a client elected not to work with me on the basis of my disclosure. I don't know how this might be different if I were a more observant and religiously active Jew rather than a spiritually oriented, cultural Jew.

THERAPIST AS SECULAR RABBI

There are other ways in which my Jewish upbringing has affected my work as a psychologist and therapist. Over a period of many years, I have come to view my work as a psychologist as a secular version of my father's profession. Like my father, I deal with the innermost dimensions of people's lives. The women, men, and transgendered people who seek my counsel do so to be understood, to find a place of compassionate acceptance, to experience a sense of belonging in a more intimate context than that provided by the larger culture. My father tended to the physically ill, the spiritually ailing and, whether with awareness or not, he no doubt dealt with all manner of emotional and psychological difficulties among his congregants. He provided a safe space, a sacred space, for coming into contact with one's self and with something greater than one's self. I feel my work as a psychologist to be a calling of the same depth and clarity as most clergy would assert their calling to serve God.

I perceive my role as healer in this culture to be a contemporary version of the roles traditionally filled by clergy of all denominations. In a secular culture, we tend to access our spirituality in secular ways. Priests, ministers, and rabbis no longer serve the culture and families in the same way they once did in more religious times. The sexism of organized religion during my growing up years and the conflicted messages I received about religion from my parents and their involvement in religious organizations made it impossible for me to choose the path of rabbi, though there was a time when I did briefly consider it.

THE PERSONAL IS SPIRITUAL

I have come to terms with the fact that I am a Jew and a rabbi's daughter. What remains is how I choose to deal with these identities in my work as a psychologist and in my relational life. Partnering over the years with women and with men in both monogamous and polyamorous configurations has turned out to be equally complicated in differing ways. I have almost never dated other Jews. Yet, in spite of my struggles with my own Jewish identity, I have found that it matters to me on some primal level to affirm my Jewishness, perhaps especially within my relationships with non-Jews. It would be easier on some inarticulate spiritual level—and on the level of familial acceptance and support—to partner with a Jew rather than a non-Jew, to partner with a man rather than a woman.

Five years ago, I married a non-Jewish man in an inclusive, queer wedding ceremony conducted by a rabbi who was also a psychologist. Although the marriage lasted only two years, the experience gave me a rare opportunity to confront my own conflicts about my Jewish identity. The richness of this work became evident in an epic dream I had shortly before my wedding about myself in relation to my Judaism and my place in the lineage of generations of Jewish women in my family.

TELLING THE DREAM

This was a dream that was more than a dream. It was a dream that was, for me, a spiritual experience. In this dream, I saw my deceased mother (may she rest in peace) and danced with my aging and declining father. My mother held me in an embrace so vivid that I woke up still feeling the touch of her skin on mine. In the dream I also met my grandmother and my great-grandmother, and my great-grandmother told me the dates of her birth and death and her Hebrew name, which I had never known. There was a sense of celebration and inclusion, of joining a long line of my maternal Jewish relatives in this process of making the decision to join in partnership.

In the dream, my mother met my partner and gave us her blessing. On the sacred altar of a tray I held in my arms, a candle burst spontaneously into flame without being lit by the fire of any match. It was my great-grandmother who ignited the flame, and the miracle of this event was not lost on me. In the dream I worshipped across the wall from non-Jewish worshippers, yet when I looked to the front of the sanctuary, I saw that we were all worshipping at the same sacred altar. I felt ecstasy.

In the final part of the dream, I discovered a house full of treasures: old furniture, a wooden armoire, and many smaller objects of sacred significance. They were family treasures of Jewish origin. Both my mother's German Jewish heritage and my father's Russian Jewish heritage were represented among these treasures. This was my inheritance, the treasure of my lost connection to my own Judaism rediscovered. I felt the connection to my heritage and the lineage of Jewish women from whom I emerged and to whom I am reconnecting in joining the flow of life as I enter creative and committed partnership with a partner of my choosing.

I awoke elated.

FINDING MY WAY HOME

My journey is not over. Far from it. In fact, my journey has only begun. I still have a long way to go in healing my connection to my Judaism. I still don't know how much formal expression I wish to give to that; whether I wish to pursue the lost dream of being bat mitzvah or mastering the intricacies of the beautiful Hebrew language, or whether I will ever wish to be known by my Hebrew name, Breilah, again in my everyday life, as I once did in my youth. In successfully threading the needle of creating a beautiful and meaningful queer affirmative relationship I have yet to understand all of the implications of that which I am undertaking. My ongoing challenge shall be discovering how to weave together the multicolored, multitextured fabric of a queer affirmative life and a committed partnership, regardless of whether that partnership is with a man or with a woman.

I know that my Judaism will continue to be an important part of this weaving and that I can abandon no part of my complete identity without harming every aspect of who I am. There are few questions as large as those that religion attempts to answer and few lives that that are not powerfully shaped by the faith tradition (or absence of faith) that clothed us in our upbringing. I used to believe that there was not enough room for me in Judaism, that it would always be a choice between my Judaism and my commitment to the authentic flowering of myself. I no longer believe this. I now believe that there is room within Judaism for all of me, and I believe that there is now room within me for Judaism as well. I am the rabbi's daughter, and beyond all that this may mean, I am also myself.

How I Lost My Yiddische Kop and Found It Again: The Un-M-Bellished Truth

MARNY HALL

"Isn't this Staffordshire dog elegant?" My sister is holding up one of the family "heirlooms"—a chipped piece of china acquired by our mother at an auction. Without waiting for my response, Elizabeth puts the cracked spaniel back in the antique hutch and proceeds, docent-like, to extol the finer points of its immediate neighbors. I am prompted to admire, in turn, a Victorian moustache cup, a porcelain platter of uncertain provenance, and a silver tea service monogrammed with someone else's initials. With their wannabe pedigrees, these items exude a decidedly un-Sotheby's aura.

"Did Mother ever spend more than fifty cents for any of these tchotchkes?"

Twin veils, opaque as cataracts, descend over my sister's eyes. "What does that mean? I've never heard that word before."

My sister is a sophisticated woman, a polyglot who crosses language borders on regular pillaging expeditions. Any organization she dislikes is a *junta*, any mystery stew a *bouillabaisse*. But mention *tchotchkes, latkes*, or even *goy* and a familiar scrim of determined ignorance descends.

"Oh come on, Elizabeth."

She pauses, creasing her brow, as if searching her memory. "I've heard of Hotchkiss, not tchotchkes." I picture the ivy-covered Gothic splendor of Hotchkiss, a New England boarding school, and resist, with some difficulty, singsonging, "Hotchkiss-not-tchotchkes." I don't want to wrangle with my sister. She'll be 85 next year and I love her dearly. Besides, I made a promise, long ago, never to be "Jewish" around her or her offspring. The rest of her living room tour passes without incident.

THE QUEST FOR THE MISSING MOTHER-TONGUE OR
MAMA-LOSHEN, SHAINAH MAMA-LOSHEN, WO BIS DU?

The passage from shtetl to Staffordshire, from tchotchtkes to Hotchkiss, has taken about three generations to complete. The ethnic scrubbing started by my mother in the 1930s has been so thorough that the family's Jewish identity has been—if not erased—so diluted that it is, today, largely irrelevant. My sister, the only propagating member of our small clan, is "not Jewish." Her children don't know they have a heritage to disown and if her grandchildren find out, their reaction may be a collective yawn. After generations of determined intermarriage, they are only fractionally Jewish.

My birth, in 1943, occurred after the constructing of a Christian family identity was well underway. The zeal with which my mother undertook this conversion is evident in my baby book. Whenever I take it out of my desk, its contents—childish scribbles, baby pictures, old report cards—tumble out in disorder. But one item is so thoroughly glued in that it never falls out. Tenacious as flypaper, the baptismal announcement of Marjory Ann Hunt Hall in St. Paul's Episcopal Church is clearly intended to stick with me 'til Judgment Day. As I child, I went to Sunday school and said "Our Father who art in heaven" every night before bedtime. Even though I had morphed into an atheist by my teens, I still identified as a WASP.

Sadly, I never had a chance to talk to my parents about my counterfeit identity. My father, a heavy smoker, died of heart disease when I was a toddler. My mother died when I was 23 and still thought of myself as a White Anglo-Saxon Protestant. My brother Richard and sister Elizabeth knew otherwise. Respectively 17 and 18 years older than I, they remembered the metamorphosis from Hirshfeld to Hall. In fact it was Elizabeth, during a confessional spasm that she has regretted ever since, who told me the truth about the family background. Or at least part of the truth. Not until I searched the archives in Austin (where my mother was born in 1905) and, through the Internet, reclaimed relatives I didn't know I had, did I begin to sense that reinvention was as much a part of my family heritage as was its long-hidden Jewishness.

FINDING ZION ON THE RIO GRANDE

When did the family's talent for reinvention begin? It is immediately evident that there is no clear starting point. No particular event—no Rhineland rampage during a twelfth-century crusade, no mass garroting by Spanish inquisitors—primed the secret conversion. Not even Kristallnacht and the events it presaged can account for it. Rather, all of these events and a thousand others never recorded prompted my predecessors' revisionism. Therefore, I will use an arbitrary starting point for family metamorphoses: my first encounter with my great-great-grandfather in the Texas American History Archives.

I discovered that Great-Great-Grandpa Seth Melawskr (1790–1860) was a peddler. Such a vocation must have entailed constant shifts of identity. Perhaps at one point on his journeys he was an expert in sharp implements, at another, a cloth merchant and, at all times, a shrewd judge of character. His ability to change languages and to bargain in different currencies must have been second nature. Even if he hadn't been a traveling salesman, he would have been a chronic (if inadvertent) border-crosser. Thanks to the geopolitics of the nineteenth century, his native village was claimed, at certain times, by Prussia, during other intervals by Poland, and still later by Russia. When these sea changes occurred, did his identity change, too? Was he, depending on the historical moment, a Prussian, a Pole, or a Russian? Or was he simply a Jew? It seems certain that, toward the end of his life, he was a member of a persecuted minority.

When I surf the Net, zoom to historical records from shortly before his death, in the 1850s, I find multiple accounts of inflamed nationalism and contested borders. I also find texts of repressive laws passed by the anti-Semitic xenophobe Czar Nicholas. Under these laws, Jewish peddlers and merchants were routinely prosecuted as smugglers and spies. Perhaps this legal harassment prompted Seth's sons to emigrate. Perhaps they feared conscription into an army being slaughtered in the Crimea. Or maybe they had word from relatives already settled in America that Texas was a promising new territory. Did they arrive penniless, or loaded with marketable merchandise? I can find no record of their native tongue. I don't know if they spoke Russian or Hebrew, Polish or Yiddish, or an indeterminate patois. Nothing in the library, and no hints from long-lost relatives, can fill in these blanks. But there are examples of reinvention scattered among the archives. The obituary of an émigré named Bernard—Seth's son and my great grandfather—notes his service as a Confederate soldier. In the archives I find his own description of this military service in a letter to a relative: "My rank was sergeant.... Our field of operations was Louisiana. The battles I took part in were as follows: Blair's Landing on Red Pines, La. where my regiment lost 65 men killed as also Gen'l Tom Green. We fought for several months around Alexandria up to the 'Yellow Bayou.'"

His handwriting is carefully executed, his spelling and punctuation impeccable—perhaps painstaking attempts to sound like a native-born American. As for those battles he "took part in," he must have wielded a mean skillet. Civil War records show he was the regiment's cook, a fact he omits from an otherwise punctilious letter. This (dis)information, along with a photo of him looking clownish in Masonic getup, tells me my great-grandfather was more chameleon than Confederate. Posing as a Southern partisan, or a member of the secret society of Masons, he did what was necessary to create the illusion of belonging.

Perhaps Bernard learned assimilationist tactics from brothers and uncles. Perhaps he saw parallels between prior and current circumstances. Despite differences in *causi belli*, continents, and climates, nineteenth century Texas, with its internecine struggles, battles over borders, and dislocation of Mexican residents and indigenous peoples, wasn't so different from the conflict-wracked Europe he had left. But for him and other Jews arriving in the newly annexed frontier, it was a propitious move, Southern defeat and Reconstruction agonies notwithstanding. This time they'd end up on the winning side. Or at least, camouflaged as native sons, they would prove themselves useful enough to be tolerated.

Bernard and his wife, Golda, had eight children. I find a photo of their house, rather grand, which the librarian tells me has been razed to make way for a parking lot. In the 1880 Austin City Directory, his name has been Anglicized: "Bernard Melasky and Son" are purveyors of "dry goods, clothing, boots, and shoes." One of Bernard's daughters, Lili, married Carl Belish, another European refugee. They had two daughters. The younger of the two was my mother.

In the Austin 1900 directory, I see *Belish Furniture* in big print. My grandfather sold "carpets, matting, stoves, pianos, organs, and sewing machines" and is one of the few merchants with a telephone listing. Old family photos showed scenes of comfort and affluence: corseted women in bombazine and big brimmed hats lean on portly, mustachioed men. The Belish girls, my mother and her sister with long banana curls beribboned, posed primly next to a pony and cart.

Stories passed down emphasized the contradictions between bourgeois privilege and anti-Semitism. My newly discovered Texas relatives told me that schoolmates shouting "Christ killers!" regularly chased the Belish girls home from school. And the Ku Klux Klan was prevented from burning a cross on my great-grandfather's lawn by locals who, intervening in the nick of time, testified to his honorable Confederate service. If such narrow-escape stories are still circulating among family members a century later, the events they describe must have been both terrifying and commonplace, perhaps standard dinner time conversation, while my mother was growing up.

MESCHUMAD (RHYMES WITH DILUTED): A WILLING CONVERT

Here, then, are some of the ingredients in the family's recipe for reinvention: deracination and relocation in potentially inimical territory, keen sensitivity to dominant cultural rules and roles, the ability to adjust quickly when they change, the perception that success depends on assimilation, and, finally, the self-objectification that comes from repeated exposure to representations of Self as Other.

My mother's "otherness" was apparently reinforced by fiction popular at the time. I have unearthed one of her school notebooks. In it she wrote, "Medieval history was fascinating to me primarily because of my extensive reading of historic novels." Her favorites were, not surprisingly, Walter Scott's *Ivanhoe* and George Eliot's *Daniel Deronda*. Both novels feature Jewish women who, keenly aware of their "otherness," struggled to transcend the social barriers that circumscribe their worlds.

My mother's first attempt to reinvent herself failed. She applied to Radcliffe. In her mad dash through high school (she'd graduated at 14) she hadn't taken the Latin courses that (the rejection letter informed her) were required for admission. She settled for the University of Pennsylvania, the only Ivy League school that had the admission door slightly ajar for Latinless Jewish girls from Texas. She left after a year, unhappy with the school's rigid social stratification, a sort of apartheid system designed to separate Christians and Jews. Back home, she finished her bachelor's degree at the University of Texas. She moved to New York, where she was introduced to a distant cousin from another of Austin's mercantile families. After a short engagement, Irving Hirshfeld and Marjory Belish were married.

Shortly after my sister and brother were born, in 1925 and 1926, my mother got a job as a reporter for the *New York Evening Post*, a Hearst tabloid. Yellowed clippings in an old trunk showed her byline morphing from M. Belish to Margery Rex to Margaret Bolton. In an article titled "A Sob Sister Speaks Out" she wrote,

> To get my story I lie, I cheat, I commit a prize assortment of crimes against fairness, honor, human decency...I eavesdrop, I violate trusts. Posing as a social worker, a payer of insurance claims, a government employee, I swindle naive mothers out of damning information about scapegoat sons or love-scorched daughters.... Call me faithless, dishonest, indecent. I have only one principle, one faith, one god: Get That Story.

By 1938, her credo had changed to Rewrite That Story. M. Bellish was ready to contstruct (*em*bellish) her own chronicle, a fabrication that would in time evolve into a de facto truth. The original family names, the religion, the old neighborhoods, and any relatives who wouldn't keep the secret would disappear.

FARTOOTST: FROM THE GERMAN *VERDUTZT*—THE STATE OF BEING BEWILDERED, DISORIENTED, DISCOMBOBULATED

When I look back on childhood and adolescence, I see a number of unconnected dots which, had I been more canny, I might have connected: my mother's perturbation when a local boy, unhappy with his pay for chores, called my family "a bunch of Jews"; my brother's disgust when I came back from boarding school prattling about "Jew canoes" (the preferred term among my peers for Cadillacs); his dismay when the Social-Register-parents of a school pal dropped by to pick her up and asked if we were related to "Judge Hall" from Darien.

I remember the hushed conversations between my mother and her sister, the abrupt shift in tone when I'd enter a room, the odd smells of dishes prepared and consumed late at night, after my bedtime. I recall, as well, the comment my mother made, repeated so often it became a refrain, that prejudice against "Negroes" would cease only after scientists found a way to change skin color.

Finally, there is the matter of my given name, Marjory. Christian mothers rarely name their daughters after themselves. But for Ashkenazi Jews, such a matronymic practice would be unthinkable, disrespectful to those dead relatives who, according to custom, provide a perfectly fine reservoir of names for the new generation. In hindsight, the cover-up is flawed—its violation of tradition so dramatic that its very overzealousness almost renders it transparent.

In spite of an abundance of such clues, I was unable to solve the mystery on my own. Or, at least, not correctly. Home from college one Thanksgiving, I glimpsed a word that looked like *abogado* on some family papers. Connecting this with my mother's olive skin and Texas background, my suspicion, previously inchoate, acquired weight and form. "My grandfather was Mexican, wasn't he?" I shrieked, triumphant. She smiled her you-found-me-out smile. For years I thought I was part Latina.

When my sister finally leaked the secret on my 30th birthday, I had a sickish sweet feeling. All those fuzzy, unconnected dots swam into focus. Assembled at last, they formed a constellation of ugly stereotypes, of shame, of *Aha, M. Belish, gotcha at last.* Then, after a wistful *hasta la vista* to my Mexican heritage, a strange realignment began. My best friends in high school and college had been Jews. My lover at the time was Jewish. Even as a presumptive Christian (albeit part Mexican), I had somehow always felt ever so slightly superior to "them." Being intimate with them, I had imagined myself racking up points on some cosmic scoreboard of broad-mindedness. The sudden evaporation of my Christian cachet exposed my particular brand of liberal elitism. When I came home with the news that night, my lover, Freda, gazed at me serenely and paused. After a moment, she said "I always thought you had a *Yiddische kop.*"

At first, my Jewish identity was an abstraction, more proclaimed and insisted on than felt or understood. Gradually, over the years, I have pulled it on like a sort of under-the-skin garment, one sleeve, one leg at a time. Part of this pulling, tugging, and patting in place has been an examination of the ways in which my family's secret Jewishness has informed my work as a psychotherapist. After brief reflection, I've concluded that the stigmatized, underground identity operating in my family created the ideal therapy internship.

GESHMAT, FROM THE HEBREW FOR ANNIHILATION

Geshmat is Yiddish for a Jew masquerading as a Christian. There's an old joke about Mssrs. Ginsberg and Grabow, both *geshmat*. When they open their business they decide, for practical reasons, to call it O'Neill and O'Neill. On their first day, a customer asks to see Mr. O'Neill.

"Which Mr. O'Neill do you want?" says the secretary. "Ginsberg or Grabow?"

I grew up in a theater of not quite convincing make-believe. Hints and half-truths, cover-ups and switchbacks, elisions and secret codes, are much more familiar, and oddly enough, more trustworthy, than certitude, straightforward assertions, and monolithic facts. As a result, the practice of therapy, with its ambiguities and contradictions, conflation of fantasy and reality, admixture of surface and depth, is where I feel most at home.

If I grew up in a sort of theater, the therapy office is the (un)dressing room, the zone where the mask can be acknowledged, even fiddled with. In this liminal space, I am allowed—even expected—to indulge in my favorite childhood activities: eavesdropping, peeking, and prodding. Instead of being scolded for listening at vents or slyly picking up the phone extension to monitor a conversation-in-progress, I am finally licensed to spy. Behind the scenes at last, faint murmurs are audible and spurious posturing, intelligible. For me the pleasures of such legitimate prying border on bliss.

The familial charade determined my career in another way. Growing up under the sway of a master storyteller, I too have become a skilled revisionist or, in contemporary lingo, an ardent social constructivist and narrative therapist. And I seem to have absorbed my mother's history-rewriting chutzpah. Instead of narrating myself into the dominant culture, however, I have become a zealous inventor/fabulist of subversive tales for my particular tribe: queer dykes.

I recast heterocentric fables, conventional wisdom about "normal" relationships, and pseudo-science about "healthy" sexuality. Clients and I replace these master narratives with idiosyncratic stories of rapture and rupture, of chosen families and select solitudes, of gender-flex and silly sex. We then find ways to certify and celebrate these unique truths—our truths. Because, during this process, clients are actually excavating and rehabilitating the disowned parts of their own stories, and their feelings of shame, guilt, and anxiety usually dissolve. Working with them on these reclamation projects helps me counteract the shame, distortions, and losses attendant on my own family secret.

L'CHAIM, MAZEL TOV, SHOLEM ALEICHEM. TO BE CONTINUED

The family reinventions have never stopped. Here are the latest iterations:

Before she died, my mother got her PhD in clinical psychology. Her dissertation, "Masculinity of Boys as Related to Family Variables," marked her transition from family propagandist to psycho-historian. Her research on the correlation between high socioeconomic status and "gender deviance" proved that queer children—the majority of *her* children—were as much a class act as china *tchotchkes*.

My brother Richard, who detested the Christian charade, wrote a tell-all before dying from AIDS. *Family Fictions* (Viking, 1991), his best novel, sold modestly, and is now out of print. An occasional copy can occasionally be spotted, peeking out of remaindered piles in used bookstores.

To Elizabeth's chagrin, her oldest son divorced his Baptist wife and married a fabulous Jewish woman. She thinks she has married into a Christian family.

I, too, have continued the family tradition of revision. In honor of my 60th birthday, my friends gave me a *bris* and a *bar* [sic] *mitzvah* at a local park. First the designated-*moile*-for-a-day sliced the foreskin off my chocolate penis cake. Then, my friends donned wigs, prayer shawls, and name tags. Impersonating my long-dead relatives, they encircled me and declared me a man. Seth, Bernie, Lili, and Carl started humming "Hava Nagillah." Picking up the tempo, they began to dance dervishlike around me, improvising wildly improbable lyrics. Part pidgin Hebrew, part Lesbianese, their *mama-loshen bouillabaisse* was utterly tasty to my ears—however unsettling to mainstream picnickers at adjacent tables who stared, slackjawed, in disbelief.

Journey to the Start of Day: Ancestry, Ethnicity, and My Work as a Clinical Psychologist

SHANEE STEPAKOFF

An old rabbi once asked his pupils how they could tell when the night had ended and the day had begun. "Could it be," asked one of the students, "when you see an animal in the distance and can tell whether it's a sheep or a dog?" "No," answered the rabbi. Another asked, "Is it when you can look at a tree in the distance and can tell whether it's a fig tree or a peach tree?" "No," answered the rabbi. "Then when is it?" the pupils demanded. The rabbi said, "You can tell when the night has ended and the day has begun when you can see that the person across from you is your sister or brother."

—Martin Buber, *Tales of the Hasidim*

An image from June 2004:

I am 41 years old. I am seated at a restaurant called Savannah, one of only two restaurants in Kissidougou, a tiny town—more like a village, really—in the forest region of Guinea, West Africa, over nine hours by road from the capital. I am working as a psychologist for the Center for Victims of Torture, an organization that provides trauma counseling and mental health training for Liberian war survivors who are in refugee camps in this region. To the best of my knowledge, I am the only Jew in Guinea. Thus, when I suddenly hear two men speaking Hebrew at the table next to me, I approach them, startled, and we start to converse. They tell me that they are from Israel and were hired to direct a road construction project in Conakry and had decided to take a drive through the country. Then they turn to me, and ask, "And what's a nice Jewish girl like *you* doing in Kissidougou?"

This article represents my effort to answer that question.

WHERE I COME FROM: LEGACIES OF RESILIENCE AND LOSS

My identity as a Jewish woman working in the psychology profession has
been shaped by the experiences and values of generations that preceded me.

My Father's Mother, Gittel

My paternal grandmother, Gittel, was born in a small village near Kiev, in
what was then called "Russia" and is known now as Ukraine. When she
was 4 years old (and her older sister 6 and her younger brother 2), in
response to the persecution of Jews in Czarist Russia, her father, Samuel, emigrated to Hartford, Connecticut, where he worked as a fruit and vegetable
peddler, sending money to his wife and three children whenever he could.
Then World War I began, and for eight years the family lost contact. Money
that Samuel sent from America was never received. Sarah, my grandmother's
mother, brought Gittel and her two siblings to live in a Bolshevik children's
home where she found work as a cook. Thus, for most of her childhood
(ages 4–12), my grandmother's father was absent, and she was raised and
supported by only her mother.

After World War I ended, Samuel placed newspaper advertisements
searching for his family, but the newspapers did not reach the remote area
where my grandmother and her mother and siblings were located. A family
friend who lived in a more central location, however, saw one of the ads, and
this friend undertook the long journey to deliver the message to Sarah. Sarah
had no money, but this friend gave her money so that she could flee.

Late one night Sarah and her three children ran through the woods,
across the border into Poland. If they had been caught, they would have
been imprisoned and possibly killed. At the border, they had to give the
Polish officials all their possessions in order to gain permission to cross. Sarah
and her three children remained in Poland for a year, with a Polish Jewish
family in Rovno, while they awaited permission to enter the United States.

After Sarah received the necessary documents, she and her three children traveled to Warsaw, where a carriage driver drove off with their only
remaining possessions. They went to Danzig, Germany, and boarded a ship,
traveling third class, bound for Ellis Island, New York. They arrived in
January of 1923. My grandmother was 12 years old.

From there, they reunited with Samuel in Hartford. Gittel did not speak
a word of English: her native language, and the language of her parents and
community, was Yiddish. Nevertheless, within a few years, she learned to
speak, read, and write English fluently. She completed the 8th grade in
Hartford and was certified to go on to high school, but there was not enough
money in the family, so instead of continuing her education she went to
work in a nightgown factory in Hartford, trimming threads off of newly sewn
nightgowns. A few years later, she completed a bookkeepers training

program at a business school in Hartford and spent a few years working as a bookkeeper. After meeting my grandfather, she began working as a food server and cashier in the cafeteria of the school her two sons were attending. She continued in that job for over 25 years.

When she was 33 years old, her father was loading his truck with fruit-and-vegetable crates to take to the market. He had almost finished loading when he realized he needed one more crate. As he crossed the road, a driver sped by and hit him, then zoomed away. He died en route to the hospital. The driver was never caught.

My Father's Father, Sam

My father's father, Samuel, had a 9th grade education. He worked selling candy in theaters and at baseball games, later as a truck driver for a department store, after that a shoe salesman, and still later as a fruit peddler (like his father-in-law). Both of his parents, as well as several generations of their ancestors, came from Slutsk, a town in the midst of the vast steppes of the Byelorussia region of Russia. Sometime in the eighteenth century, my grandfather's ancestors had migrated into Slutsk from a small, rural village called Stepkovo, located several miles away. During the eighteenth century, when the czar ordered that all Jews adopt surnames (prior to that time, most Jews were known only by their first names followed by the phrase "son of" or "daughter of"), the name of my ancestral village was shaped into a surname.

Samuel's mother, Chaya Leah ("Chaya" is Hebrew for "life") Herman, was orphaned in childhood. Chaya Leah married my grandfather's father, Yasef, when they were both quite young. Yasef, too, had lost his mother in his early childhood and had left his childhood home at the age of 13. His father died when he was about 15. In Russia, Chaya Leah gave birth to one son and one daughter, both of whom died as infants, due to illness.

As a result of the massive wave of pogroms that swept Byelorussia during that era, Yasef emigrated to the United States in the 1890s. Two years later, he sent for Chaya Leah and their surviving daughter, Rose. In America, Chaya Leah was given a new first name: Ida. Yasef became known as Joseph or, to most people, "Joe."

Joe initially worked as a kosher butcher—the same profession that his forefathers had practiced in Slutsk. Later he worked as a deliveryman and house painter. In Hartford, Ida gave birth to six more children. Two daughters died in Hartford at young ages (Rose at age 12 from pneumonia, Alice at age 21 from heart disease).

Of the five children who survived beyond childhood, two, including my grandfather, had to leave school after 8th grade to help support the family. My great-grandmother reportedly had symptoms of depression during her final years of life. I doubt that she ever had the opportunity to fully express her grief over the loss of four of her children or to talk much about the psychological challenges she faced in adjusting to a new country, where she had few relatives and did not know the language or culture. In that era, most people believed they should weather their losses and go on; there was little recognition that losses that are not talked about or adequately mourned weigh heavily on the soul. She died in her middle-age years, of natural causes, when my grandfather was 18 years old.

My Mother's Mother, Eva

Jacob Lesnick, the father of my maternal grandmother, was born in Poland. In the 1880s, when he was about 10 years old, Jacob and his parents emigrated to the United States, settling in Mattapan, a Jewish neighborhood of Boston, Massachusetts. Jacob's wife, Sarah, was also an immigrant from Poland, having come to the Boston area with her mother, Esther, as a child. Sarah gave birth to three children, of which my grandmother, Eva Lillian, was the eldest. "Eva" is an English version of the Hebrew word for "life."

Jacob had a small grocery store in Boston. When he was about 50 years old, Jacob was diagnosed with syphilis. In those days, there were no antibiotics, and he developed general paresis, which was then a common complication of syphilis. The general paresis manifested as severe and progressive dementia. The fact that his dementia was caused by general paresis was a strictly held secret. Thus, most of Jacob's relatives had the erroneous belief that he had simply and inexplicably lost his sanity. After several years of mental deterioration, Jacob spent the last 25 years of his life in a state hospital in Foxboro, Massachusetts.

At the time that her father was hospitalized, my grandmother, Eva, was 21, her sister was 17, and her brother was 13. Thus, for most of her childhood and adolescence, my maternal grandmother's father was cognitively incapacitated, and throughout her adulthood he was institutionalized. My great-grandmother, Sarah, supported my grandmother and her two siblings by running the family grocery store.

All three of Jacob's and Sarah's children completed high school, though none went to college. Eva reportedly did well in high school and was accepted to Radcliffe University, but opted to get married instead. Widowed with two young daughters at the age of 33, Eva became a successful travel agent and international tour guide. She was also the first woman in her entire neighborhood who learned to drive. Part of my curiosity about and awareness of distant lands and unfamiliar cultures derives from the dolls, trinkets, and photos she brought me from the tours she led in Italy, Hong Kong, Israel, Greece, and elsewhere.

Eva was diagnosed with breast cancer when she was in her mid-60s. During her final year of life she appeared on television, as part of a panel titled "Facing Imminent Death." This was more than two decades before the era of confessional talk shows, when most Americans were still quite private about health issues and personal hardships. On the program, which was aired on a public television station, my grandmother spoke candidly about her thoughts and feelings about having a terminal illness. She acknowledged her fears and concerns and openly voiced her awareness of the fact that she was in her final year of life.

My Mother's Father, Harry

The parents of my maternal grandfather, Samuel and Sarah Steinberg, were born in Kourland, Latvia (then part of Russia), in a region near the town of Kovno. Kourland had at one point in history been part of Germany, and for that reason it was considered a more prestigious place of origin than were other parts of Latvia and Russia. Samuel and Sarah got married at a young age and soon after had a daughter, Bessie. Samuel left Russia when Bessie was four years old, intending to go to America. However, for reasons that remain unclear but are probably related to difficulties being admitted to America, Samuel instead went to South Africa. In South Africa, Samuel was recruited to fight for the British in the Anglo–Boer War of 1899–1902.

During these years in South Africa, Samuel had no contact with his wife and daughter, who had remained behind in Russia. After the Anglo–Boer war had ended, he emigrated to the United States, settling in Boston, and sent for his wife and daughter. Bessie died of a childhood illness (probably flu) at the age of 10, a few years after arriving in the United States.

Sarah went on to give birth to eight more children. One of these eight children was my mother's father, Harry. Of these eight children, five died of heart attacks or other medical conditions before they had reached their early 40s.

Samuel and Sarah ran a grocery store in Roxbury, a neighborhood of Boston. Harry became a salesman for a tobacco company. He died of a heart attack in his early 30s, leaving behind a wife and two young daughters: my maternal aunt, age seven, and my mother, who was then three years old.

My Immediate Family of Origin

I was born in Mattapan, then a predominantly Jewish neighborhood within the City of Boston. My father, Jerry, was completing his PhD in physical chemistry at Boston University. My mother was working as a quality tester at Baker's chocolate factory to help pay for my father's education. My parents met when they were both 18 and got married shortly after turning 20. My mother's formal education ended shortly after she graduated from high school.

For my first 11 years of life, we belonged to a Conservative synagogue. Though we did not keep kosher dietary laws or strictly observe the Sabbath, we observed most of the Jewish holidays and, I often attended synagogue services on Saturdays. My brother and I both attended Hebrew school two weekday afternoons plus every Sunday morning, where we learned to read and write Hebrew and learned Biblical stories and Jewish history, values, and customs.

When I was about two years old, my family moved to a suburb, Newton, which had a substantial Jewish population; our immediate neighborhood was 100% Jewish. I attended a public elementary school in which well over 75% of the children were Jewish and a public junior high and high school which also had sizable Jewish populations. All of my parents' friends, and nearly all of my friends, were Jewish and White until after I graduated from high school.

When I was nine, my mother began working as a real estate agent, partly as a way to keep herself busy and partly to supplement our family income. Soon she was earning twice as much as my father, and this discrepancy in income, given the gender-role expectations that predominated in those days, was very painful for my father. My father's Cold War job designing atomic missiles became less and less interesting and meaningful to him. He became deeply interested in music, acting (in community theater), and writing (novels, stories, plays).

Whereas my mother thrived in our White, upper-middle-class suburban milieu, my father felt isolated and unfulfilled. My parents began to realize that they actually had very little in common and they began to drift apart. Unhappy at his job as well as in his marriage, and disconnected from the poor and working-class multicultural neighborhood and large, close-knit, extended family in which he was raised, at 38 my father experienced an existential and spiritual crisis that turned into a deepening depression.

During a week when my parents had decided to try living apart for a while, my father drove home from searching for an apartment, allowed the automatic, electric garage door to close behind him, and stayed in the car too long. Though he did open the car door and try to exit the garage, it was too late—the carbon monoxide had already entered his bloodstream. There was no note, and the authorities were unable to determine with certainty whether his death was a suicide or an accident. I had just turned 12 years old. As most people in our neighborhood and at my school considered his death to have been a suicide, I have "claimed" the identity of a childhood survivor of parental suicide.

My mother is not a psychologically minded person and did not possess the inner resources to support my brother or me in processing the shattering loss of my father. My mother, brother, and I went through the next several years as solitary beings, sharing a house though seldom interacting in any meaningful way. My father's death was not spoken about at all.

That experience of silence, and the awful burden of carrying within one's soul unformulated memories and unexpressed emotions, has had a profound impact on the choices I make in my practice of psychotherapy. In particular, with my firsthand awareness of the psychological harm caused by silences about traumatic events, I have consistently tried to support clients in finding the words to speak about their feelings and experiences. I have tried my best to offer them my empathy and emotional presence so that they will feel able to connect with their truths and tell their stories.

A few months after my father died, my school, concerned about the fact that I was not visibly showing signs of mourning, arranged for me to see a clinical psychologist. Nearly 35 years later, I remember that appointment as if it were yesterday. Until I was an adult in college, he was the only person who ever asked me how I felt about my father's death. I was never sent back for a second session, apparently because everyone had the impression that I was all right. Nobody realized the actual intensity of my frozen grief. But I never forgot that a profession existed that focused on helping children survive such catastrophes. I never forgot that there was a job that consisted of asking people what they are going through, and, when they share the reality of their suffering, striving to listen and care. I never forgot that a person who undertakes this type of work is called a psychologist.

* * *

It is possible to discern some recurring themes that inform my personal and professional identity. These include the absence of husbands and fathers; the need for women to work outside the home; truncated educational opportunities and unfulfilled intellectual potential; early, sudden, and multiple losses; the role of chance occurrences as well as of the kindness and moral choices of other people in determining life paths; experiences of social and cultural marginalization; the importance of community; the impact of economic limitations and historical and political events on individual opportunities; women's capacity to endure significant practical and psychological hardships; and the investing of the unrealized hopes and dreams of one generation into the next generation, with the concomitant sense that the descendants in some manner must hold and carry forward the hopes and dreams of the ancestors.

THE IMPACT OF MY JEWISH IDENTITY ON MY PROFESSIONAL CHOICES AND PRACTICES

Here I discuss some widely held Jewish values and core components of my Jewish identity, as these pertain to my choices and practices as a clinical psychologist. For each principle of Jewish identity mentioned, I explore some of the implications for my clinical work. In a playful variation on the theme of the Ten Commandments, this section is structured with reference to 10 commandments I have consistently sought to follow in my career. My aim is to shed light on the variety of ways that my practice of psychotherapy is informed by my ancestry and ethnicity.

1. Be Kind to the Stranger, for You Were Strangers

My ethnic identity is inextricably linked with my awareness of Jews as a historically persecuted, disenfranchised, and despised people living near or among hostile and more powerful neighbors. Thus it is no accident that in making choices with regard to my practice of clinical psychology, I have been drawn primarily to oppressed populations. My professional pursuits have been mainly at the interface of clinical and community psychology. All of my practicum/externship/internship experiences in graduate school were in low-income, urban neighborhoods and focused largely on people of color.

During my career I've been urged to leave the public sector and establish a private practice. I felt very ambivalent about doing so. At the time that I was first attempting to develop a practice, I held a position at a major teaching hospital of Harvard Medical School, providing psychotherapy to people who had lost loved ones in the September 11th attacks (mostly on the two airplanes that departed from Boston). That position allowed me to work in two areas of longstanding interest to me—traumatic grief, and political violence. Despite enjoying this work I felt that something was missing. Virtually all of the September 11th survivors with whom I worked were from a middle, upper-middle, or upper socioeconomic class backgrounds, as were my private practice referrals. I felt a deep calling to work with the poor and disenfranchised.

In April of 2004, I was offered a job as a psychologist for the Center for Victims of Torture, an organization that provided mental health training and trauma counseling services to Sierra Leonean and Liberian refugees. Based in Kissidougou, the job entailed working in community mental health centers that were located in refugee camps. I saw this as a chance to reconnect with my interest in community psychology with the quality of passionate engagement I had felt in the mid-1980s while completing a practicum at an ecumenical, anti-apartheid center near Johannesburg, South Africa. During that period of severe apartheid repression, I had became familiar with the experiences of survivors of torture and other human rights violations and impressed by their courage and strength.

Since that year in CVT-Guinea, I have become more keenly aware that to feel professionally fulfilled I need to devote significant time and energy to disempowered populations. By doing so, I am giving expression to values that originate in both my family history and larger ethnic identity. Although I am sometimes faced with social disapproval for "failing" to achieve greater financial success or rise in a more mainstream psychology setting (e.g., a medical center or university), I have the sense that my work is grounded in an important part of my heritage. Empathy for, and a commitment to empowerment of, the marginalized and oppressed comes to me not only through my constitution but through my profound feelings of personal connection with a legacy of ethnic, religious, and political persecution and mass violence.

2. Respect Religious and Ethnocultural Pluralism

As a small minority in the United States and worldwide, Jews are very familiar with the feelings of discomfort, invisibility and alienation that arise when persons in positions of authority mistakenly assume that everyone is of the same religious or ethnocultural background, or engage in any form of proselytizing. In my work with clients from a wide variety of backgrounds, and particularly in the support groups I have led, I have tried hard to ensure that there is space for diverse forms of religious and ethnocultural expression. In Africa, I have facilitated counseling groups in which singing, drumming, rituals, and Christian and Muslim prayers were combined with Western approaches to healing. In the Middle East, I have worked with Iraqi clients who have chosen to utilize Koranic verses and traditional Arab proverbs as part of their recovery from war trauma.

3. Recognize the Power of Words

In the Hebrew Bible, a belief in the power of language is ever-present. Indeed, God calls the world into being via speaking. Jewish culture, likewise, places a strong value on verbal expression. The healing power of words has been a key theme in my professional practice.

I firmly believe that whatever can be named and talked about can be borne, and, conversely, that whatever is unnamed and unspoken wreaks havoc on the psyche and will manifest in emotional and behavioral problems. Beginning in graduate school and continuing to the present, a major component of my work has been helping clients find words to express what has seemed inexpressible. This has been particularly meaningful for me in my work as a cotherapist in groups for persons bereaved by the suicide of a relative.

I also started and led a therapy group for girls who had been sexually abused. For the most part, these girls had been told by their relatives and others not to speak about the abuse. In the group, my coleader and I took the opposite view: we encouraged the girls to talk about what had occurred, to share their thoughts and feelings with one another, and to tell someone immediately if anyone ever tried to abuse them again. We also invited the girls to write letters to the social caseworker and the non-offending parent. As with so many clients, we found that in overcoming familial and societal pressures toward silence, these girls felt relieved and invigorated.

Many of the traumatic experiences that people underwent in the recent Liberian and Sierra Leonean civil wars were also considered, by the survivors and their families and communities, to be unspeakable. Nearly all of the teenage and adult women had been raped and a significant number bore children as a result of these rapes. Many of these women had been captured and kept as sexual slaves for rebel commanders for months and even years at a time. Others had witnessed their loved ones being tortured, mutilated, and killed.

Regardless of how horrific the events, an important component of my treatment approach was helping the client find the words to name and describe them. In the vast majority of cases, these clients had not talked about their experiences with anyone, not even their closest relatives and friends.

During my graduate training in psychology I concurrently completed a two-year training program to become a registered biblio/poetry therapist. I have utilized expressive writing, preexisting poems, storytelling, and book-making in many of my clinical interventions with both individuals and groups, in a wide variety of professional settings. This respect for the power of language is also a reason that much of my clinical work is informed by psychoanalytic theory, for psychoanalysis is grounded in the view that it is beneficial to put memories and emotions into words. Clearly, my belief in the psychological importance of speaking is further informed by my own experience, in my family of origin, of the silence that surrounded my father's death. Yet my passion for the redemptive power of language is also strongly influenced by my Jewish identity, and the privileged place of words in Jewish religion and culture.

4. Resist Tyranny and Pursue Justice

Jewish religion and culture are characterized by a belief in the importance of resisting tyranny and pursuing justice. These values enter into my work as a psychologist in numerous ways. In fact, a basic backdrop for all of my work is my abhorrence of abuses of power and my valuing of human rights and physical and psychological liberation.

Drawing on both my Jewish and feminist identities, I attempt to support girls and women in gaining respect, equal opportunities, greater self-worth, knowledge, and wider choices with regard to their life paths. I have worked with torture survivors from a wide variety of national, ethnic, class, and cultural backgrounds and have affirmed these survivors' efforts to seek safety, reparations, and redress. As the psychologist for the United Nations war crimes tribunal in Sierra Leone (Special Court) for nearly two and a half years, I provided psychological support to victims of war crimes as they gave public testimony about their victimization. My decision to seek the position at the Special Court was rooted in my view that in the aftermath of human rights violations, justice is a crucial component of psychological and social repair.

5. Do Not Bow to False Gods

The folktales, Biblical stories, and values I was exposed to in my family, in Hebrew school, and in the wider Jewish community instilled in me an abhorrence of idol worship in its many manifestations and a conviction that I will not bow—literally or metaphorically—to anyone but the invisible, noncorporeal God. This principle has found expression in several aspects of my practice.

One of the major false gods that I have refused to bow to in my work as a clinical psychologist is mainstream psychiatry, with its heavily medical model of psychological suffering and its rigid adherence to diagnostic categorizations that oversimplify human experience and that, in many instances, inappropriately pathologize responses to intolerable situations.

6. Claim the Capacity for Chutzpah

Chutzpah is a Yiddish word with nuances of meaning that render it difficult to translate into English. Some synonyms include audacity, cheekiness, daring, nerve, effrontery, pushiness, arrogance, gall, presumption, ballsiness, brazenness, impudence, and guts. It is traditionally used as an insult (as in "what chutzpah!"), namely, when a person disregards social expectations or behaves offensively.

In contemporary American society, however, chutzpah can also refer positively to behavior that is nonconformist and gutsy. In fact, chutzpah is a characteristic that is widely respected and admired by many North American Jews. It is also a characteristic that I proudly claim as part of my legacy, transmitted across at least the past four generations of women in my family.

In many settings where I have worked, the provision of psychotherapy without simultaneous efforts to advocate on behalf of the client's larger needs would be morally and professionally questionable. In many instances, a weekly 45 minute clinical session is simply not sufficient to address the ongoing reality-based external causes of the client's suffering. Furthermore, quite often it would be irresponsible to proceed with psychotherapy without also addressing unhealthy and dangerous conditions in the client's social environment.

Thus, I have often found it helpful to bring to bear the chutzpah of my ancestors so as to better serve my clients. In the United States, this sometimes took the form of having to battle managed care companies and Medicaid so that clients could obtain the mental health services to which they were legally entitled. In Guinea and Sierra Leone, this often took the form of helping clients access food, shelter, protection, and medical care through advocating with nongovernmental organizations or the UNHCR (United Nations High Commission for Refugees).

Occasionally I find that colleagues see me as "pushy," particularly people from White, Anglo-Saxon Protestant backgrounds, who tend to be more comfortable with women who embody discreetness, moderation, and restraint. When dealing with vulnerable populations I feel it is important to have the capacity to take a stand—and in particular, a stand that presupposes an ability to challenge abuses of power and defend human rights. My practice of psychotherapy, thus, is informed by a valuing of the capacity for boldness in thought and action.

In my efforts to achieve wholeness as a person and clinician, I have benefited from the lessons taught me by clients and colleagues from other ethnic backgrounds, in which quiet acceptance, dignity, and humility are important values. Similarly, I believe, and hope, that my clients and supervisees have felt enriched by lessons I have tried to teach them about the benefits of assertive advocacy. Chutzpah can undeniably be experienced by others (particularly by non-Jews) as off-putting but when applied thoughtfully and strategically can contribute to clients' quality of life in significant ways.

7. Encourage Critical Thinking

The word "Israel," as the name of a major patriarch of the Jewish people, and as a synonym for the people as a whole, originates in the Biblical narrative in which Yaakov (Jacob, son of Isaac, grandson of Abraham) falls asleep and, in a dream, wrestles with a divine angel and prevails. This dream experience was so significant for him that he decides to change his name from "Yaakov" to "Israel," a Hebrew term that is variously translated as "he who wrestled with God and survived," "one who struggles with God," or, more simply, "God-wrestler."

This notion is a core aspect of my Jewish identity and finds expression in personal as well as professional contexts. Of course, the concept or image of struggling with God can be interpreted in a number of ways. For me, it has usually taken the form of encouraging critical thinking among clients, colleagues, trainees, and within myself.

It was only after many years of working alongside colleagues from various non-Jewish backgrounds that I truly understood the extent to which the questioning of authority and development of critical thinking are not only *not* supported but are actually strongly discouraged and condemned in many ethnocultural groups. It took me many experiences of interethnic, cross-cultural misunderstandings and tensions to realize that many individuals (and organizations) place a higher premium on social conformity, interpersonal harmony, avoidance of argumentativeness, quietness, and respect for authority than on rigorous critical analysis, challenging the status quo, and outspoken argumentation.

An example of a professional setting in which this aspect of my Jewish identity was salient was a series of 10-session counseling groups I led for Liberian clients as part of the war-trauma treatment program in Guinea, West Africa. The groups were designed to address a number of core issues faced by Liberian refugees. Sooner or later, in virtually every group, questions would arise as to how to relate—both intrapsychically, as well as externally, given that many of the perpetrators continued to live in the community—to the people who had harmed them and their loved ones during the war. Often, many of the clients' initial remarks were fairly simplistic and superficial. Typical comments were, "Well, we should just forgive them—that's what the Bible says," or "My pastor said I should forgive him." These comments, coming from victims who had endured very extreme forms of deliberate brutality and violence, usually elicited in me a feeling of discomfort and even suspicion. Through clinical experience with survivors of severe human rights violations, I sensed that there was more beneath the surface and that these statements did not adequately reflect the full range of clients' authentic emotions.

In my capacity as therapist, I had to walk a narrow line between respecting the clients' stated values and exploring their deeper feelings. Walking this line usually led to productive discussions in which clients came to think more rigorously about issues of peace, justice, forgiveness, reconciliation, reparations, and restitution. Before engaging in these explorations, most clients viewed forgiveness as the only alternative to revenge—which the clients defined as doing to the perpetrator something very similar to what the perpetrator had done to them or their loved ones (e.g., violent assault). It was as though they felt pressured to choose between two extremes—total forgiveness or absolute revenge.

Through examining these questions in the group, clients began to entertain alternative views and to pave a middle path in which forgiveness was possible, but under specific conditions. Many came to appreciate the validity of anger and indignation as natural human responses to deliberate cruelty. Many also came to consider the presence or absence of genuine remorse and of a sincere acknowledgement and apology by the perpetrator as conditions for forgiveness. Clients also became more aware of the differences between revenge and restitution and of the possibility of seeking justice through the restoration of collective legal and judicial institutions rather than via violent, direct assault. There was, in a sense, a "Talmudic" quality to this process of utilizing dialogue to develop more elaborated, nuanced positions.

Jewish ethnocultural values cause me to challenge assumptions, and to support clients in moving beyond simplistic or superficial answers toward psychological and social stances characterized by greater complexity, authenticity, and depth. This is not to imply that a belief in the importance of forgiveness is lacking in depth. On the contrary, the capacity to forgive those who have wronged one or one's family can constitute a profound spiritual attitude. In working extensively with victims, however, it became possible to differentiate between clients who had achieved that level of spiritual insight and those who professed the importance of forgiveness merely because an authority figure had told them that that was the "right" belief.

Another area in which I have sought to challenge widely accepted views and encourage critical thinking has been the Jewish tradition of circumsizing eight-day-old male infants. I consider myself to have a strong Jewish identity, I am known by a Hebrew nickname, I am fluent in Hebrew, I belong to a synagogue, and I observe many Jewish holidays and customs. Nevertheless, my opposition to circumcision, a practice that many Jews mistakenly view as a defining characteristic of Jewishness, means that a large majority of Jews would consider me not to be truly Jewish and, if made aware of my views, would not include or welcome me. It is ironic that a stance that I developed as a result of the quintessentially Jewish capacity for questioning and critical thinking would lead to ostracism by a large portion of the mainstream Jewish community.

8. Cherish Community

I am only two generations removed from my grandmother's shtetl in the forest steppes of Russia, and my sensibility has been shaped by the attitudes of ethnic bonding and respect for community ties that characterized that milieu. These social norms have been discussed at length in the books *Life is With People: A Cultural History of the Shtetl* and *World of Our Fathers*. Despite the fact that my feminism, political views, criticism of Israeli governmental policies, and opposition to circumcision sometimes cause me to feel separate from other Jews, the reality is that Jewishness always has been and remains a very salient part of my identity and my being in the world. Often I am troubled by and critical of many aspects of the mainstream American Jewish community. Nevertheless, I value opportunities to work with Jewish clients, and I believe that a shared ethnocultural heritage can strengthen the therapeutic relationship.

The norms for nonverbal communication that are common in the mainstream North American Jewish community are different from those found among many non-Jews. The former include gesturing with one's hands while talking, a fairly rapid rate of speech, a fairly loud volume, using a questioning tone even when uttering statements that are not questions, and a quality of emotional expressiveness that manifests facially, vocally, and gesturally. In my personal and professional experience, I have found that these nonverbal behaviors tend to be explicitly or covertly disdained among White Anglo-Saxon Protestants (as well as some other white non-Jewish ethnic groups). As a result of the intuitive perception of this disapproval, many Jewish clients may feel more comfortable with a Jewish (versus non-Jewish) therapist. If a non-Jewish therapist is working with a Jewish client, the possibility of a strong therapeutic relationship and a successful treatment will be enhanced if the therapist is at least familiar and comfortable with Jewish cultural and ethnic norms.

9. Engage in Honest Self-Examination

Jewish religion and culture place a high value on honest self-examination. The holiest day of the Jewish calendar (Yom Kippur) is a day during which every Jew is expected to search his or her soul so as to courageously acknowledge to himself or herself and God those times in the past year during which he or she has "missed the mark." The weeks leading up to this holiday are known as the Days of Awe, during which Jews are required to devote considerable time and energy to soul-searching and repentance. In those instances in which one has wronged another human being, it is not permitted to ask forgiveness of God until one has first apologized to the wronged person and asked for his or her forgiveness.

The value that Jews place on self-examination can also be found in secular settings. Jewish writers, poets, and singer-songwriters have tended to be quite comfortable with confessional modes of expression. Jewish painters and filmmakers have also drawn on their internal experiences in order to make art. The Jewish background of Sigmund Freud undoubtedly had some bearing on his development of a curative approach that relies on looking inward and describing one's deepest thoughts, feelings, and memories. It is also not a coincidence that in several countries (e.g., the U.S., Argentina, South Africa), Jews tend to be more comfortable with the premises and practices of psychodynamic psychotherapy than are many other ethnocultural groups. In my clinical work, this value is expressed in the soul-searching I engage in regarding my responses to clients, and in my efforts to process my thoughts and feelings about the work via discussions with colleagues, supervision, writing, and in my own psychotherapy.

10. See That the Person Across From You is Your Sister or Brother

In the Book of Genesis—the first book in the Hebrew Bible—the idea is set forth that every human being is created in the image of God. Although I don't think of this concept in purely religious terms, I do try my best to see the humanity, worth, and spiritual core of every client. This effort is, to a large extent, grounded in my Jewish identity.

According to a well-known anecdote, a student approached a Jewish sage and, in a rather provocative attitude, asked the sage to teach him the whole of Judaism while he (the student) was standing on one foot. As the student held one foot in the air precariously, the sage replied, "Do unto others as you would have them do unto you, and that which is hateful to you, do not do unto others. All the rest is commentary: go and learn it."

This "golden rule" is a crucial component of my practice of psychotherapy. Even when the client is from a very different background from mine, it is possible to find a way to behave toward him or her in a manner similar to that which you would wish for yourself or your loved one(s) if you or someone in your family were in need of psychological care. This requires empathic attunement and a genuine willingness to imagine how the situation is experienced by the client from within his or her own frame of reference.

Sometimes, in order to generate a richer quality of connection with a client, I will visualize a kind of thread extending between that person and me, linking us together in our common humanity. Other times, through becoming aware of the depth and pace of my breathing and consequently relaxing the area of my chest cavity, I am able to experience a physical sensation that corresponds to the notion of "opening the heart." I have found that regardless of behavior or circumstances, if I truly concentrate, it is possible to feel a genuine sense of respect and compassion for virtually any member of the human species.

I have had the opportunity to test this belief in a wide variety of settings. These include a clinic for torture survivors located in an Arab country in the Middle East, a community mental health center in a refugee camp in Guinea, a long-term inpatient unit at a state hospital in Washington, DC, a public school for low-income children in New York, and a stretch of land, in Sierra Leone, that is inhabited by individuals who lost an arm or a leg in that country's long civil war. In several situations I was able to engage in successful advocacy and networking that resulted in refugee individuals or families being accepted for resettlement in the United States.

Though sometimes these efforts resulted from my moral principles, more often I looked into the eyes of the man, woman, or child in need and truly had the feeling that I was seeing one of my own relatives, even if the skin color and features and accent and dress were unlike those of anyone in my family. Perhaps, as suggested by the rabbi in the Hasidic tale recounted by Buber, I was seeing the face of a brother or sister, but more likely, the face that I saw was that of my grandmother, Gittel, who came on a ship, across the Atlantic ocean, to Ellis Island, when she was 12 years old.

* * *

An image from October 2005:

My uncle Joel calls from Atlanta to tell me that my grandmother, Gittel, 95, is in her final week of life. I have to make a decision about whether to fly home immediately or delay my return home by one day so that I can fulfill my professional commitments as the psychologist for the United Nations war crimes tribunal in Sierra Leone, where my job is to be present in the courtroom to support vulnerable witnesses while they testify. Today is the final day of the AFRC prosecution, and this is the final witness. He is a man whose wife was raped and killed in his presence and whose arm was deliberately amputated.

As I sit in the courtroom listening to his testimony, my mind keeps wandering back to my grandmother, Gittel. The Hebrew Home in Hartford Connecticut seems so far away, such a different world from this courtroom in West Africa. The vast Atlantic Ocean stretches between us. My awareness keeps alternating between the two locations, trying to hold the two realities simultaneously in mind: this man showing the judges the stump where his arm was amputated by renegade soldiers, and my grandmother on her deathbed at the nursing home in Connecticut.

Then, gradually, the guilt I have been feeling about delaying my return begins to fade. I have a deep sense that I am exactly where I am supposed to be, doing precisely what I am supposed to be doing. I start to feel that here in this courtroom, as I strive to support this bearing of witness, I am honoring my grandmother's life. I am being true to her legacy.

I flew from Freetown to Boston the next day and drove to Hartford as fast as I could. My grandmother died four days later, in my presence. Born and raised in a small village near Kiev, she was my most direct link to the land of my foremothers and forefathers, my closest connection to the Yiddish-speaking, Eastern European shtetl communities in which those forms of Jewish ethnic identity that most strongly influence my psychotherapy practice, my international humanitarian activities, and my overall life journey were forged.

May her soul rest in peace. May her spirit continue to inform my work. And may her memory be for a blessing.

Growing up Jewish: The Shaping of One Activist

PAULA J. CAPLAN

FREUD'S MOTHER AND MY GRAM

In a few minutes in 1996, all in a rush, I wrote a monologue for the character of Amalia Freud, Sigmund's mother, for my play *Call Me Crazy*. While raising my children, I had foregone the temptation to continue the acting I had loved as a child and teenager, and after obtaining my PhD in 1973 had worked as a clinical psychologist and activist and spent years teaching psychology to undergraduates and graduate students. After both of my children had left home, I returned to theater as an actor (while continuing to work as a psychologist and activist) and then decided to try my hand at playwriting. *Call Me Crazy* was my first play, and from the moment I imagined writing Amalia's monologue I saw her as my mother's mother, Esther Milner Karchmer. Esther was a dear heart of a woman, tiny, sparkly, mischievous, smart as a whip, and utterly unassuming. The more I read about Amalia Freud, the more I learned about her life, the more I imagined my Gram in her place. When I learned that Amalia died at the age of 95, it struck me that she had lived to see her son become famous, and then I tried to imagine how she might have felt about his fame and his theories, many of which were misogynist or otherwise perhaps simply embarrassing to a woman of her era. The monologue thus reflects not only the facts of Amalia's life but also much of Gram's manner as well as her attitudes and values. Amalia, after listening with growing impatience to some of the horrible nonsense spoken by some of today's worst psychotherapists can stay silent no longer and breaks into the play:

(*AMALIA FREUD enters, dancing, to "The Blue Danube," then speaks to the audience*)
AMALIA: Thank you for coming. I'm Amalia Freud. Amalia Nathanson Freud. I lived to be 95 years old. I wanted people to know my son was the great psychoanalyst, winner of the Goethe Prize for literature, but behind

their polite smiles I saw the thought, "This is the mother whose son discovered that all little boys want to have sex with their mothers". Discovered. Ha!

And about girls and their mothers what did he "discover"? That our daughters resent us for not having had the courtesy to provide them a penis. I had five daughters. How do you think his words made me feel? I love my Sigmund, but this is too much.

He told people he felt all of his life like a conqueror because he was my "indisputable favorite." Ha! So he thought. The truth is I adored all of my children. How could I not? Sigmund was my firstborn. I loved my daughters, also but kept needing to have more—five in all—until Jacob got one more son. Most of the time Sigmund was growing up his father and all of the other children and I shared three bedrooms, but he had his own. He needed to study. He complained that his sister Anna's piano lessons were noisy when he was trying to study. We got rid of the piano. Anna and I were sad but not angry. We understood. Maybe he had too much. And he decided who was normal.

You know, he threw up his hands and said, "What do women want?" What's not to understand? Is it healthy to take a mother's love or a wife's love and make it seem so complicated?

Normal, shmormal. Oh, I realize some people have to be put away—they can hurt themselves, or someone else, but it's a tough problem. You start putting people away, and somebody's going to decide who gets put away, somebody's going to choose the rules. Is what these guys decide any better than what my son decided? Thinking about it makes my head hurt.

But I'll tell you what I have noticed. Who decides is who has the power. And somehow, they seem to decide the people most like them are the normal ones, the good, the healthy, the deserving. It's the others who are derided, called dangerous, sent away. Of my five daughters, one went to New York, three were gassed in Auschwitz, and the last one starved to death in the camp at Theresienstadt.

Thank you for listening.

(*AMALIA turns and walks off, as "The Blue Danube" plays*)

Amalia's monologue is imbued with the ways that growing up in a Jewish family shaped my attitudes toward life and thus toward what I have done as an activist and psychologist. I shall discuss each of these values and foci, which are: the importance of facing reality, of working for social justice, of giving love and support, of learning and teaching and of acknowledging the limitations of my knowledge, and of joy. It's not to say that what I learned because of being raised as a Jew and in my specific family is not also learned by people not raised as Jews and not in my family, of course. But for me, it is impossible to separate a great deal of what I learned growing up from being Jewish and from being raised by my parents and in close relationships with other members of my family.

THE IMPORTANCE OF FACING REALITY AND OF WORKING FOR SOCIAL JUSTICE

Only after the importance of facing reality had become a fundamental organizing principle of my being did I hear a rabbi speak about facing reality being an important part of Judaism. However, facing reality was woven into my upbringing in myriad ways, because in my home and in my extended family, conversations and storytelling were essential parts of our lives, and they dealt with everything from our family and friends to local, national, and global politics and the arts. The local political aspect was intensified when my mother's father, Nathan Karchmer (Esther's husband), ran for mayor of our hometown of Springfield, Missouri, and was unexpectedly (to him) elected, and by the largest majority any mayoral candidate had ever received there; he was the only Jewish mayor Springfield has ever had. For me, as a psychologist and a critic of much of what happens in the mental health establishment, facing reality has included my need to hack through jargon and theory that distort and pathologize the experiences and feelings of the people who come to therapists for help. And the value of defending and empowering the oppressed, which I learned through my Jewish family and the larger Jewish community, gives added force to that. I see how immersed I was in these values while growing up when I look back at the early support that Nathan Karchmer gave to the Anti-Defamation League; my parents' palpable hatred of racism and the ways they acted on those principles; the service of both my mother, Theda Ann (Tac) Karchmer Caplan, and my uncle, William H. Karchmer, on the Springfield, Missouri, Human Rights Commission; the frequency with which my father, Jerome Arnold Caplan, urged always to "do the right thing" and had posted on his office wall, for as long as I can remember, the motto, "Be kind, because everyone you meet is fighting a hard battle," a motto by which he has always lived; and the dislike my paternal grandfather, William Caplan, had for regimentation and his support of socialist candidate for president, Norman Thomas. Furthermore, my mother, even before the 1954 *Brown v. Board of Education* decision that separate educational facilities are not equal, took it on herself to hire an attorney to plead the case of a young, Black woman who wanted to attend the state teachers' college in Springfield. The attorney went before the college's board of regents, who rejected the request on the grounds that she could travel to Lincoln University, which was for Black people but was very far away. Within the past couple of years, my mother said she had just realized that when the regents refused the request, she felt she should have told the attorney to take the case into the courts and doesn't know why she didn't. I pointed out to her that it was quite unusual for a White woman in a small Missouri city in the early 1950s to do what she had done, and before the *Brown* decision, who would have thought to take such a case into the courts?

In combination, the importance of facing reality and of working for social justice have profoundly affected my work. I have always chafed at the use of jargon—even feminist jargon—because it strikes me both as clouding the view of reality and as elitist, because it shuts out of the loop those who are not familiar with it, making it harder for them to understand what is being recommended or done to them by therapists, teachers, or anyone else. This same combination of concerns has set me free when I have been trying to help someone who was suffering and who came to me as a professional and, someone in authority used either jargon or an unthinking, unquestioning psychodynamic interpretation in harmful ways. For instance, at the Toronto Family Court Clinic where I worked and where some therapists were excellent, I had a psychiatrist supervising me as I worked with an aboriginal woman whose child (who had a severe disability) had been unfairly taken from her by the Children's Aid Society. I told my supervisor that part of what I was doing with her was to try to keep up her confidence in her fine, caring mothering ability while helping her navigate the court and child welfare system that was keeping her child from her. He gave the totally baseless reply that what I should instead be doing was to help her acknowledge what had to be the negative side of her "obvious" ambivalence about having a child with a disability, so she could willingly give her up. After realizing that he was making me feel inadequate as a psychologist for not having followed his preferred approach, it struck me how appalling was his recommendation, and of course I refused to follow it.

IMPORTANCE OF IMMENSE LOVE AND SUPPORT

Esther Milner Karchmer and my other grandmother, Gertrude Gorbach Caplan, who expressed through their different personalities the importance they placed on the giving of love and support to and the defending and protecting of their immediate families, also oriented me toward doing this in larger communities as well as within the family. So did the loving care of my parents, my uncle Bill Karchmer, and my grandfathers in their more reserved ways of showing care and respect for others. For me as a therapist and an often-critical writer about psychology and psychiatry, this has kept foremost in my mind the importance of offering human warmth and respect to those who seek our help, as well as of remembering that they are people, not diagnostic categories and not hangers on which to place thin pictures of patients-as-pathologies.

The combination of valuing social justice and love have also led, for me, to a need to struggle against elitism. So, for instance, the value in feminist therapy of trying to reduce the power differential between client and therapist found a welcome home in me. This was especially the case, because so many (though not all) of the people who seek therapy are those who do so because they believe erroneously that something is wrong with them when in fact what is wrong is that they live in one or more oppressive systems or are exposed to violent or demeaning treatment and have feelings or conflicts that understandably result from oppression and violence. As a therapist, then, when I think that people who seek my help are mistaken in pathologizing themselves, I tell them this, and I describe a variety of things that I have known to be helpful to people who are in similar situations and who are having similar feelings. I am wary about agreeing to do psycho-therapy in these instances, because I have found that, no matter how hard I try to reduce the therapist–client power imbalance, it is never as effective as I would wish, and no matter how hard I try to convey my view that their problems do not originate as individual, intrapsychic ones, the clients almost invariably have tremendous difficulty getting away from self-blame and self-pathologizing.

LEARNING AND TEACHING AS SACRED TRUSTS

There was a sheer, palpable joy that my family took in learning new things, meeting new people, seeing new places. Family trips were wonderful, because my parents loved to explore new places, learning and enjoying all the way. And when my parents met people for the first time, no one could draw them out and hear their life stories like my parents could. In a play I wrote called *Shades*, in which one character is modeled heavily on my father, someone says of him that when he is in the checkout line at Wal-Mart, he knows everyone's life stories by the time he reaches the front of the line. My maternal uncle, William H. Karchmer, left the business world to attend law school in his mid 30s, and this was during the early 1960s, when that was considered bizarrely old to do such a thing. As an attorney, he became known for not telling clients what to do but rather laying out the options and the pros and cons of each so that they could make informed choices. My mother, who had stayed at home while raising my brother, Bruce M. Caplan, and me, started a graduate program in counseling the same semester that I began graduate school. As a therapist, she was terrifically effective, and she did it largely on instinct and reasoning, often using unconventional tactics. This only confirmed my view that the vast majority of graduate train-ing in most programs is of little use to people who become therapists, that far more important are the therapists' personalities, capacities for empathy, and abilities to listen and think carefully and see what works rather than follow-ing doctrine. My mother, uncle, and maternal grandfather all taught as volun-teers in the small religious school our synagogue in Springfield had. My paternal grandmother worked at a cosmetics counter in Sage-Allen's depart-ment store in Hartford, Connecticut, for years, at a time when women who did not absolutely have to work usually avoided doing so. She loved advising people about effective products and relished the chances to meet more people all of the time. My maternal grandmother had worked as a driver for the Red Cross during World War II, but, sadly for her, then followed the stay-at-home track, a waste of her sharp mind and clever wit. Late in life, however, she began playing the stock market from her home and loved learning about which stocks were likely to be good investments.

So the first time I heard someone say that teaching and learning are sacred trusts, it powerfully hit home for me. When people have come to me asking for psychotherapy, what I have often found myself doing in large measure is teaching, including but not limited to the unscientific nature of psychiatric diagnosis; the overemphasis of the mental health system on attributing emotional pain to individual, intrapsychic, and even allegedly biochemical or other brain-based phenomena without regard for social and other external causes; the dangers as well as the often temporary benefits of psychotropic medications; and the poor quality of much research that is bruited about and that may have given them wrong impressions about what is happening to them and what will help them. I have spent a lot of time demystifying therapy for clients and practitioners, acknowledging the limitations of therapists' ability to help, teaching clients psychological theories and their limitations, and seeing therapy as jointly learning with the client about the client and myself.

ACKNOWLEDGING THE LIMITS OF MY KNOWLEDGE AND MY IMPERFECTIONS

One of the ways that the principle that learning is a sacred trust was lived out by the members of my family was their readiness and comfort in acknowledging what they didn't know and with their limitations in general. This did a great deal to make me feel comfortable as a professor, an expert witness, a public speaker, and a therapist, for in each of those roles I have been struck by how many of my colleagues expend enormous energy and feel tremendous fear that is essentially based on their assumption that they ought to know all the answers. In fact, in every one of those roles, I have found that my credibility was actually enhanced when I acknowledged what I did not know. For instance, a couple brought their young child to see me after taking him to many other therapists as they sought an answer about why he did not speak even though he was preschool age, and had no identifiable, physical reasons for not speaking and seemed to have no other significant problems. When, after a prolonged, intensive assessment, I had to tell them that I did not consider him to have autism or developmental disabilities or elective mutism, that I had no idea what was causing him not to speak, and that all I could recommend was that they monitor what he was able to do and encourage that while also monitoring whether he became able to speak, I feared that they would be terribly disappointed and upset.

It seemed to me that all I had to offer them was common sense but no explanations, no solutions I could promise, not even a hint of a prognosis. But they said they were immensely grateful because they had already read everything they could find about speech problems and had been unable to find a description that matched their son, so in an important way, they already knew that no one really had *the* answer for them; as a result, when other professionals had focused on diagnoses and recommendations that they already knew made no sense, this was not helpful to them. Living in such a psychiatrically and technologically oriented age, they had been uncomfortable trusting their own perceptions and judgement about their son, and it turned out that my acknowledgement of the limitations of my knowledge enabled them to feel more confident about acting on their own judgement. In the absence of known solutions for their child's inability to speak, that increase in their confidence allayed a considerable amount of their fear and anxiety about not being able to be good parents, and one thing on which mental health professionals can agree is that reduction of the fear and anxiety that people bring to their interactions with their children is good.

Another arena in which my family's message that to be flawed and to fail is part of being human has given me great strength and resilience has come into play in my teaching and public speaking. I had been kicked out of my doctoral program in clinical psychology in 1970, and some years afterward, when I had partially recovered from the devastation and the crazy-making nature of that experience, I decided to speak about it briefly, to illustrate some point or other in an invited lecture I was giving at a university I was visiting. I was amazed when several women came up afterward for the specific purpose of saying that that mention had instantly caused a huge shift in their perspective on their experiences as graduate students. They had been having difficult times in their programs but had faulted themselves. Hearing that someone who had gone on to get an advanced degree and write some books after having an experience somewhat like theirs suggested to them that perhaps the fault was not in them but in the systemic sexism and, for some, the systemic racism, ageism, or homophobia within academia. Those kinds of responses resonated with what my family had taught me about the importance of connection and of helping the oppressed. So when, to my amazement, I was asked to write something for a book (also published as a special issue of *Women and Therapy*) called *Feminist Foremothers*, I chose being kicked out of my clinical program as the core of my article (Caplan, 1995).

Writing what have sometimes been called self-help works (Caplan 1989, 1995, 1997, 2000), I have tried to make sure that readers do not assume that there are "ten easy steps to" whatever, that they understand that, if they try to apply the theory I set out or the practical suggestions I make and do not find that they work, they should not assume that there is something wrong with them.

IMPORTANCE OF JOY

In my family, we learned about joy and the importance of relishing every moment possible. Many members of my family loved and love theater, music, and art. There is too little joy in the world, whether in my clients or loved ones, and I think that work with suffering people should include not only the reduction of suffering but also the increase of joy.

GROWING UP JEWISH IN SPRINGFIELD, MISSOURI

I spent the years kindergarten through 12th grade in Greenwood Laboratory School, growing up as a member of one of 40 Jewish families in a city of about 80,000 people at the time. Springfield was the home of at least four fundamentalist Bible colleges and the international headquarters of the Assemblies of God's Gospel Publishing House, so when my brother and I went to the town square to go shopping, we were constantly accosted by practice preachers, students from the Bible colleges who had to spend hours trying to bring people to Jesus. My brother and I always suspected that they got more points if they could convert the Jews, but it didn't work with us. I loved my school, including the fact that there were only 30 kids in each grade, and my graduating class included 15 of us who had been together since kindergarten. I thought I knew the other Greenwood students so well, felt as though many were almost siblings to me, but until my senior year, I never realized that they—every one of whom was some sort of Protestant or Catholic—had any feelings at all about my being Jewish. In fact, until one summer in Connecticut at a beach with other Jewish kids, I never realized that my last name signaled that I was Jewish any more than did my classmates' last names like Rich, Mitchell, or McCurry signaled that they were not. The first sign that other Greenwood students thought anything of my being Jewish came one day when I was a junior, in an honor roll study hall I shared with most of the boys in my grade and the one above. (The other girls on the honor roll were putting together the school yearbook at the time.) We were studying for a physics test, and I saw one of my closest male friends whisper something to another boy; they looked at me and laughed. I said, "Come on, guys, what are you saying about me?" They looked extremely uncomfortable, and only when I continued to press them did my friend say, "We were saying we'd pray to the minister, and we'd have Paula pray to the rabbi, and we'd see who gets the best grade on the physics test." I thought that was really silly—and uninformed, because of course we don't pray to rabbis—but not objectionable, so I laughed and thought that was the end of it. Apparently, word shot around that I had laughed about and was okay with something someone said that was related to my being Jewish. The floodgates opened, and out came many remarks that had apparently been bottled up for years or spoken only in my absence. For example, a close female friend started calling me "Joan [my middle name] Jew" and said she had always thought that even though I was Jewish, I was the best Christian she knew, because I was such a nice person. It wasn't even that anything horribly anti-Semitic came out, but I was stunned and troubled to think that my assumption that we all knew each other so well and could talk to each other about anything had been so wrong. For heaven's sake, the boys used to ask me pretty intimate things for our ages and era, like, "Do girls like it when boys kiss their ears?" But my being Jewish had created an until-then invisible (to me) barrier between them and me. As you can imagine, this added to my feeling of being an outsider, something I had already felt to some extent because of being a girl who got good grades and because of being so uncool as to take it seriously when other kids were mocked for whatever reason (both characteristics, of course, being informed by Jewish traditions). That sense of being an outsider in many contexts has never left me, and although I suspect that hardly anyone ever truly and deeply feels like an insider (it's amazing how many people, including me, will tell you they were always the last kid picked for sports teams in school), being Jewish has for better and for worse contributed to that feeling. It has certainly made me want to help others learn that they may feel more like an outsider than others think they are and that sometimes, as in relation to oppressive systems, being outside is the best place to be.

REFERENCES

Caplan, P. J. (1989, January–February). More than Mother's Day: What real honor means. *Reconstructionist, 4*, 25–27, 34.

Caplan, P. J. (1995). "Weak ego boundaries": One developing feminist's story. In P. Chesler, E. D. Rothblum, & E. Cole (Eds.), *Feminist foremothers in women's studies, psychology, and mental health*, (pp. 113–123). Binghamton, NY: The Haworth Press.

Caplan, P. J. (1997). Mothers, Judaism, and true honor. In R. J. Siegel, & E. Cole (Eds.), *Celebrating the lives of Jewish women: Patterns in a feminist sampler*, (pp. 39–44). Binghamton, NY: The Haworth Press.

Caplan, P. J. (2000). Seeking serenity as a single Jewish mother. In R. J. Siegel, E. Cole, & S. Steinberg-Oren (Eds.), *Jewish mothers tell their stories: Acts of love and courage*, (pp. 237–242). Binghamton, NY: The Haworth Press.

My Names

RACHEL JOSEFOWITZ SIEGEL

The story of my names can tell you who I am and how I grew into the feminist *alte Yiddene* (old Jewish woman) of today. It is a story of Jewish migrations, of a close family clan scattered over four continents, of a family's richly varied approaches to being Jewish, and of the Jewish choices I have made during 85 years of defining and redefining my Jewish identity.

My children call me Mom. My first grandson named me Grandma Shell, and now they all do. My sister and her grandchildren call me Rochale or *Doda* Rachel, with the harsh, guttural "ch." Rochale is my Yiddish name. In Hebrew, Rachel is pronounced with the long ah, guttural ch and accent on the last syllable. *Doda* means aunt. My two brothers, two sisters, and other adults in my extended family call me Rachel, as said in French, accent on the first syllable, and "ch" pronounced as "sh." At home in Ithaca, New York, and among my professional colleagues, I am known as Roshelle, but because I continue to spell my name Rachel, I am often called Rachel, as in English, "Ra" like "Ray." Are you confused enough yet? When I attended first grade in Berlin, my teacher called me Rahel, the German name with a soft h. A year later, in 1930, due to my father's awareness that anti-Semitism was becoming more overt and virulent in Germany, our family moved to Lausanne, in the French speaking part of Switzerland.

I was six years old when confronted with the need to quickly learn French. Here I embraced the French pronunciation of Rachel, which is still my favorite and most comfortable appellation. I came to love the softness of the language, the beauty of the city, the lake, and the French Alps. I felt free to identify with the democratic values expressed in Swiss schools. I sensed the absence of the kind of anti-Semitism that I had not even been aware of in Germany, and we all felt a bit less on guard in this haven of neutrality.

Like a chameleon, responding to any given linguistic environment, I continue to answer to each of these pronunciations, but for a long time I wondered which was my one, true name.

A MINYAN OF WOMEN

Dateline Tel Aviv, December 28, 2003, the Great Synagogue, Noam's Bar Mitzvah. Noam is my sister Fenni's Israeli born oldest grandson. As I sat in the cold upstairs women's gallery, looking down and listening to the Torah service in the main sanctuary, I was deeply touched by the multigenerational, multilingual drama. Noam's father Dori had celebrated his bar mitzvah at this bimah, his grandfather had prayed here every week. The grandfather, long dead, had been one of the founders of the congregation who built this simple yet elegant stone structure on Dizengoff Street in the 1920s, when Tel Aviv was but a small town. The Orthodox congregation, now reduced to some 30 elderly regulars, had not celebrated a bar mitzvah in years and was eager and excited to welcome even a nonobservant, secular family for this coming-of-age ritual. Our own extended family, assembled here in Israel for the happy occasion, had wandered the world, had experienced and moved away from many of the old Jewish Ashkenazi traditions, and had participated in the enormous changes brought about by the Holocaust, the birth of Israel as a nation, and the impact of humanism and feminism on Jewish observance.

For me, it was one of those moments of clarity that cannot easily be put into words. Just as my names reflect the multiple strands of my Jewish identity, so did this Shabbat morning in Tel Aviv feel like a coming together of important aspects of myself.

I was born in Berlin in 1924, the fourth child and second daughter in a family of Lithuanian Jews who had fled that country because of famine and anti-Semitism. My mother was still grieving her own mother's untimely death. The night before she was to have aborted me, she dreamt that I would be a girl who would carry her departed mother's name. She called off the abortion and named me Rochel Gitel. Grandmother Rochel Gitel's large sepia photograph hung in my parent's bedroom in an oval frame, next to and matching the one of grandfather Rav Eliahu Dov Shur. Her beautiful face conveyed to me a sense of inner peace and goodness that engraved itself into my Jewish consciousness. Did I not owe my life to her? Was I not destined to become the carrier of Jewish tradition and values in my family?

My parents spoke German among Germans and Yiddish or Russian to each other and at times to us. My father's loud quarrels with his brothers were always in Russian. Our nanny spoke German, which I considered my first language. Within the family, we called one another by our Yiddish diminutives: sister Rose was Raisale, brother David was Dodik or Dodale, brother Samuel answered to Shmulik or Mulik. When sister Fenni was born, we called her Feigale. Strangely enough, we called our parents Pappa and Mutti, the German names for Dad and Mom. Only in later years when they became sick or elderly would we call them Pappale and Mammale. We were not a religiously observant family. My mother kept a kosher kitchen as long as her father was alive, should he ever come for a visit. We went to services on the High Holidays, father in his top hat and all of us in new garments, and we always celebrated a festive family seder. Jewishness pervaded our home in tense and worried conversations about the fate of other Jews, in social interactions with Jews, and in acts of rescue and caring for Jews less fortunate than ourselves. We felt a heightened sense of alertness or even preparedness for potential anti-Semitism, verging at times on paranoia. We learned and tried to conform to the social norms of our host country as best we knew how. Unlike other Western European Jews of that period, however, our family took pride in identifying ourselves as Jews. Furthermore, my parents claimed a distinguished Jewish ancestry, based on generations of rabbis on my mother's side and successful merchants on the side of my father. They relished telling us that both sets of parents had disapproved of their marriage because Pappa was not *frum* enough for Rabbi Shur's blessing and Mutti was not rich enough to please Grandfather Josefowitz.

I was told that I had a *yiddishe neshoma*, a Jewish soul; I wondered what that meant but was happy to claim it. In school I was nearly always the only Jew in my class. I had non-Jewish friends, joined the Girl Scouts, but our family never interacted with their families. I yearned to be and to be considered Swiss as well as Jewish, but I knew that we were aliens, not even immigrants, whose residence permits could be revoked at any time. Tales of German atrocities drifted into our temporary haven, and Jewish refugees frequently sought shelter in our home. As the feeling of impending war escalated, my family began to plan our own exodus to America. We arrived in New York in March of 1939.

Fast-forward. One of the things that attracted me to the American born Jewish man that I married at age 19 was that with him, I would somehow "belong," both as a Jew and as an American. No more wandering, no more feeling like an alien, an immigrant. With him I could live my version of the American dream, become a Jewish American wife and mother, a member of the Jewish community, conveying Jewish values and American norms to our future children. I joined him in his strong Zionism and active Jewish observance. Yet even then, in the first years of our life together, I bristled at his imposition of certain restrictions on my customary Saturday activities. He was openly disapproving of my going downtown with friends to shop and to a movie on the Sabbath. He refused invitations on Friday evenings, insisted on having our own Friday night observance at home. We muddled through these early signs of disagreement, not letting them interfere with the strength of our love and desire for one another.

Together we created a conservatively observant Jewish home for our children. I kept a kosher kitchen, I studied Hebrew, and we joined the Conservative Temple in Ithaca, New York, as soon as we arrived in what was to be our permanent home. I became active in the local Hadassah chapter. Our closest friends were more observant than we had been, as well as Jewishly far more educated and knowledgeable. I tried hard to catch up and fit in, and I also joined and took on leadership roles in the non-Jewish world of community organizations like the PTA, Cornell Campus Club, and Engineering Women's Club.

My life as a Jewish mother, faculty wife, and community volunteer was rich in rewards, personal connections, Jewish traditions, and intellectual stimulation. So why the migraines, the bouts of depression? Looking back, I know now that no one, including myself, had ever acknowledged the trauma of my early uprootings, of not knowing which of my names was my real name. Nor had I been aware that I lived in a gilded cage, well fed, well loved, but caged just the same. I wore gloves that made me feel warm and connected, but they were tight and did not always let my hands be free or fully expressive. Shades of Carol Gilligan (1982) and Jean Baker Miller (1976), I needed to connect, to belong, to be accepted, but I had lost—or rather never developed—the connection to my own identity. In the 1950s and 1960s, my male psychotherapist was Freudian and male-centered; I did learn to take myself more seriously, but we did not address the "disease that had no name" (Betty Friedan, 1963), which held for me a core Jewish component.

When did I change? When did I realize that our marriage could tolerate open disagreement instead of subversive resistance and that I could develop my own ideas, my own preferences? It was after Ben's first heart attack and after the children left home. It was in the early 1970s while I was back in graduate school. It was when my now adult daughter shocked me into feminist awareness. It was definitely when the women's movement became part of my consciousness. It was when I began my professional career, started to write, and found my own voice.

I began to read the works of women, to attend conferences, to meet and talk with other emerging feminists. Within this early feminist sisterhood, I found the courage to look inward, to recognize the overlapping nature of all oppressions, and to act on overcoming my own prejudices. I realized a strong need to understand my own experience of otherness. It was an exciting, tumultuous time. Being Jewish and female was at the center of my feminist awakening. My first published article was titled "The Jew As a Woman" (1975).

My husband Ben was a man of letters, he believed in the written word. At first, he was unable to hear me when I ranted and raved about my discontent with Jewish discrimination against women. It was only when my words were written and published that he began to understand what I had been saying. He became my ally, presenting the case for women's inclusion in the Torah service to our temple board at a time when there were no women on that board.

While becoming a therapist, working with women who were far less privileged and more oppressed than I, I gradually acquired the feminist lens that I could now focus on the condition of Jewish women. I was inspired and encouraged by my colleagues at the Jewish caucuses of AWP, the Association for Women in Psychology, and NWSA, the National Women's Studies Association. At the annual FTI, the Feminist Therapy Institute conferences, I became more openly vocal as a Jew, a feminist, and a writer, questioning male centeredness and male authorities not only on matters of psychotherapy but also more specifically on Jewish issues. I advocated for the inclusion of women in all aspects of Jewish ritual at home and in the synagogue.

I found my own voice, in my 50s, in the process of writing. It is a Jewish voice. It is the voice of a feminist therapist, an aging mother/grandmother/ great-grandmother, a widow, now a retiree, and always a Jewish woman. In collaboration with my good friend Ellen Cole (Siegel & Cole, 1991, 2000) and my niece Susan Steinberg Oren (2000), I coedited three collections of Jewish women's essays. The work of selecting and editing these personal articles was a wondrous experience. I felt, at times, that I was at the heart of a widely scattered Jewish women's community, and I relished the fullness and flavor of our connections to one another, the intimacy of sharing the Jewish aspects of our lives.

At home, and at my insistence, Ben began taking over some of the Passover preparations that I had found so burdensome. We feminized our reading of the Passover Haggadah, turned the four sons into four children, and inserted the midwives into the story. I fought for changes in prayer language and synagogue observance in my own congregation. These innovations have now became routine and are taken for granted in many Jewish homes and nearly all Conservative synagogues.

The first time that I was called to the Torah to recite the blessings preceding the Torah reading, I felt as if I was breaking an ancient taboo. Would the heavens open up to swallow me and my congregation? Or worse yet, would I commit the sin of misreading the holy words or the Hebrew chant and embarrass myself as well? I stood there, hiding my emotion, proud and tall, and trembling inside with a mixture of fear and excitement.

A strange thing happened to me after some years of Jewish advocacy. Having fought so hard to have women included in previously male enclaves of Jewish life, I began to have doubts about perpetuating those very same Jewish customs and traditions. I found so much that was contrary to my own humanitarian and feminist values. Now that we got in, is that where we wanted to be? Unlike many of my sister Jewish feminists who took every opportunity to quench their thirst for Jewish learning by studying Torah, I have resisted such immersion, knowing that my anger would get in the way of genuine learning. I have only occasionally approached the ancient text and liturgy with an eye for new questions and new answers in order to present and discuss these within my temple community. While my Jewish activism has been directed at the synagogue, and I feel a strong sense of community with my congregation, my Jewish identity or activities have not been primarily focused on regular synagogue services. Now that women are full participants, I enjoy the familiar chants, the pomp and circumstance of the Torah service, but I find no personal meaning in the actual prayer language. On the High Holidays I find spiritual meaning and a sense of profound connection with *klal Israel* (the Jewish people) in celebrating the Jewish New Year in the bosom of my congregation.

Family seders have had an evolution all their own, depending on the ages of children, grandchildren, and now great-grandchildren. After my husband's death I began to lead the seder myself and to co-lead it with my grown sons and daughter (Siegel, 1997). Having established my right and my ability to do so, I am now content to sit back and enjoy the seders led by my adult children, Charles, Hyam, and Ruth. On Friday nights, I often share the meal with my friends Barbara and Nicky, both Jews by choice, whose wholehearted, enthusiastic singing fills my heart with *shabbos* spirit.

My Jewish allegiances, interests, and activities reach far and wide, beyond my family, my congregation, and my feminist sisterhood, and into the language and culture of my parents, the horrors of the Holocaust, and the complexities of Jewish life in Israel.

My connection to Israel, my love of the land, the history, and the people, became intense during the year we spent in Jerusalem, in 1961. So much has changed since then. Israel is no longer the idealistic land of early settlers and of kibbutzim, the refuge of Holocaust survivors. My unease with Israeli politics and government policies began during the war with Lebanon and has grown ever since. I weep at every suicide bombing and I weep at every Israeli retaliation. I fear for the safety of my sister and her children and grandchildren. I despair at the generations of young people on both sides learning hatred and cruelty. And I feel frustrated by my own powerlessness.

After some 50 years of avoiding films and literature about the Holocaust, my work with Holocaust survivors and their children has led me to an immersion in Holocaust literature. In a deliberate process of desensitization, I have read many women's memoirs of that period and have learned to tolerate more of the agony. In 1997, during a trip to Eastern Europe, I stood at the mass grave in the Warsaw Jewish cemetery, unable to cry. I returned from Theresienstadt unable to speak of what I had seen and felt. On Rosh Hashanah of that year, I said kaddish for the six million Jews, the gypsies, the gays, and the others who had been so savagely murdered.

My Jewish life has become more secular as I get older. Now in late life, I feel a strong pull to reconnect with my Jewish roots and to convey some of my cultural and linguistic Jewish inheritance to my middle-aged children and grandchildren. I have traveled to Switzerland and Berlin with my granddaughters, revisiting the streets where I grew up. I have gathered a genealogy of my extended family, bridging seven generations, from my great-grandparents to great-grandchildren. My *mishpochah* is scattered in Europe, Israel, North America, Australia, and South Africa. When I joined a Yiddish-speaking group, I discovered that I have retained much more of the overheard language than I was aware of, and I relish every opportunity to use it. I belong to a Jewish reading group where we read Jewish books as well as books by and about Palestinian and other Arab women. The brief vignettes and memories that I write in my weekly writing circle convey the Jewish flavor of my long life.

I now live alone, have been widowed some 20 years, and continue to make subtle changes in my expressions of Jewish identity. I feel less bound by the earlier influences of family, spouse, and social environment. It is not easy for me to name the components of my Jewish identity other than to say that it keeps changing and growing. I continue to find more sources of pleasure, more puzzles, more arguments in my engagement with being a Jewish woman. My names embody the paths and detours of my Jewish wanderings, the connections and disconnections with Jewish and non-Jewish cultures, the complex relationships with Jewish and non-Jewish friends, colleagues, and family members. Each of my names carries colorful associations and memories. I no longer worry about who I am, which of my names is my true name; they all are.

I've come a long way in my Jewish journey, and it is not over. I have found, within feminism and feminist therapy, the tools and training to fully appreciate my Jewish history and identity. I relish the kaleidoscope of Jewish memories and images. My heritage of acute Jewish pain has been tempered by the cultural, humorous, and spiritual richness of that same heritage. I have been conscious of being Jewish all of my life, have never ignored it or taken it for granted. I have made deliberate choices and actively questioned my Jewish decisions, yet much of my Jewish experiences, activities, and attitudes come from a place of habit, familiarity, nostalgia, and even sentimentality, which defy conscious analysis.

REFERENCES

Friedan, B. (1963). *The feminine mystique.* New York: W. W. Norton.
Gillian, C. (1982). *A different voice: Psychological theory and women's development.* Cambridge: Harvard University Press.
Miller, J. B. (1976). *Toward a new psychology of women.* Boston: Beacon Press.
Siegel, R. J. (1977). The Jew as a woman. *Jewish Spectator, 42*(4), 40–42.
Siegel, R. J. (1997). Who will lead the seder, now that I stand alone? In S. Berrin (Ed.), *A heart of wisdom: Making the Jewish journey from midlife through the elder years* (pp. 215–219). Woodstock, VT: Jewish Lights.
Siegel, R. J., & Cole, E. (Eds.). (1991). *Jewish women in therapy: Seen but not heard.* Binghamton, NY: The Haworth Press.

Siegel, R. J., & Cole, E. (Eds.). (1997). *Celebrating the lives of Jewish Women: Patterns in a feminist sampler.* Binghamton, NY: The Haworth Press.

Siegel, R. J., Cole, E., & Steinberg Oren, S. (Eds.). (2000). *Jewish mothers tell their stories: Acts of love and courage.* Binghamton, NY: The Haworth Press.

GLOSSARY

alte yiddene: Old Jewish woman (Yiddish).

bar mitzvah: Coming of age ritual (Hebrew).

bimah: Pulpit-like platform for Torah readings (Hebrew).

frum: Religiously observant (Yiddish).

doda: Aunt (Hebrew).

haggadah: Story of Egyptian exodus read during Passover seder (Hebrew).

kaddish: Mourner's prayer (Hebrew).

Klal Israel: World community of Jewish people (Hebrew).

mishpochah: Extended family (Yiddish).

Rosh Hashanah: Jewish New Year (Hebrew).

seder: Ritual Passover meal (Hebrew).

Shabbos: Jewish Sabbath (Yiddish).

Torah: Five books of Moses on parchment scrolls (Hebrew).

yiddishe neshoma: Jewish soul (Yiddish).

On Being and Not Being Jewish: From Pink Diapers to Social Activist/Feminist

IRIS GOLDSTEIN FODOR

"I have found that my own womanhood is a very important factor in my work as a therapist.... I do know how it is, I have been there and I am still there"

—Miriam Polster (1972, pp. 261–262)

I was a pink diaper baby, born in the Bronx in the depression to two young parents. My parents, Helen and Jack, were part of a generation that labeled itself as "progressive," a term used then for anyone with left/socialist ideology. My parents, and most of their friends, were not active in any left organizations, and they made it clear to distinguish themselves from "communists" who belonged to secret cells. During my childhood, which was also marked by World War II, I never received any formal religious training or cultural history about being Jewish. The few times I went into a synagogue it was to look for my grandmother, an old lady immigrant from Poland who spoke only Yiddish, to fetch her for dinner on the Jewish holidays. The shul was in a tenement building, cramped, full of women sitting in a back room, muttering in Yiddish, a language I could not understand. When my brother turned 12, my parents decided he needed a bar mitzvah. Saul, the father of my aunt's husband, an old White bearded man wearing a skull cap, came into the house to prepare him. I was excluded from this instruction. The bar mitzvah was more of a big party than a religious ceremony for the relatives and my parents' friends. I was 14 and wore a red formal dress. No one in my neighborhood ever considered a ceremony or party for the girls when they turned 13.

However, we did have a family secret, which I am somewhat reluctant to reveal in this piece. It always lurked in the family background. While my father's parents were working class and I was raised in a working class, immigrant Bronx neighborhood, my mother's parents were educated and upper middle class, which was a big deal in the Bronx in those days. My mother's older sister went to college and got a trip to Europe as a graduation present. When my mother was 19 her parents who were Russian moved back to Russia to work for the great socialist experiment, the Soviet Union. My mother refused to go and my father, age 21, gallantly agreed to marry her so she wouldn't have to go. At the age of 19 my mother watched her parents sail off to Russia, with two of her siblings as well. She never saw her parents again.

Hence, while I grew up in a typical working class Jewish family, the family religion as espoused by my mother's idealistic memories of her wonderful social activist parents was Marxism. Such phrases as "we are working class" and "never make money out of someone else's labor" were family creeds. The greed of the rich and capitalists and the need for a reorganization of society that spoke of people working together to share the profits of their own labor formed my own schema of values. During the war, Roosevelt was our much beloved hero, and given that Russia was our ally and my grandparents were in Russia, to a lesser extent Stalin.

The newspapers that came to the house were the *Daily Worker* and *PM* (a new York liberal daily). The books on our shelf were from the Book Find Club, a progressive book of the month club that featured the writings of Howard Fast and left writers. I had no idea at that time how off center my own readings were. I did most of my book reports at Roosevelt High School in the Bronx on books by Howard Fast. I learned about Judaism from his history of the Jewish people published in 1941. Books with titles like *Igor's Summer* (a Russian children's book), *Stalin Must Have Peace, Citizen Tom Payne*, and the Lanny Budd series of Upton Sinclair were my primers. (The latter fanned my fantasy of leading an adventurous life.)

Despite the left ideology, my own nuclear family was very traditional. My father worked long hours as a radio repair man in a store owned by a wealthier family while my mother stayed home. Given the Depression and the war that followed, we lived in the same apartment house, about 99% Jewish for my entire childhood, and my family pattern of the man as a hard worker and breadwinner and the wife as "housewife" was the norm in our apartment house.

The women in our building worked hard at housekeeping, shopping, cooking, and at cleaning. They wore flowered cotton housedresses, hair in curlers during the day until it was time for their hardworking husbands to come home for dinner. Then they dressed, put on makeup and lipstick and nice dresses. My father too often went back to work after dinner and always worked on Saturdays. My mother considered my father an exploited worker. He did not make much money, and all of the profits went to the boss, who "was rich." My father was always promised a piece of the business, which never happened. When my father and the boss's son finally began their own television business in the late 1950s, the "boss" continued to extract from them a percentage of each old customer they continued to service. Even though a couple owned the store, the "boss" was Ruth, a large, strong woman, dominant over her three grown children and husband who worked in the store and my father. She was my first role model of a "working woman," and it was not positive.

My father was young, good-looking, smart, clearly in charge of our family. He could fix anything, even as he got older. He could carry air-conditioners and refrigerators on his back up the stairs in walk-ups, and he loved baseball. On his one free day, Sunday during my childhood, he played for the Ritz Rangers, a sandlot ball team, and the Yankee game during the season was always on the radio. He was also a good dancer who loved parties. He was smarter than most and was often critical and intolerant of incompetence. He was very hard on me and held me and my brother up to high standards.

My young mother was very beautiful, tall, and dark. My parents were a striking couple. My mother loved to shop and found lovely clothes at bargain prices or wholesale, which they wore when they went out or to parties or "affairs" (weddings, bar mitzvahs). As my mother got older, it became apparent that she became more and more dependent on my father. She was often ill. So, my parents were in traditional roles, she shopped, cooked, managed the money amazingly well, and looked attractive. They were never in debt and always saved. He worked long hours, fixed and lifted heavy stuff, and drove. My father was the disciplinarian, "Wait 'til your father comes home" was the phrase used when we were in trouble. My father could become quite angry, and when he seethed I was careful not to "aggravate" him or bring up unpleasant topics at the dinner table.

My father's biggest regret was that he was not drafted during WWII. My mother would not let him enlist. Most of his friends went off to war, and we all followed the war closely. During dinner we listened to the news, and my father read everything about the war. As he grew older he amassed a collection of books on WWII. He died six years ago at 92 and I inherited the family book collection. When news of the Holocaust emerged during the war and afterward we had many sad and thoughtful conversations about the plight of the Jews in Europe. Throughout my father's life he continued to be very interested in and able to discuss world events. He became more of a mainstream Democrat as he got older. The day after his 92nd birthday we watched the beginning of the Gulf War on television together. My father lived in Florida and was enraged at what happened there in the 2000 presidential elections. He used the butterfly ballot correctly and could not understand how the "idiot voters" made mistakes. As he got older, after my mother died, in Florida, my father became more connected to Jewish customs. He very much enjoyed the Friday night services and singing.

When I was two years old my brother was born. My mother continued a love affair with him, my brother, until the end of her life. He could do no wrong, yet he became the classic "bad boy." I had to be the good girl. He was dark and I was a fair blonde with curly hair. We shared a room, and I hated him. He was hyperactive, always into my things, and he never got punished. He was expected to become an engineer, like my mother's father, when he grew up, and my father taught him to fix things. He never had to help wash/wipe the dishes, wash laundry, or go to the grocery story for errands. Since my mother was sick a lot, I had a lot of these chores to do.

My Jewish identity was shaped by growing up in the border street between the Jewish and Italian neighborhoods. While I was not socialized as Jewish in my own family, it was wartime, the Nazis were persecuting the Jews and Italy was run by Mussolini. I went to public school with the Italians and was also a part of a small Jewish minority in the class. On a daily basis I was always made aware of how different I was. There was no confirmation in a white dress, no going into St. Agnes or St. Carmel, the neighborhood churches. My parents were young Americans. Their parents were older immigrants from Naples and Sorrento, many of whom did not speak English. As I got older I went to PS 45 and Roosevelt High School, in the heart of what is still Little Italy, with all of the handsome Neapolitan boys. A forbidden no-no was to date them. No wonder that one of the great loves of my later life was an Italian. I was beaten up in high school because I did not sign up for Italian. The tough girls taunted, "Ain't it good enough for you Jew?" Ironically, I was sorry later I didn't study Italian, but who knew from my childhood experience that Italian was the language of culture and art and how fantastic Italy and Italian men really were. My daughter minored in Italian studies at Wesleyan. I named my Jewish son Anthony.

My roots of feminism lie in growing up in a traditional family with stereotypic gender roles. My father was a macho man who loved me and whom I loved but who was quite controlling. My brother was my mother's favorite. I did all of the errands, took care of her during her many illnesses, tried to be "good," but he was clearly the special male. Both parents expected my brother to go college. My father wanted me to marry my Jewish boyfriend from the neighborhood who enlisted in the Marines and who later became a cop.

My mother loved to tell me stories about her parents, their political activism, interesting friends and adventures. I longed to know my missing grandmother. As I got older, my mother told me I reminded her of her mother who could do everything. However, there was a sadness and bitterness about the tragic price her family paid for her parent's idealism and adventurous behavior, given the war and Soviet-era repression. My father was angry about their leaving and called them her "crazy" parents.

Because I was attractive, my mother thought I could be a model and then become an actress. She enrolled me at age 16 in the Barbizon School of Modeling. That was my first professional degree. In modeling school, I learned how to dress for jobs, walk runway walk in spiked heels, apply makeup, etc. My teachers were "beautiful," thin, and not Jewish. This made most of us 16-year-olds feel we were not attractive enough. My lifelong interest in women's body image was fermented by the long hours spent in front of the models mirrored vanities comparing my facial features and body with the other aspiring models who had small noses, more perfect features, and straight hair.

But I did not want to be a model. I wanted to go to college. Luckily City College of the City University of New York (CCNY) was free, so I could go. I earned my college money by donning my high heels, large brim hat, gloves, and patent leather round model's bag, making the round of garment center showrooms. I found work as a show room model for winter coats each summer in the garment center. Sitting in the models room between showings, meeting non-Jewish "beautiful girls" who played up to the buyers and talked about their sexual experiences was an eye opener for this unschooled Jewish virgin. My own lifelong feelings of not being attractive enough had their roots in this modeling experience.

I was the second class of "girls" at CCNY and had only two female professors. One of them was a child psychologist and the other an anthropologist. The psychology professor, Gertrude Schmeidler, became my role model, although I wished I had the courage to be like the anthropologist and travel the world. I also loved history but was told that it was not a field for women. CCNY had a first rate psychology department, and I was fascinated with these courses. I volunteered to work for Gertrude Schmeidler at her home (doing research on ESP). For the first time I got to know a working woman with a husband and children. I decided to become a child psychologist.

My first taste of political activism was in college in the McCarthy era. The HUAC (House Un-American Activities Committee) came to CCNY. I was a student leader who participated in sit-ins. At that time I was a young democrat, wanting to work for change within the system.

I graduated from college six months earlier to work to save money for graduate school. I became a welfare worker in the South Bronx in the area later known at Fort Apache. Moving beyond my Jewish neighborhood further north I experienced firsthand during the home visits the dire poverty and dilapidated tenement neighborhoods of extremely poor Puerto Ricans and Black single mothers.

After college, in opposition to my parents, I went to an "out of town school" in Boston to study psychology. My father said I was not to leave the house until I was married. I left anyway, but did not have enough money to last the year. I asked for financial aid or a fellowship from the Department Chair, Dr. Nathan Maccoby (the husband of Eleanor from Harvard) and he asked if I could type. I said yes, so I started the master's program at Boston University as the fill-in Psychology Department Secretary in exchange for the tuition. It was $600 a year.

The Psychology Department faculty was all male at that time (Rose Caron came in my second year). I was "pretty," blonde, and flirted with and was loved by them all. I typed, filed, did errands, and learned about administrating a psychology department. These skills later came in handy when I ran a program at NYU. Nathan Maccoby was my mentor and he encouraged me to go on for a PhD. I meet Eleanor as well and was accepted for the PhD in clinical at BU and developmental at Harvard. BU gave me more money, so I stayed.

I loved the clinical courses and training. The program was classically psychodynamic. I took in the traditional Freudian view of women and never questioned what I now see as a rather sexualized, sexist Rorschach course. I even wrote a Freudian paper on sex role identification for Rose Caron's course. I was thrilled to get an internship at Children's Hospital in Boston where all of my supervisors were Freudian analysts. I was offered a staff psychologist position following the internship and worked at Children's for two years, testing (writing up reports from a Freudian perspective) and treating children and adolescents, supervised by the Freudian psychiatrists while the social workers worked with their mothers. We were not encouraged to discuss our treatment with the mother's therapist. Fathers were almost never seen. I accepted all of this.

FIRST MARRIAGE

I was a boy crazy teen. I loved to date, neck, have crushes, and go steady for awhile. In my first year of graduate school living in an undergraduate dorm, I was one of the few "girls" not pinned or engaged. I felt like an old maid at 21 and worried that there would be no one left to marry. In my second year of graduate school I got engaged and a year later married a graduate student at Princeton, who, while Jewish, looked Italian to me. I thus freed myself from my ethnic Jewish name of Goldstein. Since my degree and all of my work experience is in the name of Fodor, it is the name I still hold until this day, even though there have been other husbands.

The move to Boston to graduate school was a culture shock. Everyone in this predominately Irish city perceived me as Jewish. I discovered my Jewish heritage in graduate school with roommates who were raised in the Jewish tradition. I went with them to religious services but felt alienated from the religious rituals and teachings. I did not observe Jewish rituals until I said kaddish for my mother 25 years later.

I was attracted to my first husband because he was the most interesting man I had ever dated. He was handsome, self-confident, intellectual, and quite sophisticated. He was also quite aesthetic and, like my modeling school mentors, cared about how I looked and advised me on fashion. He had a car, could fix things, and I loved hanging out with his clever, witty friends in Cambridge. In our marriage, he was the important person who mattered, who was going to make his mark on the world. Like many women of my generation, I relied on his achievements and drive to provide me with an interesting life. He could be moody and had temper outbursts. I modulated my behavior to forestall these outbursts and provided support and nurturance. Despite being a PhD student and working full time, I was less self-confident and felt less smart and even less attractive. My mother's advice to me in the marriage room prior to the ceremony was "always cater to your husband," which I did. I was no different from the other Cambridge academic wives of these special men, we took pride in our cooking skills and dinner parties, chatting together in the kitchen while the men talked and argued theory.

My husband and I moved around a lot. He had many opportunities to advance his career, so I would quit my clinical jobs and moved along with him. We moved to Oxford, England, Palo Alto, California, and Urbana, Illinois, always returning to Boston. I always found new clinical work in hospital settings. Despite working and finishing my dissertation I was a traditional wife. I did the shopping, cooking, packing, arranging the moves, finding the apartment, etc. I had trouble conceiving, and we did not have a child until the 10th year of our marriage. Then, even though I still worked, I was the caregiver for the baby.

After a year in California where my husband was at a think tank (with only fellows, all male, invited at that time) we returned to Boston and bought an old house in need of renovation in an urban renewal neighborhood in the South End. In the midst of the renovation, when our son was two years old, he left me for his attractive, much younger research assistant. He moved in with her around the corner and left me with our son, the dog and most of his stuff, sports car, debts, and the mess of a house undergoing renovation.

I went to the Virgin Islands the summer of 1968, cried for six weeks, and got a divorce (in those days it was hard to get a divorce in Boston and one had to go elsewhere to establish residency). The woman left him soon after that and he wanted to come back to me. In those six weeks alone with my son I realized that my husband did not know or appreciate who I was. I still loved him, but I did not take him back. I knew I needed to be on my own, no matter how painful. We had married too young.

> "All present interpretations of the universe...are subject to revision or replacement."
> —Kelly (1955, p. 15)

In the mid-1960s, what was exciting in psychology and psychotherapy was happening outside of psychoanalysis. I was lucky enough to become active in the beginnings of two psychotherapy movements: cognitive-behavior therapy and feminist therapy. Much more so than psychoanalysis, they have remained my core.

In the first decade of my training and career as a psychologist, many of the changes that occurred in my life were not actively sought but were the results of exposure to new experiences related to the life and moves of my husband, at that time, as well as changes in the culture. Like many women of my time, our husbands' careers were more important than ours and they, not we, chose where they wanted to live and work. The most important shifts for me occurred in these circumstances. Having to change jobs resulted in my working with varied clinical populations and thus exposed me to other therapeutic modalities in settings as diverse as rural southern Illinois and Oxford, England. However, by the 1970s when I was no longer married, I was actively seeking new challenges for ways of working as a therapist.

While living in California I took a postdoctoral fellowship at the Palo Alto veteran's hospital. The year in Palo Alto was a pivotal experience that changed my life. It was the 1960s and it was California. That year I saw my first Beatle's movie, the free speech movement at Berkeley began, and the flower children of Haight-Ashbury were attracting attention.

At the hospital I was assigned to the ward Ken Kesey drew on for *One Flew over the Cuckoo's Nest*. Some of his patients were still there. On my first day, a patient tried to throw a chair through the window of the nurse's station. I knew that my previous training had not prepared me for work in this setting. We were taught behavior therapy. In addition, I was exposed to the following:

- An anti-Freudian bias. Once a week a Freudian psychiatrist would come to the case conference, and his interpretations would be cause for laughter.
- Radical psychiatry. The patients and doctors would meet together in a therapeutic community each morning to process and discuss events and decisions on the ward.
- A weekly family therapy supervision group run by Don Jackson. He taught us a systems approach to therapy, including the radical ideas of Bateson and other systems theorists.

However, the most important influence on me that year was psycho-therapy supervision with Walter Mischel, who had been a student of George Kelly. Mischel taught me about a constructivist approach to person-ality and supervised me on my psychotherapy cases. In my first encounter with adults and a constructivist perspective I found the meaning that the Freudian approach lacked, giving a person responsibility for framing their life and choices. I began to envision a way of working with clients' present-ing problems directly, which was refreshing after my previous analytic training.

Another client had profound anxiety symptoms and Mischel, a framer of social learning theory encouraged me to learn behavior therapy. Teaching the client how to relax and learning systematic desensitization was a profound change for me. I could now work with clients on what seemed most important for them, develop a plan with them, and see changes related to the therapeutic work (Fodor, 2000).

Back in Boston again I was offered a job in the inpatient unit of Massachusetts General Hospital doing traditional psychodynamic assessment. I discovered a group of other mental health professionals in Boston, all men, interested in behavior therapy. We met regularly, reading articles, teaching one another, presenting cases, working on projects together, and being a support group. Many of these men were instrumental in the further development of behavior therapy.

I began seeing clients privately for behavior therapy. My colleagues referred me mostly phobic and overweight women. The big issue in psychoanalytic Boston, as we presented our behavioral approach, was with the problem of treating symptoms. The analysts said one couldn't treat symptoms without dealing without the underlying pathology. But we did, and our treatments appeared to work to alleviate symptoms.

BEGINNINGS OF SOCIAL ACTIVISM IN THE 1960s

I came most alive in the 1960s. In the South End of Boston, a mostly African-American neighborhood, I became a social activist. I also decided to become an academic and joined the faculty at Northeastern University. Our Boston/Cambridge friends in linguistics, philosophy, and psychology were also political activists. I became part of a social activist faculty at Northeastern and my house in the South End of Boston became one of the headquarters for the draft resistance movement. The antiwar movement and later neighborhood antipoverty movement occupied more and more of life. I went to my first Seder with these friends, a leftist freedom Seder. I went to my first feminist meeting. It was held at MIT and organized by women political activist friends in 1969. I was bowled over by the obvious fact that while I and my women friends were aware of so many oppressions of other people I didn't see the most personal oppression of all, the sexism inherent in my personal life and marriage.

MARRIAGE ENDING/NEW BEGINNINGS

By the time the marriage ended my husband was a tenured professor and well known. Although we began graduate school at the same time, I was just beginning my academic career. At Northeastern I taught very large undergraduate courses at 8:00 a.m. each day. It was in contrast to the world of the "privileged, special academic" world that I was no longer connected to. I left Boston in a new rebound relationship to move back to New York, in 1970. I was lucky to get a teaching position at New York University. I went back home to new challenges, and I also began to write.

FEMINISM, FEMINIST THERAPY, AND GESTALT THERAPY

When my generation was in their early adult years, fulfilling their traditional roles, the feminist movement began and altered the lives of many of us traditionally raised women and men. For my generation, it was forging a new path with excitement, anxiety, and a good deal of personal upheaval, as the old paradigms no longer fit the life we were living. I remember Gloria Steinem say that we were becoming the men we had hoped to marry.

By the early 1970s I was living in New York, a single parent again, with a baby girl, a four-year-old son, and an academic job in the School Psychology Program at NYU. I had been hired to teach the traditional psychodynamic assessment courses and to develop a behavior therapy practicum sequence. I began to do research and writing and began a New York psychotherapy practice doing what is now called cognitive behavior therapy, mostly with anxious, phobic women.

I felt lost without the traditional script that I had been following, and I had a hard time financially. Early on, in the many lonely evenings at home with the children asleep, I read every feminist book that came out. I was particular impressed with Simone de Beauvoir's (1953) *The Second Sex*, the existential framing of woman as the "other" and descriptions of her personal struggles to become an independent woman. I began to construct a new view of myself and what my life as a woman was about. I also joined a consciousness-raising group.

Many of my women clients and students at that time were also experiencing similar struggles. At the same time, I joined with other women therapists in studying women's lives and began actively to think and write about women's mental health issues. Many of the problems of the women that I worked with appeared related to their socialization into the female role. I also joined with other women faculty to start a women's studies program at NYU, where I developed a course on women and mental health.

Almost all of my specialty areas have emerged from my own struggles. My work with women has focused on assertiveness training, weight and body image, and mother and daughter relationships. I was socialized to be unassertive and to put others' needs before my own. This was especially true in my marriages. I realized from my own personal struggles the need for women to be assertive in their relationships and to fight for their rights.

Body image and weight concerns mirrored my family's concern that I be thin and attractive and not like other overweight members of my father's family whose struggles I recalled from childhood. Coming to terms with my mother, the choices she had made for herself, and wishing to pursue a different path set me to work on these issues with other women. So many of the women I grew up with and knew seemed helpless, dependent on their husbands, feared going out in the world on their own. So I worked with these women and wrote about women's fears and phobias. When I brought my 11-year-old daughter, Jody, to a mother–daughter assertiveness workshop and identified more with the mothers than the daughters I realized I was working these issues from both sides. I raised Jody to be creative and independent. She is a now a dancer and choreographer with her own dance company. My son, primarily raised by his single parent mother, is a biologist, who with his ecologist wife coparents their two toddler daughters.

I became a leader in the feminist therapy movement even before I had a firm sense of my new identity. In New York I was a candidate in a psychoanalytic institute with the goal of integrating psychoanalysis and behavior therapy. I had gone into a personal analysis with a female Freudian analyst, but like many women of my generation, I found the traditional analytic approach at that time to be too restrictive toward the new way of thinking about women. Some of my psychoanalytic colleagues who stayed with psychoanalysis became leaders in developing the new psychology of women.

I moved further away from psychoanalysis to behavior therapy as I became a feminist. I saw behavior therapy as providing a model for women to take charge of their lives and to learn new ways of behaving. My first clinical publication in 1972 was titled "Sex Role Conflict for Women: Can Behavior Therapy Help?" I proposed a link between stereotypic female socialization—to be dependent and helpless—and the development of phobic symptomology, and I proposed that behavior therapy could help women become less fearful and more self-sufficient and assertive. I became an advocate for behavior therapy to better address women's issues and began speaking and writing about its applicability for the new generation of women seeking change (Fodor, 1972a).

During the 1970s women therapists began working together to create a feminist approach to working with women. At the same time, we began using these same techniques, with the support of other therapists in our consciousness raising groups, to reparent ourselves. I specialized in assertiveness training, in body image and self-esteem problems, and in helping women take charge of their lives and overcome their fears and phobias to move beyond the model of helpless woman. The behavior therapy community provided support for this work, and I was invited to present at conferences and universities. There was an excitement and freshness about behavior therapy at that time and I felt fortunate to be able to integrate the behavior therapy and feminist modalities. Through this work I met many creative behavior therapists, most of whom were Jewish, who influenced me and who are still my close friends.

By the 1970s behavior therapy had became more cognitive, which fit my own orientation. I brought the feminist perspective to my beginning work in cognitive therapy. I built on prior training in constructivism and saw the major change process in cognitive behavior therapy for women as cognitive restructuring, envisioning other ways of being, and then developing new behaviors for change (Fodor, 1988).

At NYU, Janet Wolfe, a graduate student in clinical psychology who was actively involved in clinical work and training at the Institute for Rational Emotive Therapy (now the Albert Ellis Institute), asked me to work with her on her dissertation, thus launching a long-term collaboration and friendship. She reintroduced me to the cognitive approach, this time in the form of rational emotive therapy (RET). We began to work together to develop, conduct, and do research on women's assertiveness groups.

We proposed that woman's lack of assertion was tied to cognitions stemming from sex role socialization messages. We suggested,

> For many women, the stereotypes about the "shoulds" and "oughts" of sex role behavior and assertiveness function as internal belief systems or schemata through which their own and other's behaviors are evaluated and when their behavior deviates from what they believe they ought to be, or from what others expect them to be, feelings of anxiety, guilt and confusion results. (Wolfe & Fodor, 1975, pp. 45–46)

Janet and I ran assertiveness training groups for women at Ys, at national and international conferences, and networked with women's groups, etc. It was exciting and fun to be at the edge of this movement. Women's assertiveness training groups in the mid-1970s became an important part of the women's movement, were adapted by the public, and contributed to women's empowerment. We also encouraged women to become social and political activists and agents of change, moving beyond the person to the political (Fodor & Epstein, 1983).

I have also brought the feminist perspective to my work with phobic women. I addressed the social context of anxiety and phobias in women, with an emphasis on socialization, as a key factor in their developing and maintaining phobic avoidance behavior. At that time I believed that behavior therapy, by developing techniques to enable women to face their fears, provided remediation for prior social conditioning (Fodor, 1972b).

In a similar vein, after failing to help overweight women lose weight with behavioral techniques and seeing low self-esteem and body image issues in too many adolescents I argued that behavior therapists need to consider the societal messages about attractiveness and weight in designing their treatments (Fodor, 1983). Body image, self-esteem, and eating behavior and media influences continue to be an ongoing interest in my therapeutic work with women (Fodor, 1996). In addition, I am now addressing the fears of aging and ageism in older women (Fodor, 1990; Fodor and Franks, 1990).

As I further focused on assertiveness issues in the mid-1970s, highlighting the interpersonal aspects and building on what I learned in relational psychodynamic therapy, I became increasing dissatisfied with what I viewed as the limitations of cognitive-behavior therapy. At that time, I began working more experientially in the assertiveness groups, to access the affective patterns and its tie-in to cognitions, and I decided to seek some Gestalt therapy training. Gestalt therapy was then outside of the psychotherapy mainstream and was taught mostly in intensive workshops or by individual trainers at Gestalt Therapy Institutes. As I discovered more about Gestalt therapy it became clear to me that Gestalt therapy was a rich, theoretically based system of therapy that addressed the very issues I felt needed further development in cognitive therapy.

Gestalt therapy, in espousing organismic self-regulation, presents a positive view of people's ability to take charge of themselves once they become aware of and own where they are, what they need, and the choices and resources available or unavailable to them. Gestalt therapists have a tradition of moving beyond personal work to social activism. The integration of CBT and Gestalt is still ongoing (Fodor, 1987, 2000).

PHOTOGRAPHY AND DIGITAL STORYTELLING

In preparing presentations on women's body image and gender stereotyping in the 1970s I began shooting photos from fashion magazines to prepare slide shows to illustrate these talks. I was not particularly good at photography in the predigital age. I decided to take a slide photography course at the International Center for Photography. As I developed photographic skills, I developed numerous slide show presentations on body image, images of aging, and gender stereotypes to present to a wide range of audiences, arguing for a move beyond the media stereotypes to enable girls and women to feel good about themselves and their bodies.

As I became more interested in photography I sought out well known photographers to study with and went on travel photography workshops. On 9/11 I witnessed the whole horror from my 16th floor picture window. I became a neighborhood photographer in the week that followed, capturing on film the memorials, gatherings, and the smoldering ruin. I took a narrative photography course and wrote a paper on photography as healing, which featured the photographs (Fodor, 2002).

Realizing the power of visual images for advocacy, I decided to work on integrating psychology and photography. Through the photography community, I met Phil Borges, a photojournalist who photographs and teaches photography to indigenous children worldwide. In the past five years I have become a mentor for his nongovernmental organization, Bridges to Understanding (e-mail:info@bridgesweb.org) and have traveled to Peru, India, and South Africa to work on Bridges projects. Moving beyond individual therapy, digital storytelling fosters resiliency in marginalized and groups in crisis by helping individuals create narrative art projects. Digital stories also serve to highlight awareness of social and cultures concerns and serve to foster social activism.

The first Bridges project I worked on was teaching Tibetan refugee children at the Tibetan Children's Village in Dharamsala, India. What is most evident working in Dharamsala is the continued experience of repression, trauma, and flight, it's as if the Holocaust has been going on for 50 years, and despite the Dalai Lama's prominence, the world stands aside. Parents send their children out of Tibet never knowing if they will see them again. The Tibetan Children's Village is an unusual boarding school for these refugee children. Our work with the photography club involved brainstorming a story idea, mentoring students to take digital photos, and working together to create a visual narrative, adding words and music to create a short digital film. My first digital movie was about Tibetan music, the second about the Baby Room where the infants and toddlers are cared for. Being Jewish, I resonated with the plight of the Tibetans (Fodor, 2009). I also volunteered at the Tibetan woman's association where I networked with Tibetan feminists and worked on a research project.

In South Africa, for the past two summers, I mentored students at a Bridges Project at an African High School (Hector Peterson School) who live in a township where the community is coping with extreme poverty, unsanitary living conditions, and a high rate of HIV infection. For our first project these African teens wanted to make a movie honoring the struggles of their single mothers in the township to show on Woman's Day, a national holiday in South Africa. Last year, Human Rights Watch selected this short digital movie for their first International Teen Festival at Lincoln center in New York City. The movie, which was pieced together from the photos these African adolescents took in their township, featured their poetic chorus, highlighting the struggles of their mothers to feed them, work, and provide for their education. It ended on an inspirational note. At the showing, their single mothers loved the movie. One of the African students selected to be part of a panel for the showing said at Lincoln Center that he made the movie to remind African men of their responsibility to the mothers of their children.

COMING HOME

In returning to New York City and living and working at a university I felt very much at home with so many Jewish faculty and students after so many years away. As a feminist therapist, I continue to work with women and mentor mostly women students. The social and economic inequities I experienced in the Bronx are still present and in working with my students on their projects I am continually challenged. The newer work on digital story-telling in cultures in crisis is ongoing, both in New York and overseas. I will be returning to India for a longer stay next year. This year I exhibited photographs in a traveling show with psychologist photographers from APA on the theme of social justice.

As I get older, I also have been faced with many losses: my mother, father, all of my aunts, uncles, and recently my husband of 20 years. Although I have not been connected to the traditions of Judaism, while visiting my father in Florida I loved going to services with him in his retirement community, seeing him and the others joy in singing Jewish songs. I appreciated the wisdom of the retired rabbi who knew how to connect to these people whose parents came from the ghettos of Eastern Europe almost one hundred years ago. I did feel a part of that community. I plan to hold on to my father's condo in Florida.

However, the Jewish religious path was not for me. Given all of the losses, I have increasingly found spiritual solace in Buddhism. From my early workshops in Gestalt therapy, where my trainers were into Vipassana meditation, to more recent work with the Tibetan community in Dharmasala, India, I have found in Buddhism what I did not find in my own religion. Ironically, many of the best American Buddhist teachers are also Jewish (Ram Dass, Jack Goldstein, Jack Kornfield, Stephen Levine, etc). I find the Buddhist teachings that focus on present centered awareness useful for remaining centered and for teaching mindfulness to clients. I am inspired by the teachings on Compassion and Loving Kindness. Meditation has enabled me to cope with the many losses and my aging. My brother and I became close friends as we dealt with my father's illness and death. Yet what is most meaningful, particularly in this stage of life, is the continuing relations I have with my women friends. These female friendships, many of them formed in feminist meetings or therapist training, remain my foundational core.

REFERENCES

de Beauvoir, S. (1953). *The second sex*. New York: Bantam Books.

Fodor, I. (1972a). The phobic syndrome in women. In V. Franks & V. Burtle (Eds.), *Women and therapy* (pp. 132–168). New York: Bruner/Mazel.

Fodor, I. (1972b). Sex role conflict and symptom formation in women: Can behavior therapy help? *Psychotherapy: Theory, Research, Practice*, *2*(1), 22–29.

Fodor, I. (1983). Behavior therapy for weight disorders: A time for reappraisal. In M. Rosenbaum & C. Franks (Eds.), *Perspectives on behavior therapy in the 80s* (pp. 378–384). New York: Springer.

Fodor, I. G. (1987). On integrating gestalt therapy to facilitate personal and interpersonal awareness. In N. Jacobson (Ed.), *Psychotherapists in clinical practice: Cognitive and behavioral perspectives* (pp. 340–410). New York: Guilford.

Fodor, I. (1988). Cognitive behavior therapy: Evaluation of theory and practice for addressing women's issues. In M. Douglas & L. Walker (Eds.), *Feminist Psychotherapies: Integration of therapeutic and feminist systems* (pp. 91–117). Glencoe, IL: Hayworth Press.

Fodor, I. (1990, February). On turning 50: No longer young/not yet old: Shifting to a new paradigm. *The Behavior Therapist, 13*(2), 39–44.

Fodor, I. (1993). A feminist framework for integrative psychotherapy: Cognitive and gestalt perceptives. In G. Stricker and J. Gold (Eds.), *Comprehensive handbook of integrative psychotherapy* (pp. 217–221). New York: Plenum Press.

Fodor, I. (1996). A woman and her body: The cycles of pride and shame. In R. Lee & G. Wheeler (Eds.), *The voice of shame: Silence and connection in psychotherapy* (pp. 229–265). San Francisco: Jossey-Bass.

Fodor, I. (2000). Making meaning of therapy: A personal narrative of change over 4 decades. In M. Goldfried (Ed.), *How therapists change: Personal and professional reflections.* Washington, DC: American Psychological Association.

Fodor, I. (2002). Photography as healing: September 11 through the lens of the viewers. *Gestalt Online, 6*(1).

Fodor, I. (2009). Digital story telling with Tibetan adolescents in Dharamsala, India. In D. Ullman & G. Wheeler (Eds.), *Cocreating the field: Intension and practice in the age of complexity* (pp. 211–223). New York: Routledge.

Fodor, I., & Epstein, R. (1983). Assertiveness training from women: Where are we failing. In P. Emmelkamp & E. Foa (Eds.), *Failures in behavior therapy* (pp. 137–158). New York: Wiley.

Fodor, I., & Franks, V. (1990). Women and midlife and beyond. The new prime of life? *Psychology of Women Quarterly, 14*(4), 445–449.

Kelly, G. (1955). *The psychology of personal constructs.* New York: Norton.

Polster, M. (1972). Gestalt therapy. In V. Franks & V. Burtle (Eds.), *Women and therapy* (pp. 247–262). New York: Brunner/Mazel.

Wolfe, J., & Fodor, I. (1975). A cognitive/behavioral approach to modifying assertive behavior in women. *The Counseling Psychologist, 5*(4), 45–52.

COMMENTARIES

We begin this section with an apocryphal tale about the famous Rabbi Hillel. Hillel and Shammai were two biblical scholars. Shammai was known for the strictness of his views and Hillel for his kindness and concern for humanity. In this tale, a non-Jew comes to Shammai and tells him that he will convert to Judaism if Shammai can teach him the whole Torah in the time that he can stand on one foot. Shammai dismisses him as foolish. The stranger posed the same question to Hillel, who responded, "That which is hateful to you, do not do to your neighbor. That is the whole Torah; the rest is commentary."

One Particular Minyan

ELENA J. EISMAN

On contemplating how I would reflect on the stories in these pages and on how to extend this dialogue, I knew right away that my response would be based on the emotions of shared experience among rich differences. There is a Zen-like experience among Jews, or at least among this Jew, feeling at once connected yet acutely aware of our different paths. The ever present unifying Jewish awareness of generations of persecution clings to most of us like a cape, and just like a cape, it can be different depending on who is wearing it. For some it covers the arms, preventing action and agency, yet for others it enables them to catch the wind and fly.

Even the jokes we tell to and about ourselves reflect these different perceptions. It begins with the unity built on survival reflected in the description of Jewish holidays: "they tried to kill us, we survived; let's eat," to the strong appreciation for our differences. The latter is reflected in the story about the rescue of the Jew marooned alone for years on a desert island showing his rescuer the structures he had built, pointing out "that's my synagogue, and over there that's the one I don't go to."

One thread that binds us together is *tikkun olam*, repairing the world. I was moved by the courage of the women in this book who so often referenced this lofty goal. If there was one consistent theme related to Jewishness in these narratives it was that. Yet how can one single person change the world? I have always been somewhat mystified and incredulous when this is discussed in temple. Is it chutzpa? Grandiosity? Fantasy? I pondered the similarity among these strong women with such different experiences all pointing to this ultimately unachievable value. It brought to mind the questions I have asked about this concept throughout my spiritual and professional journey. I believe it refers more to how one lives ones life *on the journey* rather than to actually *reaching the destination*. It is about the different routes people take even if they are heading to the same place. This is one way that we describe the work that we do as psychologists.

A MINYAN OF WOMEN

My personal reasons for embracing feminism and going into psychology most likely were conceived at one particular minyan. I was almost 13, and my 9-year-old sister had just died after a two-year battle with Leukemia. The sadness of the many days and nights of coming home to an empty house while my parents were sitting at the hospital had worn me down, and I thought that I had experienced the depth of pain, but it was nothing compared to the pain I was to encounter. It was after the funeral when we were all in my living room sitting shivah, with mirrors shrouded and hard low benches to sit on (as if we needed reminding that we shouldn't be at ease). At some point, it was time to say kaddish, the mourner's prayer for my sister, which required 10 men to comprise a minyan in order for the prayer to be chanted. The rabbi counted. My mother said that she would like to be counted among the minyan, but the rabbi said it was not allowed. It was bad enough that he wouldn't count her, but there was a risk that they would not be able to say kaddish for Amy at all unless more men showed up. It was then that my 1950s era mother, so compliant toward authority figures, changed in front of my eyes. She said again that she wanted to say it, needed to say it, it was her remembrance, and it was her daughter. However, the rabbi said it was not allowed—*he* would not allow it. I thought I had seen pain during Amy's illness and death but it was then that I first experienced the unimaginable kind of soul-wrenching, primal agony of my mother's loss. The men formed a circle and began to chant Kaddish and my mother stood on the periphery, hands over her eyes, silently mouthing the words, body heaving with tears rolling down her cheeks. I was forged that evening; I would never be the same. I realized that the world and the people in it needed repair. I vowed to be one who helped. I realized on some level that my calling in life, much like that of my sisters in this volume, was to help the world through helping the people in it. I also began my journey of understanding *tikkun olam*, that one way that you repair the world is through helping the people in it.

The stories told in this book speak to the wide variety of Jewish identities we experience. I am grateful that there are so many variations because it has allowed me, as it has others in this book, to mold the experience of my spirituality through the connection with like-minded people and communities. I shared many experiences with women in this book, taking art classes at the Henry Street Settlement House, not learning Yiddish because assimilation was the family goal, waiting for lightning to strike me when I had my first aliyah (being called up to recite the prayer before the Torah reading previously allowed only to men), hearing my parents tell of the anti-Semitism they encountered. One particularly poignant and symbolic experience was when my mother, very pregnant with me, was looking with my father for a hotel to stay in overnight in Deal, New Jersey. They were not permitted to stay "at the inn" because the Christian manager said it was "restricted," meaning that Jews were not allowed.

I also recognize many of the Jewish denominational and synagogue community variations expressed in these narratives as they remind me of my own journey trying to "shul-shop" for a synagogue community that felt right for me: egalitarian, welcoming of diversity, not too fundamentalist but also with richness of ritual, singing, spirituality, and meaning. There is a parallel between this quest and the importance of "match" for doing psychotherapy. I never worried when a patient said of our alliance that it just didn't feel like a "good match." People are different, look for different things, and seem to know what is right when they find it.

I was one of those women who needed to learn her feminism with a jump-start from enlightened men before I could learn from enlightened women. The same society that supported my mother's exclusion from the minyan and unsuccessful assertiveness worked its unmagical magic over me as well. However, I was fortunate, and I found some wonderful help. I was fortunate in my quest to attend a summer camp where there was a scholar in residence, Rabbi Mordecai Kaplan. It was not until many years later that I came to appreciate the impact of this small rotund man with a cane and white hair and beard, who would take his daily constitutional, walking up the hill between the boys' side and the girls' side of the camp. Camp leaders would talk about him with hushed reverence, but I never knew why until years after. As one of the leaders of the Conservative movement, he was the first to allow Jewish women to be called up to the Torah, beginning bat mitzvah, the rite of passage previously allowed only to men. Why? Because he had only daughters and he grew to understand. He also founded the newest branch of North American Judaism called Reconstructionism. This is where I found a home. This denomination values ritual but sees the Jewish people as a culture that must adapt teachings and practices to be meaningful for modern life such as practicing respect for all people and for the planet. The sense of being a part of a diverse egalitarian Jewish community embedded in a larger world community is what I was looking for to fit my identity. When I first went to visit the congregation during the Sukkot holiday (the traditional harvest feast of the tabernacles where Jews build shelters outdoors and eat meals under the stars) the congregation not only planned a dinner in the Sukkah but also brought in an expert to talk about the homeless to raise awareness of their plight. I was hooked. The congregation is reflective and accepting of many identities and many varieties of families—straight, lesbian and gay, interfaith, interracial, single parent, and single. Our rabbi is a lesbian and she and her wife have two children. Her sexual orientation is such a nonissue for our congregation that when she was profiled in the *Boston Globe* (Radin, 2007) as the first gay or lesbian rabbi elected to the presidency of denominational rabbinical organization (the Reconstructionist Rabbinical Association) our listserv buzzed with tongue-in cheek comments about why she was portrayed that way instead of being called the "bowling rabbi," referencing another of her identities.

This type of Judaism works for me and repairs my heart, but I can also appreciate how other Jewish women and men find meaning in more traditional forms of Judaism. I remember as an early career psychologist speaking to a psychology colleague who was one of the first feminists I ever knew. She married into an orthodox marriage and lifestyle where her husband went to study Talmud during the day leaving her to earn the money and run the house. I asked her how she could say she was happy and reconcile the two identities that *I* perceived as at war within her. She said that they did not feel disparate. She said that she loved her work, she believed that she was the better earner, ran the house and family better, and had quite a bit of freedom and recognition within her life. She was happy and fulfilled.

As a family therapist, I well appreciate that even within our own families we can find difference and assumptions about attitudes, identity, and beliefs that prove neither accurate nor well understood. In fact, much of the work of family therapy is coming to understanding, appreciation, and adaptation to these various differences. When I first married, my mother was very worried about when her mother would ask me "the question." "The question" was whether I would keep a kosher home. It had been a source of conflict and disappointment for my grandmother when my mother decided not keep kosher in her own home, and my mother was worried that this would make for tension and spoil my wedding day. With this build-up in mind, I steeled myself for the inevitable. It finally came. I took a deep breath and said, "No Bubbe (grandmother), I am not planning to." She looked at me for a minute, smiled, and said, "Good, it's too much trouble for a young girl like you." Therefore, just as the preface of this book observed, people have differences that cannot be assumed nor predicted; one needs to ask to find out.

That these beliefs about people are tightly held often without examination and that the process of recognizing what they truly are or where they come from may serve to repair the main impediment to good relating is a lesson I learned and use when I do therapy. This can be something as simple as how towels are folded. One couple argued for years about how to fold towels. Do you fold them in half then fold them over or do you do it in thirds. Each had a reason that explained why his or her way was the "right" way. Finally, one day the wife was at her mother-in-law's house and she noticed that, like her husband, her mother-in-law folded the towels in thirds, so she asked her why she did it that way. "Simple" she responded, "I have a narrow linen closet."

I believe that we need to be able to look at the assumptions we make about one another and take the time to understand how even similar experiences can be felt, interpreted, and reacted to in very different ways as well as how people can arrive at the same destination even if they do it through different routes. The words of Andrea Bergman and Carol Heffer are both talking about how their different experiences of inclusion and acceptance were answered through people who had the wisdom to step back and see the larger picture, to appreciate what was important for the human condition even if it meant bending the rules, and to accept people into their lives even if the people themselves felt like outsiders.

Hebrew is a language with a different alphabet (aleph bet) and is read from right to left. It is not uncommon in religious training to teach the reading without expecting the student to understand the language, and many prayer books have English translations on facing pages to the Hebrew. For some of us, reading fluently is a challenge, and the concept of feeling an outsider is stimulated by not being able to read along in the prayer book. Modern prayer books also include transliteration to English letters and sounds, which allows everyone to participate in the chanting of the Hebrew. It is no less understandable to read a language you do not understand through transliteration than it would be with the original Hebrew alphabet, but the experience of belonging and connection this small step achieves is so much more improved.

These narratives say something even more important than the importance of being for the other, for repairing the world. They also celebrate the beauty of diversity and creativity and perspective. They trace a sense of connection through a larger identity that leaves room for individual differences and even for the very understanding of what they are identifying with. It celebrates the creative problem solving of people holding onto a culture despite many challenges and roadblocks, threats of annihilation, and prohibitions both from without and from within. It also recognizes that not everyone can or wants to stay connected. Moreover, it speaks to a theme that if something has meaning or is important to do, wise people can find a way that works for them and they keep searching for it until they find it.

My cousin tells a story of his days in an Orthodox yeshiva in Brooklyn in the 1940s. A yeshiva is a Jewish day school where both secular and Jewish subjects are taught. A new lay teacher was hired and she made a serious mistake. It is well known by even the youngest pupil that when writing about the deity you write G-D omitting the middle "O" in the name since once it is spelled out completely becomes sacred and cannot be erased or destroyed. She, being hired to teach a secular history course was unaware and spelled out the whole name. The class emitted a collective gasp, and they worried that if a solution was not found that the blackboard could never be erased. Their solution was to call for the rabbi. He was known as a worldly individual in part because of his experiences, such as the time he served in the army as a chaplain. He had seen the world and lived at times on K-rations and he was the only one in the larger community who had tasted nonkosher food. He came in, looked thoughtful for a moment assessing the problem, stroked his beard, then adding "Arthur" to the beginning and "frey" to the end was able to erase "Arthur Godfrey" from the board.

Much creative work has been done to repair the world, but there is certainly more to do. Descriptions of how Jews were able to "pass" in this society leave out the experiences of Sephardic Jews. One of my friends is of Yemenite heritage. She is often not seen as a person of color to the ethnic-minority community but to the larger world is asked if she is a Latina, Arab, or Indian. As with everything in life there are no simple answers, and the more we find solutions, the more there are problems left to solve.

I will end my discussion with a story about my mother's funeral. Things change, and the temple of my youth is now egalitarian. I was part of the minyan and stood with my husband, daughters, and family within the circle saying kaddish. I too was crying, but my tears were of pure loss and not out of the frustration of exclusion once felt by my mother. A small part of the world had been repaired, yet there are people still crying, and we all have work to do.

REFERENCE

Radin, C. A. (2007, March 13). First openly gay rabbi elected leader. *Boston Globe.* Retrieved from www.boston.com/news/globe/city_region/breaking_news/2007/03/first_openly_ga.html

On Poets, Revolutionaries, and the Power of Naming

RUTH E. FASSINGER

What a gift my Jewish sisters have given in sharing these stories! And what an honor it is to add my voice to this conversation about identity. I believe that it is through our stories that we come to name ourselves and the truths about our lives. It is through our stories that we find the threads of connection among us in the commonalities of our joy, our pain, our struggle, and, ultimately, our triumph. In this spirit of sharing, I offer a brief story of my own. It is a story about how a lifetime of Jewish presence has helped to shape me, a non-Jew, into the person I am today.

> The beginning of wisdom is to call things by their right names.
>
> —Chinese proverb

When I was a little girl in the 1950s growing up in a small town on Long Island I thought that everyone was Jewish. I simply assumed that it had something to do with living on Long Island. Obvious religious differences didn't disturb my belief system in the least; I thought that some Jews (like myself) went to the Lutheran church, some Jews (like my best friend Kathy) went to the Catholic church, some Jews went to the Episcopal and Methodist churches, and some Jews (but certainly not any of my friends) didn't go to church at all. In retrospect, I realize that I had no idea where the real Jews did go to worship, as there was no synagogue that I knew of in my town or in any of the surrounding towns nearby.

I also thought that everyone who lived on Long Island was White. I didn't notice any people of color in my town until I was in junior high school. The pictures I saw in books convinced me that Negroes, Indians, Chinese, Aborigines, Eskimos, and other people who were not White were members of various exotic tribes who lived in foreign countries and dressed in strange costumes that had nothing to do with me. The fact that I was a girl didn't worm its way into my consciousness until age nine when my twin brothers were born. My father's giddy ecstasy over his sons and my plunge into instant mini-mothering (because my father's meager earnings compelled my mother to work) were clear signals that my presumed status as my father's favorite and my perceived freedom to play whenever I wanted were, in fact, constrained somehow by my sex. Thus, throughout much of my childhood, I named myself as Jewish, White, Lutheran, not-rich, and (later) a girl.

By adolescence, I knew that people came in many shapes and colors, but I was White and that was the best (i.e., most normal) color to be. I also had figured out that I wasn't Jewish after all, that, in fact, Jews were a religious group different from Christians. In my church preconfirmation class that I had to attend every Saturday morning through seventh and eighth grades, we learned that Lutherans were going to heaven but everyone else was going to hell. Moreover, there seemed to be a clear order to God's disdain for the unsaved, as Catholics were second from the bottom and Jews were at the absolute bottom of the list in terms of their likelihood of enjoying a sweet hereafter. We learned that Jews were godless and had either killed or rejected Jesus, depending on various versions of the story. Catholics, on the other hand, merely worshiped false gods like the Virgin Mary and the Pope, clearly preferable to killing Jesus. I worried a lot in those days about the eternal fate of my friends, as very few of them went to the Lutheran church, and I wasn't interested in heaven if my friends weren't going to be there with me. I tried to get Kathy to stop worshipping the Virgin Mary (she was my best friend, after all, and I wasn't giving up on her), but I felt deeply sorry for my Jewish friends and slowly started to distance myself from them.

During adolescence I also began babysitting and thus spending time in other people's houses without a friend to distract me. Because my family home was furnished mostly in retrievals from the town dump, other people's houses fascinated me. There were separate bedrooms for each of the children, matching furniture covered in plastic to keep it nice, bathrooms with showers, green yards with yet more matching furniture. It all seemed miraculous to me. A few of the families for whom I babysat were Jewish, and I remember that their homes seemed somehow different from other people's houses in my town. Their furniture seemed more elegant and spare, their surfaces less cluttered, and their walls more interesting, with fancy mirrors or paintings on them. I remember thinking that their refrigerators were disappointing, with strange and unappealing foods in little jars, and I assumed that this must be why the women were so thin. I felt sorry for the Jewish children for whom I babysat, both because they didn't experience the wonders of Christmas and because they were doomed to hell forever, no matter how cute or well-behaved they were.

My preoccupation with hell doubtless was due to the confusing religious phase I was going through at the time. Despite my church's teachings, I was drawn strongly to Catholicism, which I was learning from my friend Kathy. I loved the ceremony and costumes, I fervently wished that Lutherans could get ashes smeared on their foreheads on Ash Wednesday, and I was seriously thinking about becoming a nun so that I could sing all day. Now that I no longer named myself as Jewish and was having grave doubts about being Lutheran, I was beginning to wonder what, exactly, I was.

How simple a thing it seems to me that to know ourselves as we are, we must know our mothers' names.

—Alice Walker

I spoke very little to my parents, both of them children of immigrants and of the Depression, about my thoughts regarding groups of people, maybe in part because their opinions already seemed clear to me. My father, Buddy, was an uneducated, good-natured, irrepressible, endlessly optimistic, oddly compassionate bigot who would refer casually to ethnic groups in all the vile terminology of the day (spic, nigger, kike, wop, chink, etc.). However, he would give his last 75 cents (no small amount for him) to one of these people at the gas station if they needed it. I now understand him to have been fundamentally a gregarious individual who loved talk and laughter and sharing big dreams and long stories with anybody who would listen, despite his deeply ingrained prejudices. I learned from my father that talk and laughter are best expressed loudly, that people can surprise you, and that words and actions are not necessarily the same. It was from him that I also developed a strong preference for judging people by what they do, not what they say.

My mother, Mary, was very different from my father, and I often wondered what kept them together. Like many of the women described in this volume, she was an intelligent woman whose talents were severely constricted by gender and class and she longed for wit and beauty in her life. She registered people to vote, she worked toward a college degree at night, she wrote poetry about civil rights and environmental issues, and she collected the downtrodden like I collected stray cats. Thanksgiving and Sunday dinners often featured a diverse assortment of people we barely knew whom she had decided needed a good meal, and Christmas was always preceded by weeks of gathering and fixing up old toys to give to those less fortunate than we. If my siblings or I voiced anything remotely resembling resentment about these ministrations to others, my mother's admonishment was swift and clear. We were extremely blessed to have food and clothing and a roof over our heads and we were to share that abundance with others. This probably goes a long way toward explaining why I didn't recognize the full extent of my family's compromised financial circumstances until much later in my life.

My father was fun, but it was my mother who was the bedrock of the family. Often humorless, constantly worried, and full of bitterness and regret as she aged, she had the impossible task of keeping food on the table, keeping her husband anchored in reality, and keeping her children firmly on the path toward educational success and community responsibility. She didn't put much stock in religion, so my religious doubts would not have disturbed her. However, I'm certain she would have quickly attacked any negative stereotypes I was developing about groups of people, as my father's casual bigotry caused her great consternation and she constantly begged him to be careful about what he said around his children. My mother had a deep respect for the strength and power of words, and she used them proudly and judiciously. I learned from her that words matter, that they can be weapons or offerings, and that they can be used to change the world. My mother was my first poet and revolutionary, and she set me on that same path, but I realized it too late to ever thank her.

> To name oneself is the first act of both the poet and the revolutionary.
> —Erica Jong

When I left home in 1969 to attend an upstate teacher's college, my roommates at first thought I was Jewish. I was from Long Island, my name was Jewish, I was loud and opinionated, and I never made my bed (they thought I had a maid at home). Because hand-me-down clothes were the hippie rage at the time, I pretended to be stylistically nonchalant instead of poor, and this contributed to confusion about my identity. Initially, I was quick to correct perceptions that I was Jewish, but over time I became more and more comfortable at being mistaken for a member of the group I was coming to admire greatly. Thanks to my mother's influence, I was committed firmly both to learning and to human rights, and, as far as I could tell, Jews were at the leading edge on both of these fronts. I knew that Jews were supporting civil rights struggles in the South, and I noticed that many of the most exciting thinkers of the (re)emerging feminist movement were Jewish women. Even some of the fiction writers, poets, and folk singers I loved best were Jewish. Who wouldn't want to identify with leading intellectuals, artists, peacemakers, and others determined to make the world a better place?

During my first year of college I had abandoned religion consciously and deliberately, having decided that the things I had been taught, including the hierarchy of the damned, just didn't make sense given the worlds of new knowledge that were opening up to me. This was quite freeing, and I began to claim my identity as an intellectual, a free thinker, a nonconformist, and a catalyst for social change. During this growth period I continually assumed that my Jewish friends and acquaintances would be the social leaders in both opinion and action. My friend Kathy even had a Jewish boyfriend who actually had published a book.

During early adulthood, I had several important romantic relationships with Jewish men. One of them affectionately referred to me as his *shiksa*. I remember being a little ambivalent about this endearment, immensely proud that my blonde hair and blue eyes apparently accorded me a unique place in his life, but constantly reminded that I was an outsider. As fate and love would have it, I ended up marrying a radical, nonconformist man who did not identify as a Jew, but I suspected that he had Jewish roots in Eastern Europe. When his nephew developed undiagnosed medical problems that looked like Tay-Sachs disease, we tried (unsuccessfully) to convince the family to discuss this possibility with the doctor. And when his grandmother, in one flash of coherence before she died, told me her entire life story involving flights from adversity that sounded very much like pogroms to my untrained ear, we tried again (unsuccessfully) to query the family, ultimately giving up on exploring that possible part of my husband's heritage. We both had become teachers by then and we settled into a town in Western New York that was overwhelmingly Italian and Swedish. I lost my faux Jewish identity for almost a decade, but I continued to name myself a rebel, a revolutionary, trying to change the world one child at a time. My husband and I together sought to live a radical, nonconformist life and yet fit into the conservative community in which we were living, a constant social negotiation that left me, at the end of the decade, starved for intellectual stimulation, unfettered lifestyles, and activist camaraderie.

I think your mythology would call them fallen angels. War and hate are their business, and one of their chief weapons is un-Naming—making people not know who they are. If someone knows who he really is, really knows, then he doesn't need to hate. That's why we still need Namers, because there are places throughout the universe like your planet Earth. When everyone is really and truly Named, then the Echthroi will be vanquished.
—Madeleine L'Engle (*A Wrinkle in Time*)

When I entered graduate school in psychology in the early 1980s I had become impatient, and I wanted to change the world quickly and directly. I thought that psychology would give me the tools to help people more effectively than I was able to do as a classroom teacher. Graduate school felt like a homecoming to me, and I now believe that part of the reason for this sense of comfort was that I reconnected with some of my lost sense of "Jewishness"; that is, with the values and activities and self-chosen identities that I had come to associate with being Jewish.

Indeed, psychology itself, or at least the therapeutic enterprise, felt to me like a very Jewish field, not just because of obvious factors such as the ethnic roots of the major thinkers and writers but in the very idea of therapy as a healing medium. The process of therapy seemed to be about telling family stories, uncovering buried secrets, naming pain and suffering, interpreting and discussing and arguing and trying to make sense of things, learning to trust, reclaiming one's rightful place, healing the world one person at a time, and constantly learning, learning, learning. I rediscovered the joys of intellectual life and the satisfying challenge of directing one's work toward radical social change. Through my training to be a therapist I remembered what it is to name significant truths about oneself, and I developed the skills to help others name their truths as well.

I also came out as a lesbian during this time and my feminism deepened, buttressed by the women (many of them Jewish, of course), writers, teachers, role models, mentors, friends, and colleagues who helped me take on the mantle of this new identity proudly and with infinite joy. Of hundreds of memories of my Jewish feminist sisters, one stands out: It was my first American Psychological Association convention and I was a graduate student. Like many graduate students in that situation, I was overwhelmed by the crowds, worried that I wasn't dressed well enough, and wondering if I would ever fit in with all these smart, fancy people. Suddenly I was watching someone who didn't look at all like anyone else. It was the inimitable Laura Brown, dressed in overalls, her wild hair exploding around her head, strong, determined, dramatic, inspiring, marching down hallways like she owned the world. I didn't know who she was, but I wanted to be just like her. Almost 30 years later, I still do.

Women have had the power of naming stolen from us.

—Mary Daly

I am now at that professional age when the years I have spent in this particular calling as a psychologist outnumber the years I spent prior to it. I would like to believe that my professional work over the past several decades has, indeed, promoted social justice and change and that I have helped students, clients, and colleagues to name themselves, their experiences, and their truths. I rejoice that I am in a profession that begs me to learn about myself and others continually. And I am especially grateful when my sisters tell their stories publicly, because it is a deeply radical act that restores to women the power to name.

Every single story in this volume speaks to me in some way. The thwarted mothers, the silence and family secrets, the struggles with immigrant parents and grandparents, the issues over appearance and socioeconomic background, the ambivalence about religion in one's life, the insider–outsider conflicts, the problem of being defined by others, and the fierce desire to name oneself and one's path, all of these themes have found their ways into my life as well. In reading these stories, I remembered events that I hadn't thought about in a very long time, and I was able to give words to feelings that had resided only dimly on the edge of my consciousness. In short, these stories have encouraged me to name truths about myself and how I came to be the person that I am. Profound thanks to this minyan of women—poets and revolutionaries, all of them.

Looking Beneath the Surface: Trauma, Invisibility, and the Negotiation of Identity in the Minyan

PRATYUSHA TUMMALA-NARRA

When I first moved to the United States as a child, I considered my home to be my birthplace in India where I lived with my family for seven years. Later in adolescence, I developed the sense that my home is the in the United States. Since migrating to the United States, I have been periodically asked by Americans of various ethnic backgrounds about the place of my origin, my home. It is the visibility of my physical features, such as my dark skin color, that largely propels this question, which has become a reminder of difference. This question regarding home is one that is perhaps too often asked of people who look physically different in some way from mainstream White Americans and too little of those who bear more resemblance to White Americans. The authors of the minyan collection bring to our attention the nature of invisibility in the experience of many Jewish Americans while the physical and psychological notions of home and identity are transformed, sometimes dramatically, throughout their lives. These women reflect on their life journeys with honesty and depth and welcome the reader to experience the complex ways in which identity is shaped by trauma, persecution, strength and adversity within family dynamics, and resiliency. While each essay contains a unique perspective that illustrates the diversity within the experiences of Jewish American women, two overlapping themes were particularly salient for me, including the experience of trauma and related silence and the influence of migration on identity and invisibility. I am mindful of the fact that my commentary on these narratives is developed against the backdrop of my own experiences as a Hindu, Indian American woman, and psychologist. I deeply appreciate the opportunity to read these narratives as they inform us not only of the nuances of Jewish identity in contemporary times but also raise important questions about identity transformation for those of us who negotiate multiple identities.

TRAUMA AND SILENCE

Several authors describe memories of the Nazi Holocaust (both those recalled by themselves or their family members), the murder of family members, displacement from their homes, the loss of belongings, and exile. In considering the horrors of the Holocaust, the pogroms of the pre-Holocaust era in Europe, and anti-Semitism in the new, adopted country, silence about these traumatic experiences within the family and larger society is profound. Some families, as Marny Hall describes her experience, erased their Jewish identities and adopted new, more acceptable religious and cultural identities as a way to stay safe. Sophia Richman's narrative illustrates the ways in which silence was essential to survival both through the Holocaust and to their adjustment to their forced migration away from home. Richman describes how she and her family had to assume a Christian identity in order to survive death in the Holocaust. This transplantation of identity is an experience shared by many of the authors in this volume. Dorith Brodbar elaborates the point about silence through her discussion of her mother's pain and guilt related to losing family members in the Holocaust, and Judith Glassgold states that the descendants of Holocaust survivors must "accept the gift of life, of not having endured the fate of so many others." These narratives demonstrate the intense impact of survivor guilt across generations, sometimes leaving the younger members of the family confused and anxious. Laura Brown's narrative illustrates the complexity of traumatic experience within the family in the face of negotiating the persecution of Jews on a broader scale.

Dorith Brodbar points out that the silence about the Holocaust does not preclude the internalization of pain among the descendants of Holocaust victims and survivors. Kogan (1993), an Israeli psychoanalyst, has written about the collective memories of the Nazi Holocaust as contributing to a "second generation" of survivors, where many children of Holocaust survivors re-create their parents' traumatic experiences and related affects in their own lives. This dynamic is particularly important in the ways that Jewish Americans negotiate identity, fluctuating from silence of past traumas to vigilance about safety in their present home.

Several authors in this volume extend the silence of trauma to the disavowal of religious identity within the practice of psychotherapy, which has its roots in psychoanalysis. Richman makes the point that the silence about the Holocaust lifted since the 1970s, when survivors were encouraged to tell their stories more publicly. The crisis experienced by Jews around the loss of safety during the decades following the Holocaust is related to the concealment of religious identity in the development of American psychoanalysis and psychotherapy. Freud viewed the participation of the psychoanalytic movement in religion as dangerous and as a threat to the creation of a positivistic discipline (Aaron, 2004; Akhtar & Tummala-Narra, 2005).

Nevertheless, Freud's psychoanalytic theory and technique, as suggested by the minyan authors, is steeped in Jewish cultural traditions, including the practices of dialogue and interpretation. Interestingly, despite the overt dismissal of religiosity by Freud and his early followers, many Jewish psychotherapists have found in psychoanalysis, as Sarah Zarem states, "a secular Jewish home." Other authors in this volume indicate feeling conflicted about psychoanalytic theory but still integrate Jewish values such as the importance of dialogue, critical thinking, and social activism in their feminist understandings of psychological and social problems and, more broadly, into their psychotherapeutic practice. For example, Laura Brown describes the way that *tikkun olam*, the belief in healing the world, as a critical motivator for her professional work. Barbara Sang discusses the influence of the Jewish values of curiosity and learning on her eclectic approach to psychotherapeutic work.

MIGRATION, INVISIBILITY, AND IDENTITY

There are numerous ways in which migration influences the negotiation of identity. The minyan narratives in particular raise issues of loss, marginality, and redefining cultural and religious identity in the adopted land. The traumatic circumstances that surrounded much of the migration of Jews to the United States in part define dilemmas concerning visibility versus invisibility and the experience of alienation versus belonging. These dilemmas are connected to the wish and need to assimilate and to maintaining safety. The narratives speak to how "successful" assimilation often comes at a price, with the loss of connection to culture and history. For instance, Sara Zarem writes about her cultural identifications as a Jew and her disconnection from and her longing for her religious identity. Carol Heffer describes giving up speaking in Yiddish as a way of coping with associations to oppression prior to migration and of easing the assimilation to living in the United States. As I read Zarem's and Heffer's narratives, I was reminded of how I struggled with choosing Indian names for my children, wanting the names to be pronounceable to non-Indians in an attempt to help my children's transitions to mainstream life. At the same time as I was considering these "easier to pronounce" names, I felt resentful about having to potentially compromise my desire to give them names that held deeper, more personal meanings in Sanskrit. The path to belonging is indeed wrought with conflict.

Several of the authors describe their experiences of marginality and feeling like the outsider sometimes within the Jewish community and within mainstream Christian White contexts. The issue of invisibility complicates this experience. Sari Dworkin, in describing an experience of family messages about social activism, writes of her mother's conflict with how much she both wished for her to pursue her activist goals and remain less visible. Concerns about safety in the face of anti-Semitism and assimilation profoundly impact many of the authors' experiences and those of their families, particularly their parents. Kornelia Harari adds that a key means to surviving hatred and discrimination was to be "smarter, stronger, and more successful." This struggle then potentially contributes to conflicts concerning the extent to which one can be visible with academic or professional success but remain invisible with regard to the practice of one's cultural and religious traditions. While Jewish Americans have not been considered by many people of color to be ethnic minorities, the label of *model minority* that is applied to Asian Americans, comes to mind as we consider the duality of Jewish Americans' overt success in mainstream society and the invisibility of loss and conflict.

The issue of invisibility is even more pronounced in the case of negotiating multiple social identities and privilege. The minyan authors raise our attention to the complex intersectionality that characterizes identity as shaped by culture, religion, language, gender, sexual orientation, race, and social class and often across different geographical areas and time periods. In a sense, retaining one's identity inclines the individual toward being seen by others as different while assimilating to mainstream context implicates invisibility. The experience as the "other" is one that pervades many of the authors' experiences within and outside the Jewish community. The authors highlight conflicts around trusting others that are rooted in historical persecution of Jews and ongoing anti-Semitism. Ellen Cole, in her description of being Jewish in Arizona and Alaska, notes her unconscious and conscious attempts to "scan" her surroundings for other Jewish people. The seeking out of others from familiar cultural backgrounds is salient for many groups, indicating a need for "refueling" (Akhtar, 1999).

Several authors in this volume suggest that their Jewish identity feels more salient in certain contexts, while less relevant or outside of conscious awareness in other contexts. These contexts include physical spaces, peer interactions, and intimate relationships. Many of the authors discuss the difficulty of separating their Jewish identity from their lesbian identity, as they are identified with both even when social circumstances demand that they privilege one aspect of identity over another. Geographical location is also relevant, as Julie Ancis in her narrative offers her experience of being Jewish as notably different while living in New York City when compared with living in the South. The presence or absence of Jewish identity is further connected to privilege, which contributes to the problem of invisibility. In her narrative, Louise Silverstein describes her experience as an adolescent of being berated for showing romantic interest in an African-American boy and subsequently avoiding this friend to manage her own feelings as an outsider. Her understanding of this experience as one that involved her choice as a White woman with privilege contributed to her later interests in racism and sexism in her professional work. In this sense, the experience of invisibility becomes suppressed with the adoption of White identity and accompanying privilege.

In a similar vein, the narratives raise questions about changing constructions of race and racial groups in the United States. The authors speak to a largely conscious awareness of race and privilege as important to their developing identities as Jewish woman and psychotherapists. The notion of race, in contrast to culture, is precarious, as suggested by Carol Heffer, who points out the use of race as a rationale for the Holocaust. Race is perhaps a category that has been both consciously and unconsciously avoided in coping with the aftermath of collective trauma and the stress of assimilation. As with other minorities, the degree to which race is experienced as significant can vary with physical features. Minyan authors, Judith Glassgold, Sari Dworkin, and Sophia Richman highlight how skin tones and hair textures either serve to protect Jewish women or contribute to increased vulnerability to be physically and psychologically harmed.

The privilege of carrying the distinction between race and culture is unavailable to most people of color in the United States and has complicated the ways in which Jewish Americans are categorized by others. In recent years, several Jewish psychotherapists have challenged the collusion of Jewish cultural identity with mainstream, White Christian cultural values. Langman (1997) suggested that the practice of psychotherapy has erroneously been viewed as originating in White cultural context. He pointed out that Jews and Jewish culture has been noticeably absent from literature on the history of psychotherapy. Friedman, Friedlander, and Blustein (2005) elaborate on the absence of Jewish perspectives in the multicultural counseling literature. The minyan narratives highlight this issue of the Jewish experience remaining invisible despite it's the pervasive influence in psychotherapy practice. It is worth noting that several of the minyan authors reveal an interest in reconnecting with Jewish aspects of identity in more recent years, as have other Jewish psychologists who have discussed the relevance of their Jewish identity in their therapeutic practices later in their careers (Aron, 2004). Perhaps, revealing these truths is only possible later in one's career or in particular time period, reflective of concerns about safety, which I mentioned earlier. The interest in reconnecting with cultural and religious identity may also be seen as an extension of negotiating insider and outsider experiences and finding a sense of professional and personal belonging within the realm of multicultural psychology.

Inherent to this negotiation is one's connection to home. Several of the authors in this volume recall wishing to connect with their Jewish identity throughout their childhood, and one of the important factors in finding this connection involved the identification of home. The search for such a home may have been especially salient in light of the multiple displacements from home faced by many of the authors and their families. The narratives reflect diverse attempts to establish a sense of home and belonging, including visiting Israel, connecting with other Jewish Americans, passing on Jewish cultural and religious practices to children, and finding professional home institutions where one can interact with other Jewish people. Perhaps the authors in the task of writing these narratives have found another way of reconnecting with home and have discovered aspects of their identity that has remained largely out of conscious awareness. The narratives remind us of the importance of this notion of home and how fantasies of home and the re-creation of home are central to the experience of immigrants and their families in facing the challenges of separation from country of origin, related trauma, coping with discrimination, and negotiating multiple new identifications in the adopted land (Tummala-Narra, 2009).

CONCLUDING THOUGHTS

One of the most remarkable features of these narratives involves the resiliency of the authors and their family members. The multidimensional nature of resilience is represented in the narratives, as each author describes a unique approach to coping with loss, separation, and social injustice. For many of these women, participation in social justice efforts and activism are rooted in Jewish culture and history. For others, developing a personal relationship with God is experienced as empowering. The search for identity through a connection with Judaism is thought to be critical for many of the women in this volume. It is also worth noting that the minyan authors have worked to actively define their faith through an integration of culture, religious beliefs, and feminism. This plurality of perspective that defines religion and spirituality is echoed in the experiences of women psychotherapists of various spiritual traditions (Rayburn & Comas-Diaz, 2008). Finding one's feminist voice amid difficult social and family adjustments is an important source of resilience for these women. I found it interesting that the encouragement of dialogue within the family context and a sense of rebelliousness fostered by parents seemed to contribute to a sense of liberation and choice in the experience of many of the authors. There are numerous examples of resilience in the face of adverse and traumatic experiences across the narratives, most of which are connected with legacies of parents, grandparents, children, and extended family. Each of the narratives illustrates the fluid nature of identity transformation and the individual and collective resiliency that shapes identity.

A striking aspect of each author's professional life involves her relationship with clients in psychotherapy. Several authors share their dilemmas about self-disclosure about being Jewish, the focus on difference versus similarity between themselves and the client, and the relevance of faith in the therapeutic process. Andrea Bergman writes of her dual identity as an eclectic psychotherapist, feeling like an outsider in both psychodynamic and cognitive-behavioral circles. The question of belonging persists for many of the authors. At the same time, the feeling of being an outsider has also provided insight into and the desire to inquire into the experience of marginalized others (Jews and non-Jews), beyond the surface. Mourning connected with trauma, immigration, and its intergenerational impact is a continual process for these psychotherapists, as their Jewish identity is further transformed through their interactions with their clients. The dilemmas related to invisibility and identity mentioned earlier are relevant to the therapist's interactions with clients, especially when we consider that the subjective experiences of the client and the therapist shape the process and outcome of psychotherapy (Aron, 2004).

The minyan narratives challenge us to reconsider our constructions of identity as more complex than what we experience on the surface, the lasting effects of collective trauma on individual experience and the ways in which dialogue about these experiences is either embraced or dismissed. The authors provide us with a unique opportunity to engage with the diversity of Jewish identity and as such raise important questions about the invisibility and visibility of difference.

REFERENCES

Akhtar, S. (1999). *Immigration and identity: Turmoil, treatment, and transformation*. Northvale, NJ: Jason Aronson.

Akhtar, S., & Tummala-Narra, P. (2005). Psychoanalysis in India. In S. Akhtar (Ed.), *Freud along the Ganges* (3–28). New York: Other Press.

Aron, L. (2004). God's influence on my psychoanalytic vision and values. *Psychoanalytic Psychology, 21*(3), 442–451.

Friedman, M. L., Friedlander, M. L., & Blustein, D. L. (2005). Toward an understanding of Jewish identity: A phenomenological study. *Journal of Counseling Psychology, 52*(1), 77–83.

Kogan, I. (1993). Curative factors in the psychoanalyses of Holocaust survivors' offspring before and after the Gulf War. *International Journal of Psychoanalysis, 74*, 803–814.

Langman, P. F. (1997). White culture, Jewish culture, and the origins of psychotherapy. *Psychotherapy, 34*(2), 207–218.

Rayburn, C. A., & Comas-Diaz, L. (2008). *Woman soul: The inner life of women's spirituality*. Westport, CT: Praeger.

Tummala-Narra, P. (2009). The immigrant's real and imagined return home. *Psychoanalysis, Culture & Society, 14*(3), 237–252.

Leah with an "H" or How I am Jewish, But Not Really

LEAH M. FYGETAKIS

To the wonderful minyan of women who looked within yourselves to write your stories, I have to say, "You had me at hello." To be honest though, you've had me at hello for a very long time.

If Sara Zarem of Chapter 1 is the yin, I am her yang. I begin my commentary with a remembrance of my college fencing days where 3 of my teammates (out of 12) were Jewish. On the very first day that we met as a newly selected team, a teammate said to me, "It's pretty cool to have more than one Jew on the team. I know Lisa and Gail are, and you are, too, right?" I replied, "Well, no, actually I'm Greek." "But your name is Leah." "Yes, it is. I was named after my grandmother, Evangelia," I answered. "But you spell your name with an 'h'?" "Yes," I said. "Well, that's not Greek, that's a Hebrew name!" She was emphatic about it. While this was news to me, from the perspective of being Greek, she had a very good point. Every other Greek woman who I had known to be named Evangelia, or with another name that ended in "lia," spelled the shortened version, "Lia." There was no "h."

Over the years there have been other times when people have assumed that I am Jewish because of my name (or could it be something else)? As the story went, my older cousin convinced my immigrant parents to spell it that way because a three-letter name would be too short and Leah would provide a spelling that was "more American." I now know that her insistence was likely due to her discomfort in having an identifiable "Greasy Greek" name herself, which had cost her entrance to such groups as the Junior League to which she had aspired to join. If she could erase the Greekness of one of my names, perhaps her younger cousin would stand a better chance at being able to move in the right social circles, especially if I were to marry a Smith or a Jones and take his last name.

I identify very strongly with my Greek ethnicity. I have presented at the American Psychological Association and I have written about the complexity of holding multiple identities for those who are female, Greek, and lesbian. In a chapter titled "Greek-American Lesbians: Identity

Odysseys of Honorable Good Girls" (Fygetakis, 1997), I began with a story describing my attendance at a lecture in 1984 by Evelyn Torton Beck, editor of *Nice Jewish Girls: A Lesbian Anthology* (1982). After her lecture, I happened to exit the auditorium at about the same time as her. Immediately she was rushed and encircled by the Jewish lesbians in attendance. There I was in the midst of such joy, energy, excitement, and a cacophony of laughter and conversation. It had the warm, loving feel of belonging to a group of one's own people. It was the feeling I used to enjoy being among other Greeks before things got complicated by identifying as a lesbian. I so wanted to bask in the joy of that feeling again, but I knew that I did not really belong.

Now, 25 years later, that longing remains. When the editors of this little tome gave me a sneak preview of this book, within the first couple of hours of reading, I sent an e-mail to them. I couldn't put it down. It had me laughing and crying and it brought me back to my age old question "Where are *my* peeps, damn it?!" What I would give to have a dinner table of Greek feminist friends to discuss the variations in our families, our cultural experiences, and how this informs our work. In Judaism, there are Orthodox, Conservative, Reform, and Reconstructionist approaches for religious thought and expression. For Greeks, there is only orthodoxy. For Greek Americans, in order to have access to one's people outside of family, it usually means going to church. Greek American communities are mostly centered around their churches. In orthodoxy, traditional sex roles remain in place. In this context, it is rare to find feminists. It is rarer still to find lesbians who will come out, even only a little so that we may find one another. Oh, to dream that Greeks like me could have the equivalent of that which is possible for Jews, to have enough variation in Greekness as there is in Jewishness that I could find an easier way to meet kindred spirits in feminist thought and in agape (genuine affection, love). The editors' response to my enthusiasm was to invite me as a late addition to the commentary, giving me a one-week deadline to read the book in its entirety and to write my piece. So, most likely, what I write will be published close to raw, original form. Perhaps, in this case though, it is better to speak from the uncensored heart than from schooled intellect.

Every therapist in this book has engaged in the self-reflective journey elicited by the questions "What does it mean to be Jewish" and "How am I Jewish?" From the perspective of a non-Jew, I started musing on my own variations of the theme. Can Jewishness be claimed outright on the basis of coming into the world through the birthing-blood of the mother who is Jewish? Is that necessary and/or sufficient in making one Jewish? My children were borne from the loins of an agnostic Jew and the seed of an anonymous Greek donor, a decision my partner and I made together. She gave me her permission (to say she gave me her "blessing" would not be quite accurate in this case) to have them baptized in the Greek Orthodox Church. Another question: can Jewishness truly be claimed through religious conversion? Some Christians convert to Judaism. When this occurs, does this make them Jewish? Alternatively, is it possible that one who is not Jewish can feel and claim Jewishness through a similarity in experiences and a sensibility with the Jewish people? If so, then I may be Jewish.

MY FAMILY HISTORY OR "THE GREEK CHORUS" TO THE JEWISH EXPERIENCE

What is a "Greek Chorus?" Wikipedia informs us that

> plays of the ancient Greek theatre always included a chorus that offered a variety of background and summary information to help the audience follow the performance. The Greek chorus comments on themes, and shows how an audience might react to the drama. The chorus also represents, on stage, the general population of the particular story. In many of these plays, the chorus expressed to the audience what the main characters could not say, such as their hidden fears or secrets. The chorus often provided other characters with the insight they needed. (http://en.wikipedia.org/wiki/Greek_chorus)

All four of my grandparents were Greek. My mother's parents decided to give the land of opportunity a try and so it came to be that my uncle and then one year later my mother were born in the United States. However, within a few short years, my grandparents felt homesick for Greece and decided that they would prefer to return. My mother was about three or four years old. After their return, another two siblings were born.

The family lived in Thessaloniki (Salonika), Greece. This is a port city in the northern part of the mainland. It is second in size to Athens. Prior to World War II, the city's cultural makeup was an interesting blend of cultures, still evident by some of the old architecture that remains. In some areas, one can see churches, mosques (from the 400-year Turkish-Ottoman reign), and buildings marked with the Star of David all in close proximity to one another. In the Spanish expulsion of the Sephardic Jews in 1492, Salonika became one of the major areas of their resettlement. My mother had Jewish classmates and girlfriends whom she felt close to. She does not recall any tensions between Christians and Jews. Life was good, and then the German army arrived. Even today, I sometimes have to shake off the feelings of disbelief over what happened next. However, it did happen, and with the help of a Jewish feminist therapist I came to understand my mother and myself with greater clarity.

What follows is not in any particular chronological order. It is a collection of the bits and pieces of oral family history as told by my mother over time and in conversation with my cousins. For context, it was helpful to me when I realized that developmentally, my mother was the same age as Anne Frank.

When my mother was in her midtwenties she returned to the United States for her brother's wedding. While here, she met my father and they married. During my childhood, whenever we visited my grandparents in Greece, there was the ongoing mystery of "The Door." My grandparent's home was the middle flat of a three-family building. One of the bedrooms had a door that remained locked and unused. "Where does it lead?" my cousins, younger sister, and I would ask. We never got a satisfactory answer. As we got older, we realized that the door led to the inner landing and staircase. We thought it was the oddest thing. Why should a bedroom have a direct entrance and exit to the outside?

As we eventually learned, soon after the army's arrival, a German officer decided to appropriate a room in my grandparent's flat as his own for the duration. In some ways, the family was lucky in that he did not kick them out into the street as had happened to some others. With the language gap between a German and a Greek, my grandfather tried to convey that they had lived in America and asked the officer if he spoke any English to see if they could communicate more easily. The rest of the family held its collective breath as the German bellowed, "There will be no English spoken in this house. Verboten!"

The Germans rerouted the family's electric lines to feed them across the street to the barracks that had been set up. The family was forbidden from using any electricity. However, an exception was made for the doctor who lived on the first floor so that he could continue to see patients. In quiet resistance, while the German officer was away, my grandfather continued to teach his children English and on the back side of the apartment. He rigged a line up through the doctor's office window to his bedroom so that he could listen to the BBC and the Voice of America on his radio. My grandmother and the children were terrified that the officer would find out. While that never happened, there were other narrow escapes.

One evening, my grandfather received word that his store was on fire. Curfews were in effect and it was understood that to break curfew put one at risk of being shot on sight. He took that risk and was seen and detained. In the randomness of luck, the soldiers who stopped him were willing to return to his store to check out his story, that he had broken curfew to fight the fire. The other close call involved my mother. Soon after the Germans arrived, they started to gather the Jews into fenced and tented holding areas. One day, my mother and a couple of her girlfriends decided that they should try to find and visit their Jewish girlfriends. Remarkably, they somehow got through a gate unchallenged. They found one of their friends and were happy to be together. Leaving was not as easy. Shouts of "Halt!" rang out and weapons were drawn. Again, in the randomness of luck, a Greek man who was making deliveries recognized the children as ones he knew from the neighborhood and was able to convince the soldiers that they were fool-ish little girls for entering but that they were not Jewish. While both my grandfather and mother were spared, death still befell the family when my mother's younger brother went blind and died of typhus.

As the war went on, everyone was hungry. There was famine, with people begging for food and dying on the streets. Each morning, the German officer would step out and return with food. Then he would leave for his day's work. He expected my grandmother to cook for him and have his dinner ready upon his return each evening. My mother being the eldest daughter helped my grandmother in the kitchen. Psychologically, it was complicated. Sometimes he brought only enough food for his meal. Some-times he brought extra for the family. He ate his meals at the dining room table. However, they never ate together.

Fast-forward to my childhood in Ohio. For years, I could not under-stand why my mother would get so worked up before our extended family arrived for a holiday meal. Being the eldest daughter, I was expected to hold sentry by her side to help her prepare. As the arrival time neared, the greater the tension became. It was very unpleasant. My mother would start yelling at me over things that seemed inconsequential. In turn, at some point, I would explode, "Why do you get so worked up? You act as if it's a matter of life or death. Nobody cares if we eat ten minutes later or if one of your recipes doesn't turn out perfectly. For G-d's sake, it's just family!" Now I know. If I grew up with a gun-carrying oppressor in my home who expected me to feed him a timely and tasty meal each evening, would I feel any differently? As for that mysterious door, apparently it was a point of negotiation between my grandfather and the German officer. The officer began to bring "prostitutes" home for his pleasure and my grandfather did not want his children to witness any of it, so a new egress was constructed. Personally, I suspect that the so-called prostitutes were likely desperate mothers who were trying to find a way to feed their hungry children. Thus, my mother's formative years of sexual awareness were within earshot of a nightly brothel.

I have often wondered how my mother felt in the dead of night while she sat under the dining room table with a shaking floor and rattling furni-ture from the bombs of allies falling? Did she root for the allies to keep returning with their bombs to chase the Germans away, or did she wish for them to stop out of fear that she could die? My mother scared me some-times. Deep in sleep, I would sometimes awaken to the silhouette of my mother hanging her head outside of my bedroom window, gasping for breath. In the beginning I would ask her what was wrong. Her answer was typically along the lines of "I can't breathe, but I'll be fine. I'm here because I don't want to wake up your father. He has to work tomorrow." She didn't sound fine, but what does a child know about panic attacks and posttraumatic stress?

As for my father, he was a quiet, gentle soul. The little he disclosed about the war consists of two pieces of information. One was to tell me that a cousin was taken to a concentration camp and survived to be emancipated. She was not Jewish and he did not know why she was taken there, but he had seen her number on her arm. The other was a tearful admission that while he was apprenticing with a tailor on the island of Rhodes, they were sought out by many Jews to sew their money beneath their coat linings and to hide their gold coins in the halved hollows of large buttons. Everyone knew that the upcoming mandatory "boat trips" planned by Mussolini's Italian soldiers held an aura of foreboding, but everyone went through the motions of preparing, nonetheless.

WHAT WOULD ONE EXPECT FROM ALL THIS *MISHEGAS?*

It was many years before I was able to connect the dots and realize that my mother's wartime experiences had plenty to do with my behavior. Teasing it all out was confusing. My mother isn't Jewish. She was never in a concentration camp. Neither one of us would go so far as to claim that she is a Holocaust survivor. Yet, the outcome and my transgenerational inheritance of her experience vibrate within us as woeful as the sound of two parallel violin strings from a musical score of Schindler's list. My mother did not experience the degradation of the Jewish people but she did suffer from other losses: the loss of safety, the loss of a carefree childhood, the freedom of movement, the freedom of speech, and the death of her brother from the same scourge prevalent in the concentration camps. While most of these losses can be attributed to the war in general, they were further accentuated within the home by the fact that she had no choice but to live imprisoned (psychologically) under the presence of a Nazi, his gun, and his rules. Similar to what Kornelia Harari describes in her essay, because I knew my mother suffered so much, I tried very hard to be good and not to do anything that might cause her heartache. Like Ellyn Kaschak, I quickly learned that curfews were not to be broken. Does this have a familiar ring?

HOW HAS THIS INFORMED MY WORK AS A THERAPIST?

My lessons are similar to those that have been expressed by others. To be an effective therapist, one must first and continually work on her own person. It was important for me to walk up and touch the elephant of pain from many different angles to understand my mother, myself, and our relationship. Could I have come to my understanding of that pain and my newfound respect for my mother's strength and resiliency without a Jewish therapist?

Would a non-Jewish therapist have spotted and understood the magnitude of importance to keep me going back to that place of darkness for as long as it was necessary? Perhaps, but not as likely. I also believe that by having a Jewish therapist I could trust her repeated refrain that I should not minimize this because it was not on the same level of suffering and the price paid by the Jewish people. I was repeatedly reminded that I had the right and in some ways the responsibility to explore my family's story and my family's pain, for in the end, we are all one humanity.

I can directly point to that piece of personal work as informing my work as a therapist. I think about how I was able to help a Bosnian refugee with a deep-felt survivor's guilt over the annihilation of her village. She broke through to be able to claim her right to be happy and she permitted herself to celebrate her extraordinary success in the United States. My personal work helped me understand a college student struggling with having his father held as a political prisoner by a new regime, and it guided my instincts in pursing many less dramatic but equally important stories woven in the lives of my clients.

FINAL THOUGHTS

In closing, I feel a great affinity for Jewish people. Beyond the beckoning feelings of having some similarity in history, I have other points of connection as well. In my dating history with women, my most significant and promising relationships have been with Jewish women, including my partner of 18 years. Her extended family hails from the Borscht Belt of the Catskills. The warmth, the storytelling, the humor, and the teasing that I experience with them fills my heart.

I also know that I am drawn to the driving force of the Jewish woman who lives in the spirit of *tikkun olam*. I am happy to be in the presence of other women who strongly identify in their ethnicity as it creates the space for me to contemplate and express my own. During those times when Jewish lesbians are not trying to carve out some "alone together" time, I stand with them. I revel and soak up what I can to soften the feelings of longing for the existence of an equivalent Greek lesbian community to which I could belong, and sometimes it is enough.

REFERENCE

Fygetakis, L. M. (1997). Greek-American lesbians: Identity odysseys of honorable good girls. In B. Greene (Ed.), *Ethnic and cultural diversity among lesbians and gay men: Psychological perspectives on lesbian and gay issues* (Vol. 3). Thousand Oaks, CA: Sage Publications.

Speaking Truth to Power in the Minyan

JANIS SANCHEZ-HUCLES

Ellen Kaschak states that writings by women therapists who are Jewish are not ordinary. It is easy to agree as these essays are extraordinary. They capture the diverse experiences of women with ancestors from Europe and Israel as they were raised in the United States. The intricate paths are traced along the lines of identity to families, religion, and culture. Most of these authors acknowledge their cultural ties to being Jewish, but several surprise themselves in realizing how strong an impact the Jewish philosophies have had in shaping their therapeutic styles. These women comment on how they now better understand the weavings of gender, ethnicity, race, sexual identity, class, and other dynamics in their lives and in their clients. They express a strong allegiance to social justice, *tikkun olam* (helping people), and feminism. Many cite secrets in their family histories, and they are committed to knowing, to remembering, and to questioning. They are rescuers, caretakers, and self-healers and have complex relationships with their mothers, fathers, siblings, and grandparents.

I found myself intrigued by these stories because I grew up in a suburb of New York City with a strong Jewish population. School was not held on Jewish holidays, and I was given a wonderful education on the Jewish faith from a series of child publications that my mother secured for me to read. I had Jewish friends throughout my schooling and we traversed bar mitzvah's, bat mitzvah's, and sweet 16 parties together. I also took 4 years of Latin with a class of Jewish men. But despite this exposure and friendship, we rarely talked about what being Jewish was like or what being African American meant even during the confrontations of the late 1960s and early 1970s.

My sense of self was related to my family, and I came from a large family. I became the eldest of six children when my older brother died at the age of three, when I was two. My parents added two sisters and three brothers to our family. Each of my parents came from a family of six with three females and three males. Life was filled with family gatherings at my grandmother's house or at one of my aunts' homes. My identity was also related to being Episcopalian, as my grandmother helped start the Black Episcopal

Church in my home city. I grew up with weekly attendance at Sunday School followed by church with communion and catechism every Wednesday.

My racial identity ranged from understanding that I was "Colored," "Negro," "Black," and African American. There have been discussions all of my life on the meaning of my skin tone, facial features, shape of body parts and facial features, and hair texture and length. There were ways in which I was different from the diverse White friends I had in how I styled my hair, what I ate, and a sense of my history as an African American. I knew that other people noted my skin color and often made assumptions. Interestingly, this happened across race with a Black substitute teacher asserting that I would eventually have a "houseful of children" and a Spanish professor noting that many minority students would not be successful in college because they came from deprived backgrounds. I learned early on to develop my own sense of self to protect myself from the projections of others.

It was during the time period when I was in college that my own identity was being shaped into the African American activist who joined "sit-ins" for important causes. During this time I was also exposed to the sexism of the Civil Rights movement, which I initially accepted, albeit with some reservations. The move to embrace feminism, for me, took years and was helped considerably by Nancy Bazin at Old Dominion University who persisted in inviting me to speak to her Woman's Studies classes. My own journey into a deeper appreciation of my multiethnic consciousness as African American and Cuban, my rejection of sexism by all men and women, and my identification with feminism occurred over many years and deep soul searching. It was therefore fascinating to read about these women's quest to understand their identity as Jewish from multiple perspectives.

In this short commentary, several important themes are discussed. I will explore the authors' views on Jewish identity from a cultural, ethnic, and religious perspective. The focus is on how being Jewish, in whatever form, has had an impact on the therapist's life and style of conducting therapy. I also explore how ideas on social justice and feminism are reflected in their perceptions on healing. Finally, I will touch on the relationships of these therapists to their families and how the dynamics of these arrangements have influenced therapeutic styles.

JEWISH IDENTITY

It was startling to observe how many of the therapists in this volume began their essay with the introduction that they identify culturally with being Jewish but not religiously. These identifications are important as they shape therapeutic styles, relationships with clients, and strategies for conducting therapy.

How does Jewishness affect therapeutic styles? Many of these therapists articulate a sense of Jewish philosophy, values, and way of life. For a large segment of these authors their parents and grandparents were free thinkers, Marxist, or activists in leftist organizations. Several of these women ascribe to a secular humanism in which God does not play a part, but ethical, social, and ethnic traditions are highly valued. There was also a strong sentiment that all were children of God and that Jewish individuals had a unique sense of ethical fairness.

For Dorith Brodbar, becoming a psychologist fulfilled her passion to "listen to stories" as she did growing up hearing Jewish relatives. Her mother's stories of the war and of having her war trauma dismissed because she survived strengthened Brodbar's resolve to listen to the voices of clients who are often silenced around their pain. Kornelia Harari and her brother became more identified with the Jewish faith than either of their parents. Harari was strongly affected by her mother's care for her parents after the Holocaust and her father's perfectionism. For her, her career as a therapist models a repetition of her mother's caring and her father's issues of perfectionism. A sense of Jewish identity was delayed for Marny Hall who did not learn that she was Jewish until age 30, but she asserts that this secretive identity prepared her well to be a therapist. She has become a social constructivist and a narrative therapist.

Shanee Stepakoff talks about her life as a therapist from the context of the relatives who preceded her. Most poignantly, her father died of an apparent suicide attempt and she, her brother, and mother did not talk about her father's death. Stepakoff brings these firsthand experiences of silence with her as a therapist to help clients speak truth from their traumas. Silence about trauma is a theme that resonates throughout the stories.

Sara Zarem observes that Jewishness first imparted a "reverence for learning and education" that led her to secure a doctorate, but her practice of therapy was deeply affected by her mother's silences about her past, her relatives, and what they endured. This has set up a unique tension for Zarem as she seeks to both know and not know her clients. Zarem's work has led to a very diverse and fluid style of therapy and to help clients think for themselves. Barbara Sang describes herself as following the Jewish traditions of education for herself, questioning things, and of giving back to others. This began early for her and allowed her to use her writing, presentations, and clinical practice to challenge the notion that lesbian or gay sexual orientation was a disease.

For Sari Dworkin everything was connected to her Jewish identity and she observes that many Jewish youth had communist or socialist parents as she did. She learned from her father to donate to charity by placing money from her allowance into the Tzadaka box and thus embarked on a commitment to give to those less fortunate and to develop a career that helped others.

Facing reality, storytelling, and conversations were important parts of Paula Caplan's upbringing. She learned from the larger Jewish community the importance of social justice and to advocate on the behalf of those who were oppressed. Caplan was personally inspired by her parents who were community activists.

Some of these therapists encountered a disconnect in their attempts to adopt the Jewish religion. For Rachel Siegel, it wasn't until her children were grown that she connected with feminism, began writing, and questioned male dominance in Jewishness and psychotherapy. She has helped change roles in Jewish services that were restricted in the past to men and she practices feminist psychotherapy.

Ellen Kaschak learned to embrace Jewish ethnicity and culture but believes that the religion historically belonged to men. She now practices Buddhism as her spiritual practice but she is deeply committed to social justice (*mitten drinnen*), psychology, and feminism. Iris Goldstein Fodor indicates that her brother was the favored child but she was able to persist in her schooling and earn a doctorate. From a career as a model she emerged as a feminist in the late 1960s and began writing about women's issues. Today, she also practices Buddhism and recognizes that many of her teachers are Jewish.

INSIDER–OUTSIDER STATUS AND MULTIPLE IDENTITIES

Many of these therapists have felt like outsiders, on the margins and periphery because they were unlike other Jewish individuals or unlike the majority group of Christians. Barbara Sang was an outsider who did not follow gender stereotypes for girls, was very different from her brother, recognized class and racial differences and insensitivity, and did not eat Jewish food. Despite not feeling as though she belonged, she learned to trust her own instincts and developed an eclectic and fluid therapy model. Her process-oriented education and the Jewish tradition promotes a practice in which she gives back to others. For Andrea Bergman, she feels both affiliation and alienation with her sense of Jewish identity that mediated her decision to become a clinical psychologist straddling two theoretical orientations. In relationships to clients she is both connected and an outsider.

The advantages of marginality were touted by Hannah Lerman as she was able to observe the largely Christian world that she operates in from a distance. Lerman comments that this perspective of looking into a world as an outsider is critical as a therapist. Sophia Richman and her mother pretended to be Catholic to avoid persecution during World War II. This definitely introduced a sense of "otherness." Richman believes that these complex roles of concealment versus disclosure has led many survivors of the Holocaust generation into the mental health field as rescuers, caretakers, and self-healers.

For Louise Silverstein, her quest for "insider status" to deal with growing up as French, Catholic, and Jewish, has helped her accept the ambiguity and complexity of life and of doing therapy. She has learned to block blame, focus on self, and take responsibility to mobilize the power to change. The feeling of being an outsider, the dynamics of affiliation and alienation, and of being the keeper of secrets were key to the career path of a clinical psychologist for Andrea Bergman. Carol Heffer also notes her outsider status, issues of trust with others as a therapist, her pride in being Jewish and her quest for learning and knowledge as survival tools and part of her Jewish inheritance. Heffer recognized that always asking *why* was part of her heritage. Barbara Rodriguez asks if she is Jewish, despite a long lineage of Jewish forbears. She learned respect for learning, to use her skills in the service of others, and to better humankind but challenges those aspects of Jewish traditions that she feels marginalize people of color, brought home to her as the mother of mixed race children and the wife of a man of color.

Laura Brown notes that Jewishness informs her ways of relating to knowledge and how she conducts herself as a therapist, feminist, and lesbian. But because she is an outsider in so many ways, she cannot "otherize" her clients. Instead, she creates an "inside" in which therapy can happen. The ability to tolerate conflicts of identity is critical according to Judith Glassgold. She reflects that each individual must build on the spaces of their combined experiences, be they social justice or lesbian identities and to act in spite of fear. Marsha Mirkin exhorts therapists to help individuals to speak truth to power and reminds us that women must question both what is spoken and not spoken.

Julie Ancis brings regionalism to her discussion of a Jewish identity. Being Jewish from the Northeast is different from practicing this religion in the South. Her identity is made more complex by adding that she is a world traveler, a feminist, liberal, a mother, and a multicultural scholar and teacher who wonders how others will understand her identities. Ancis often also feels like "the other" because of her multiple identities. She is able to note parallels and differences among experiences that she has versus those of others and builds on these experiences to teach multicultural competence. Ellen Cole, like Ancis, grew up in New York surrounded by other Jewish individuals. But as she moved from larger Jewish population centers she became more interested in connecting with other Jewish women and other outsiders. Cole notes that a Jewish identity becomes more important to her and her work in cities where the population of Jewish people is limited.

Claire Holzman acknowledges the diverse definitions of Jewishness in her quest to understand her identity and discuses the areas of persecution, ethnicity, religion, and race. She quotes Kantrowitz (1992) in asserting that Jewish individuals are the closest of the "coloreds" to White or the closest of the Whites to "coloreds". Her thoughts on different races led to her famous work on White privilege. Holzman read of the parallels between her faith and the traditions of psychoanalysis and continues to be engrossed in helping clients decipher the stories of their lives. She is able to ask taboo questions, bring up banned topics, and help individuals better understand what is not clear.

Beth Firestein asserts that her status as the rabbi's daughter has colored her positions in life. She identifies as Jewish, bisexual, and a feminist. Firestein observes that there appears to be a high Jewish representation in feminist organizations that she believes reflects *tikkun olam*. It is interesting that working as a psychologist appears to Firestein to be similar to her father's work as a rabbi. She counsels, accepts, and provides a respite to allow people to accept self and divinity. This journey of identity has allowed her to reclaim and integrate her own Jewish identity.

SOCIAL JUSTICE AND FEMINISM

The majority of the authors in this volume self-identify as feminists, and many are involved in feminist therapy. In fact, they believe that Jewish women are overrepresented as the espousers of progressive values. A commitment to social justice and feminism is in accord with intellectual values and curiosities. Several note that in feminism and feminist therapy that they have the tools and training to better appreciate their Jewish history and identity. This orientation stems from a dedication to *tikkun olam* and to fight against any form of discrimination. Many learned from their parents and grandparents to be activists and to fight racism, classism, sexism, homophobia, and anti-Semitism.

These women were also nontraditional and often followed their mother's or grandmother's pattern. They grew up on cultural stories of joy, pain, and struggle that were transformed into sagas of feminine strength and endurance. Many felt that they were "not a typical" girl. Some were tomboys, while others felt unconstrained by convention to choose whom they would love: males, females, or both; Jewish, Christian, or neither. The sense of "otherness" led them to think about whom they could trust and to a desire to learn and ask why as a first step toward wisdom. The Orthodox faith supports religion and education for boys. In some cases the fact that male children were preferred gave these women the push to secure their own educational goals and to pursue a quest for a more spiritual orientation.

Some of these therapists had mothers, fathers, and other family members who suffered from depression, anxiety, personality disorders, schizophrenia, and even suicide. Their experiences with these individuals also helped guide them into work as therapists. For one therapist, her work has led to providing aid to international and marginalized individuals who are often the victims of torture. This represents her way of pursuing social justice for many in need through her work as a therapist.

Many of these authors grew up in women-centered worlds where male impact was minimal or absent. They learned that women were powerful and competent and they were deeply affected by their mothers. They learned to "know and remember" as a protection from loss and trauma. For others, it was a strong male figure who influenced their development, and they sometimes identified with their father and his interests. Some internalized their father's ethics and felt morally obligated to find higher paths. We also can see that for some of these women, it was the keeping of secrets about the father's and grandfather's violence or of the fluctuation of concealment and disclosure that affected their careers and views of feminism.

Another interesting aspect of identity is derived from how these women appeared to others. For some with blonde hair and Eurocentric features it was easy to pass as non-Jewish. Other women looked ambiguous, Lebanese, Arab, Latina, or mixed race. It was interesting to note that several women have become actively involved in the "Be Present" movement that was originally started by Black women but is now open to all.

A unique perspective is noted by one author that being Jewish made it easier for her to be a lesbian. She has learned to tolerate conflicts between identities and to create her own spaces. Another woman notes that she has always been able to reject projected shame about her sexual orientation and believes that being different is a source of pride and celebration. Another perspective is that Judaism was invisible in the lesbian community, and lesbianism is often invisible in the mainstream Jewish community.

There were also wide divergences among siblings with respect to identifying as Jewish. For some families, Jewish identity became a secret. But others noted that there was something about their Jewish identity that drew them to others like them and to those who were "other" by some type of minority status. This feeling also increases with age as women view their selves and their relationships and look for deeper meanings. The Jewish tradition of asking questions led many of these women to the desire to be both a feminist and a therapist.

This discussion has focused on how the diverse experiences and understandings of being Jewish have affected the orientations of these women as therapists. I also examined how relationships with relatives have had an impact on the philosophies and styles of therapy that were adopted. I focused on how perspectives on social justice and feminism are reflected in commitments to health and healing. These women differ in their identification with the Jewish faith with respect to religiosity and culture. They share a belief in making the world a better place and advocating for the ideals of feminism and social justice. Most confess to a sense of being an "outsider." But given the multiple oppressive systems that we as women face, perhaps, as Paula Caplan notes, being outside is the best place to be.

REFERENCE

Kantrowitz, M. (1992). *The issue is power: Essays on women, Jews, violence, and resistance* (1st ed.). San Francisco, CA: Aunt Lute Books.

Healing the Self, Healing the World:
A Feminist Journey

LILLIAN COMAS-DÍAZ

> The best teachers of humanity are the lives of great (wo)men.
> —Charles H. Fowles (in Cook, 1997)

The memoirs in this anthology narrate stories of loss, uprooting, connection, and transformation. As these women struggle, they find strength; as they mourn, they find meaning. The essays in this collection take us through a healing course where identity evolves out of context. These are the stories of women who embark on a feminist journey to heal themselves and heal their world.

These women struggle against patriarchy, anti-Semitism, classism, sexism, heterosexism, homophobia, xenophobia, and other forms of oppression. Several women experienced what Adrienne Rich (1967) called the split at the root—the fragmentation of a Jewish female identity. To illustrate, Louise Silverstein discussed her identity development while negotiating two different sets of families—a split between being Jewish and Catholic. Likewise, Sari Dworkin experienced a dichotomy between being a Jew and a lesbian. Andrea Berman reported feeling like an outsider but also feeling connected. Moreover, as she described the geography of her life, Ellyn Kaschak asserted that while visiting Costa Rica, locals asked her whether she was a Jew or an American. Likewise Rachel Josefowitz Seigal provided a dramatic example of being split at the root. She was called different names according to her migration context.

Cultural traumatic oppression negates females their right to name themselves. A cultural trauma results from a history of collective oppression leading to ungrieved losses, internalized oppression, and learned helplessness (Duran, 2006). Unfortunately, cultural trauma can graduate into post-traumatic stress disorder. Along these lines, Hannah Lerman asserted that post-traumatic stress disorder is a most significant diagnostic category in the American Psychiatric Association's *Diagnostic and Statistical Manual of Mental Disorders* (APA, 2000).

The narrations in this collection highlight the interaction of context with trauma. For example, cultural trauma can bear adaptive fruits, such as socio-political activism. Several of the women in this collection, among them Paula Caplan and Barbara Levine Rodriguez, identified their working class background as a preamble to their development of a Marxist consciousness. Likewise, passing as a member of another ethnicity is a survivalist response to cultural trauma. Some women in this collection, such as Sophia Richman, whose mother hid her Jewish ancestry and passed Richman as a Catholic during the World War II, described how she survived by passing as a non-Jew. Additionally, passing is a response to a societal pressure to conform. For instance, Sari Dworkin stated that she straightened her curly hair to appear less ethnic. Adrienne Rich (1967) noted that some women straighten their hair to modify their Jewish look.

The contributors in this anthology reexamined their lives as they narrate their trauma stories. Regardless of their diverse backgrounds, these women followed a healing path. They renamed themselves psychotherapists. Indeed, the power to choose our own name is the first sign of liberation (Castillo, 1994). For example, Kornelia Harari, empowered herself when early in her life she decided to become a psychotherapist. Women like Paula Caplan, Ellen Cole, and Shanee Stepakoff empowered themselves through the healing power of words. Specifically, Marny Hall highlighted the healing benefits of storytelling by using narrative approaches in her therapeutic practice. "Writing is sweet," observed Marsha Pradver Mirkin. Likewise, Iris Goldstein Fodor envisioned writing as a process of consciousness and evolution. Indeed, many women in this anthology identified their professional writing as an instrument for social justice.

As I read these women's stories, I witness a feminist identity development. Simply put, these women reformulated their identity going through (a) passive acceptance (being unconscious of oppression), (b) revelation (becoming aware of oppression), (c) embeddedness/emanation, (d) synthesis, and (e) active commitment (Downing & Roush, 1985). Most of these women reach the stage of active commitment through their commitment to *tikkun olam*, the effort to heal the world. Accordingly, Laura Brown expanded her pledge to *tikkun olam* by accepting responsibility toward the Other. Indeed, these women's Jewish cultural legacy of having been strangers in Egypt, taught them to embrace the Other.

The goal of a feminist identity journey is to heal the self and to repair the world. Similar to the wounded healer's journey, the women in this anthology heal after overcoming the injuries of oppression. Such journey rewards women with the development of cultural consciousness. This process entails an awareness, reclaiming, and celebration of an oppressed ethnicity and culture (Comas-Diaz, 2007). For example, Carol R. Heffer reminded us that when women embark on a healing voyage they navigate the waters of their culture. Consequently, cultural consciousness facilitates females' reconnection with their cultural strengths. To illustrate, Beth Firestein discussed how she learned to transform the injury of a stigmatized identity into a source of cultural pride and a celebration of difference. Likewise, Claire Holzman reported feeling proud of her Jewish community's achievements.

Many of the women in this anthology contributed to the evolution of feminism. For instance, Paula Caplan asserted that learning and teaching are sacred trusts. Likewise, Laura Brown examined the meeting of feminism and spirituality. Moreover, Sara E. Zarem analyzed her countertransference through a multicultural lens. Similarly, Louise Silverstein reframed her insider/outsider status as an asset in her multicultural therapeutic work. Indeed, the marriage of feminism and multiculturalism is a natural evolution. It is not surprising that Barbara Sang, Marsha Pravder Mirkin, and Julie Ancis identified themselves as being multicultural and feminist psychotherapists. Certainly, the collaboration between multiculturalism and feminism promotes healing. The work of Laura Brown, Sari Dworkin, and many others in this anthology attests to this assertion. A daughter of multicultural feminism, Judith Glassgold, subscribed to a liberation therapeutic practice involving Paulo Freire's (1970) critical consciousness and Ignacio Martin Baro's (Aron & Corne, 1994) psychology of liberation. These liberation practices affirm cultural strengths and help women to reconnect with ethnic healing practices.

The *synthesis* feminist developmental stage facilitates the integration of diverse healing approaches into an empowering psychotherapy. To elaborate, Iris Goldstein Fodor discussed how her feminist consciousness helped her to expand her psychodynamic therapeutic framework. First, she embraced behavior therapy and later she added cognitive behavior therapy as female empowerment tools into her psychotherapeutic practice. Afterward, Fodor integrated rational emotive therapy, Gestalt therapy and mind–body approaches into her feminist therapy practice.

I believe that the next developmental stage for feminist therapy will be the incorporation of spirituality into its practice. A spiritual dimension helps women to become whole (Murdock, 1990) and to heal an identity that is split at the root. *The personal is spiritual.* Some of the women in this collection identified themselves as being ethnically Jewish, religiously Jewish, culturally Jewish, and or a combination of these categories. Notwithstanding their self-identification, most of these women seemed to share a spiritual connection. Judith Glassgold identified the role in spirituality as the struggle to find meaning in the midst of chaos and oppression. In a similar vein, Beth Firestein described therapy as a sacred space where clients connect with something larger than themselves. Moreover, Ellyn Kaschak wrote that she sees Buddhist spirituality as an antidote and a way to reduce her inherited cultural sorrow and terror. Likewise, Iris Goldstein Fodor reported finding solace in Buddhism. Based on her interest in Eastern philosophies, Barbara Sang incorporated mindfulness into her therapeutic practice.

Equally, Shanee Stepakoff described her healing work with torture victims as an opening of the heart.

The opening the heart is a spiritual practice. In Buddhism this practice is known as the opening of the heart chakra—the unfolding of love and compassion toward self and other. Besides fostering healing, an open heart welcomes creativity. Interestingly, many of the women in this anthology have resorted to creativity to balance their lives. To illustrate, Shanee Stepakoff writes poetry and is involved in visual and performing arts. Iris Goldstein Fodor uses photography aiming to heal the self and the world. This anthology is replete with more examples.

In conclusion, the women in this anthology are my sisters. A feminist DNA links us. This is an ancient connection, dating back to the Old Testament. To me, the biblical Jewish women are more vibrant, assertive, and courageous than the pious female saints from my Latino Catholic upbringing. As I read their tales, my consciousness was awakened. Consequently, I decided to imitate Judith's bravery, to learn from Queen Esther's diplomacy, and to emulate Miriam's service to her community.

The narrations of the women in this collection take me home. I join them in a feminist celebration where we sing songs of loss, connection, and redemption. As we rejoice, we dance the hora. Dorith Brodbar described the hora as a festive gathering where people join hands and create collective dances passed down from their diverse ethnic ancestries. The guest of honor in this celebration is *solidarity*. My collectivistic culture taught me to extend solidarity to all oppressed groups. As I embrace my own *tikkun olam*, I hear Reverend Martin Niemoller's (1946) words:

> First they came for the communists, and I did not speak out
> because I was not a communist.
> Then they came for the trade unionists, and I did not speak out
> because I was not a trade unionist.
> Then they came for the Jews, and I did not speak out
> because I was not a Jew.
> Then they came for me
> and there was no one left to speak out.

REFERENCES

American Psychiatric Association. (2000). *Diagnostic and statistical manual of mental disorders* (4th ed., text revision). Washington, DC: Author.

Aron, A., & Corne, S. (Eds.). (1994). *Writings for a liberation psychology: Ignacio Martín-Baró*. Cambridge, MA: Harvard University Press.

Castillo, A. (1994). *Massacre of the dreamers: Essays on Xicanisma*. New York: Penguin.

Comas-Diaz, L. (2007). Ethnopolitical psychology: Healing and transformation. In E. Aldarondo (Ed.), *Promoting social justice in mental health practice*, (pp. 91–118). Mahwah, NJ: Lawrence Erlbaum.

Cook, J. (Ed.). (1997). *The book of positive quotations*. Minneapolis: Fairview Press.

Downing, N., & Roush, K. (1985). Form passive acceptance to active commitment: A model of feminist identity development for women. *The Counseling Psychologist, 13*(4), 695–709. DOI 10.1177/0011000085134013

Duran, E. (2006). *Healing the soul wound: Counseling with American Indians and other Native People*. New York: Teachers College Press.

Freire, P. (1970). *Pedagogy of the oppressed*. New York: The Seabury Press.

Murdock, M. (1990). *The heroine's journey: Woman's quest for wholeness*. Boston: Shambhala Publications.

Niemoller, M. (1946). *First they came*. Retrieved on January 6, 2010, from http://en.wikipedia.org/wiki/First_they_came

Rich, A. (1967). *Split at the root: An essay on Jewish identity, Snapshots* (pp. 35–40). New York: W. W. Norton.

Memories, Reflections, and Questions

KAREN FRASER WYCHE

I have been asked to do two things. The first is to comment on these rich narratives of self-disclosure related to these authors' identity as Jewish women as it impacts their lives and their work as psychotherapists. The second is to reflect on what I gained from these stories of identity. As an outsider, an African-American woman, reading these stories I am struck by similarities and differences in how, as women, we chose to construct our identities within our "group" and the distinctions that come from being a Jewish woman versus an African American racial minority woman, an identity I share with other contributors to the commentary of this volume. For this reason, my narrative will focus on issues related to women's identity, those of the Jewish woman in this book, and of my own. I will not discuss issues related to how being a Jewish woman influenced being a psychotherapist, for I thought those narratives were similar.

This is the second time I have contributed to a book about women's discussions of their Jewish identity. The book *Daughter's of Kings: Growing Up as a Jewish Women in America* (Brody, 2007) was the brainchild of Leslie Brody. All contributors were fellows (1995–1996) at the Bunting Institute of Radcliffe College (now subsumed under the Radcliffe Institute for Advanced Study at Harvard). My Bunting sisters who were not Jewish wrote about our interactions with Jewish people that shaped our understanding of the complexity of Jewish women's identity. Then and now I am surprised to read about some of the ambiguity or continued journey regarding Jewish identity among some of the authors both in this book and among my Bunting sisters. In both books, some women articulate no ambiguity. Am I surprised because all of the Jewish women I know seem so confident, smart, assertive, and self-assured? Do I equate these qualities with having a clear picture of what Jewish identity means to them? Is it that my idea of a Jewish woman is a New York woman who happens to be Jewish? I am not sure.

Reading these narratives triggered memories regarding some of the ways my own identity development was shaped. My guess is that the authors in this book thought also about people, situations, family stories, and other life events that vividly became flashbacks of memory once they began to write about themselves as Jewish women. This focus of attention seems less salient for some of the authors whose narrative about themselves as therapists were more elaborate than the narrative about families of origin influencing who they are as Jewish women today. This should not be interpreted as a negative. It is only an observation as a reader. Reading multiple stories of the developmental pathways traveled to reach the current lived experience as Jewish women made me reflect on the pathways that converged to form my identity as an African-American woman. I view my identity as a racial/ethnic woman, an African-American woman. The culture of African Americans (in all of its many permutations and definitions) is subsumed under my ethnicity as a racial minority woman in the United States. This self-identity description is different from the ways these women discuss their Jewish identity. They make a distinction between being a cultural and/or religious Jew.

I enjoyed reading about the family journeys to America, especially to New York City. I started to think about my own family's journey and how that influences my identity. First let me say that on my mother's side, my brother and I were the fourth generation to be born in New York City. My great grandmother was born there (her mother was from Georgia), her children, their children, and my brother and me. My grandmother (DOB 1898) and great-aunt (DOB 1896) were born at 341 West 41st Street in a tenement and a neighborhood that had Black residents at the time. This structure is long gone, but during one of my grandmother's hospitalizations (at Roosevelt Hospital in the same neighborhood), in her mid-90s and with increasingly senility, she kept asking to go home to that address although she had lived in Harlem for over 65 years. Most Whites assume that African Americans, unless from the Caribbean, have migrated to New York from the South. Many have seen Jacob Lawrence's famous paintings of the *Great Migration* series (1916–1919) that depicts Blacks moving in crowds toward trains going to Chicago, St. Louis, and New York. My father and his siblings (8 out of 11) were part of that great migration journey from Georgetown, South Carolina, to New York City. They left for a better life, to escape institutional and noninstitutional racism, and in many situations to save their lives. This was the city of opportunity where African Americans (first called coloreds and then Negroes at that time) could get work and dream about a better future. It was also an exciting place. As one of my uncles told me when I was an adult: "Sugar, you could hear the grass grow in Georgetown." The journey was not on a ship that went through Ellis Island as was the case for the families of the authors in this book. Rather, the journey was on a Greyhound bus with money only for a ticket and to take the A train to Harlem or Bedford Stuyvesant and a phone number for a family member or friend who would house them until work was found. This journey for freedom was experienced by the relatives of the women in this book. All who migrated/emigrated went to ethnic ghettos, as that is where they were allowed to live.

A MINYAN OF WOMEN

The stories of being a Jewish in a Jewish neighborhood had a common theme. Everyone who lived in these neighborhoods knew they were Jewish. How they were Jewish differed based on religion, politics, or behaviors. These distinctions are made salient in the chapters and discussed as part of identifying the variety of ways identity was shaped growing up as Jewish girls and later women. However, to the outside world (Italians, WASPs, Greeks, etc.), the neighborhood was Jewish and the families homogeneous. I lived in a Black, segregated neighborhood in Harlem, but I had many contacts with Jewish merchants who owned stores in Harlem. I was a scholarship student to Ethical Culture School from kindergarten through fifth grade where the Jewish families were the middle and upper class progressive liberals and in living in New York City. As a school-aged child, I saw social class differences between the Jewish community (I assumed all were as wealthy as those in my school or as the merchants who must go home to big prewar apartments at night). My parents lived with my grandparents, uncle, and the renters in my grandmothers' house. To me Jewish people were the successful ones in New York City as I didn't have interactions with other minority or majority groups. In the sixth grade my family moved to rural eastern Long Island so that I could attend public school. Money was tight and my family was told that I wasn't academically strong enough to go to Fieldston, the high school of Ethnical Culture School that I was attending. We were one of the few African-American families who lived there all year round. There I learned of anti-Semitism and experienced a blatant type of racism toward African Americans in this White, working-class factory town with Polish, German, and Italian descendents. I was an outsider on many levels, but especially because I was African American, from the city, and had Jewish friends.

Another common theme for the authors was that of families who had economic resources leaving the ghetto neighborhood for better opportunities in the suburbs. The escape to the suburbs often resulted in the loss of family togetherness (with tension at times) that reinforces ethnic identity for the younger members of any family. I too remember this loss when my parents moved to this rural community. The regular doses of loving social support from the network of grandparents, aunts, uncles, and cousins disappeared. The cultural fabric of intergenerational teaching was minimized. For my nuclear family, there was no longer a buffer for the marital problems of my parents. Their divorce eventually followed. The visits to family in Harlem were scheduled, not spontaneous. As a parent, I attempted to re-create this loss of family comfort and identity inoculation with my own children. It was hard. We lived far away from New York and so I tried to expose our children to their extended family during summers and holidays. It wasn't until my great aunt came to live with us, from New York City of course, at age 95 that my sons really got the intergenerational transmission of ethnic and cultural identity that comes from those who tell the stories of identity within the cultural lens of their life and time.

Outsider status was discussed by many of the authors. It was framed in who knows I am Jewish, should I tell others, should I pass, or are there alternative types of choices that could be made? Generally, most racial minorities cannot pass because they aren't White. Physiognomic features, hair, skin tones, or other visible signs are obvious to the observer who seeks a label to place on people. However there is a history of "passing" among African Americans to find or keep jobs. (Nella Larsen a Harlem Renaissance writer wrote a fascinating book on this titled *Passing* in 1939.) My family's racial minority status was known and viewed as suspect, different, and therefore deviant in the years of my youth. We were too many different shades of skin tones, or hair texture, or eye color, a reminder of slavery's genetic stamp. As a racial minority woman, one's ethnic identity status becomes constructed based on this reality. Family socialization messages are to be proud, be strong, recognize that racism exists, don't be loud or crude, and be respectful. These themes of survival still exist today for parental warnings. What were the parental warnings about being a Jewish woman for the authors? I wanted to know more.

The intergeneration transmission of female Jewish identity differed among the authors. In my reading of these stories the grandmothers were the ones who modeled what a Jewish woman was at their historical time. Mothers were strong, fluid, ambivalent, or secretive in how they thought or behaved as Jewish women, and this conflict still remains for some of the authors. As an African-American woman, the intergenerational transmission of what is my racial and ethnic minority identity as a woman was clear and the teaching deliberate and strategic. I was raised by race women. They socialized me to be proud of my people, to be strong, to strive to achieve my goals, but to remember that the hill would be steep. They wanted me to be more successful than they had been. They told me I could achieve and that I would have to work harder because I was Black and not White. They were right. And "still we rise" continues to be an apt saying for me and my people.

The salience of ethnic identity was discussed by those who have lived where the Jewish community is tiny or practically not existent. One becomes more attuned to finding those like you when there are few of you around. I resonate to this as it has been typical of my experience as an African-American woman in academia. Size matters when you don't see anyone who looks like you on campus. You become aware of the homogeneity and the insularity of much of the United States. Many times, as the only woman of color on the faculty, it is the Jewish women in the university who are my kindred spirits. I know what the High Holy days are they know what Kwanza is. Neither of us has to observe these celebrations; it is the knowing that is important.

The women in this book were asked who they are as Jewish women. So who am I? I am an African-American woman. My racial category is first. That is the category that has the sociohistorical and political salience for my people. Unlike most of the Jewish women in this book, religion doesn't define African Americans as a group; however, it does not define all of the Jewish women either. Race influences my life profoundly, where I have been and where I have yet to journey. Sure, it is figure and ground sometimes. In a room of strangers of only men I am aware that I am the only woman, but then I look to see how many men of color are there. Sometimes I am counted twice for other's gain. In affirmative action hiring forms I can be checked off in the category "woman" and "African American/Black." Both African American and Jewish women are victims of discrimination and stereotyping. However, our identity searches are uniquely ours. There are no right or wrong answers. We reflect, looking back to look forward. These stories have much to offer in self-reflection.

REFERENCE

Brody, L. (2007). *Daughters of kings: Growing up as a Jewish woman in America.* Winchester, MA: Faber and Faber.

The Minyan: Through the Lens of a Black Child of Harlem

FRANCES K. TROTMAN

I have never understood why Black/African American people all look alike to people who are not group members. There are multitudes of different combinations of various colors, tones, shapes, and styles that make up and differentiate the people defined by the "one drop rule" as Negroes. As this wonderful and similarly varied collection of "Jewish" histories, events, life-styles, and relationship to Judaism attests, knowing that someone is Jewish tells us both very little as well as, potentially, a great deal about her. These stories of and by brilliant, thoughtful women, as Ellen Kaschak wished, do complicate the dominant narrative, explicating the connections between family dynamics, the development and consolidation of one's identity, and the effects of that identity on their psychotherapy practices. As the editors intended, by expanding the minyan to include multiple women's voices, this volume illuminates a wide spectrum of ways to experience oneself. Each contributor has examined her personal journey to the present understanding of who she is as a Jewish woman and what kinds of experiences were salient in shaping her. Their collective brilliance, thoughtfulness, and simplicity encourage all psychotherapist to explore our own journeys while shedding light on every reader's understanding of what it means to be Jewish.

Beverly Greene's description of her childhood implies a cultural pride that I did not experience in my 1940s and 1950s childhood in Harlem. My Harlem childhood was darker, more filled with anger, shame, and self-hatred. The only history that I remember overhearing about was the stories about the lynchings, abuse, mutilations, and degradation of Negroes, atrocities that we (Negroes) were somehow responsible for. Corporal punishment, as practiced and passed down from the slave master, was very much a part of a Harlem Negro child's experiences during the 1940s and 1950s. Just as Beverly and I can be very similar and share a common heritage yet grow up with very different visions of what that heritage is and what it means, this volume illustrates that the Jewish women who share these stories have different visions of their heritage despite common cultural bonds.

I am a medium/light-skinned, heterosexual, African American psychotherapist. Although I was baptized in my youth and am technically a Christian, I do not practice any formal religious faith. My hair is not kinky as is typical among African Americans but is straight in texture with natural curls. My hair texture and its very light brown to blondish color, I think, leads many people to view me as racially ambiguous, hard to pin down precisely. Yet a disproportionately large portion of my clients are combinations of women who identify themselves as White, Jewish, and I have a large number of LGBT clients. I and the larger society do not identify me with any of those categories. Other than one Jewish client who was the daughter of a very well-known prominent rabbi who came to me to "hide her therapy" from her tight-knit community, many of my clients have assumed that I shared their cultural identity or they didn't consciously think about it. However, my psychoanalytic training and underpinnings as well as my natural curiosity dictate that I examine some of the possible reasons for the attraction of my clients to me and their unfounded assumptions about similarities between us despite our differences. Certainly issues of oppression, discrimination, shame, and social justice are commonalities with which I have had to grapple. My somewhat ambiguous negritude has also often given me the privilege and responsibility of a choice about how and when I would "come out." These are obvious directions that I will follow as I continue to explore my own personal journey to who I am as a psychotherapist.

My first recollection of being confronted with an identity happened when I was four years old with my aunt Miriam. She took me on a trip to Orchard Beach in New York City (to which we had to take two busses and two trains and still seemed to walk for miles, lugging heavy equipment, food, and drinks). My aunt, who was not really my aunt but my mom's friend who grew up with her in the Negro orphanage, watched me from her beach blanket as I met a new playmate of about six or seven years old. I thought she looked like me, different from my Harlem friends. My new playmate and I played happily in the sand as she placed her arm next to mine to admire my tan. I giggled to tell her that I was not tan, I was a Negro. I still remember the look of horror on her face as she screamed and ran from me to the safety of her parents' arms. I returned to my usually kind aunt's blanket to recount the events. Her response, hiding her own shame and pain, was to angrily yell at me that I should never have told her that I was "a Negro." She and I quickly packed up all of our things and we abruptly left the beach. The possible effects on my self-esteem and identity are obvious. Similar and worse such incidents happened to many of the women in their narratives. The question that I often ask is how we survived such onslaughts to our sense of ourselves, and I wonder if such attacks actually make us stronger and help to account for our "successes."

Different than my aunt's reaction would imply, "passing" for my mother was a definite taboo. As an orphan with issues about rejection and abandonment, my mother ingrained in me that "passing" had dire consequences. It was dishonest and bad and wrong. Her favorite movies were *Imitation of Life* and *Pinky*, which we watched over and over with endless discussions about why I was never to try to "pass." She told me countless stories about people who "passed" and then regretted having to deny their family of origin. I later realized that her admonitions were more an expression of her own fears that I would forsake her for a life of White bliss, free from the degradation and oppression of being a Negro, leaving her abandoned and rejected.

I read each of the Jewish women's narratives to futilely try to discern, through my African American/Harlem/New York City lenses, how much of the influences were geographical versus religious versus familial versus gender-based versus idiosyncratic. Many of the events experienced by the authors resonated with me. Sara Zarem speaks of not comprehending Hebrew, of being a nonbeliever and nonobservant but still being touched by the music and the mood of the culture. Similarly, because my father was raised in the Midwest and my mother by the White nuns in the Negro orphanage, I did not share or grow up on the foods, language, and religion of my Southern Baptist Harlem neighbors. Yet I am very moved by gospel songs of hope amid tremendous struggle and pain. I can actually feel the pain and experience optimism as well as sadness.

African American Gospel songs are a curious mixture of references to Exodus, calling on Moses to lead them/us out of bondage and the New Testament, referring to Jesus as a friend and savior. Rarely is the God the father figure of the Old Testament ever mentioned. I have a theory about the weakened effects of the use of religion to strengthen the patriarchy among African American women as opposed to what I see as its virulence among European-American women. Because of the slave master's and slave owner's need to maintain control over the bodies and minds of enslaved African-American women, religion could not stress allegiance and obedience to a father figure or husband. This may have had the effect of having African-American women experience religion as a solace and hope of salvation but as a less virulent strain of patriarchal indoctrination than that experienced by European American women. This may have contributed to the image of African-American women as relatively strong and independent. These stories have inspired me to devote more thought and exploration to this idea.

Many of our African-American ancestors maintained their hope, resilience, sense of humor, and even patriotism despite the tremendous oppression and discrimination that they endured. The authors and their families have experienced many of the same strengths amid extreme adversity. There are many similarities. Yet there may be some differences in the overall reactions to the horrors heaped on each of the groups, African Americans and Jews. On the surface there seems to have been self-hatred and shame for each of the groups as a result of the horrors imposed on them. Not only were they victimized and brutalized but they were also made to feel responsible for it with the dire psychological consequences that this entails. With the caveat that I am a fairly ignorant outsider, it seems to me that Jewish culture analyzed and recovered (are recovering) from their shame and self-blame at a faster pace than have African Americans. Sophia Richmond's account attests to the fact that Jewish talk of the Holacaust began to surface in about the 1970s along with the slogans "never forget" and "never again." This was fewer than 30 years after the horrific trauma of the Holocaust and recovery began beginning. Yet 100 years after slavery, there still seemed to be little talk of and less public pride in African heritage. If so, reasons for such a state of affairs may have to do with the need to totally dehumanize African Americans in order to justify slavery. A land based on principles of freedom, justice, and equality for all human beings makes slavery a blatant contradiction. The only way out of the cognitive dissonance produced by this state of affairs is to convince oneself and the enslaved that they are not really human. The United States was quite effective at this. For a very long time, most Negroes preferred to not be associated with anything "Black" or "African." Shamefulness surrounded slavery and African heritage until late in the Civil Rights era, the 1960s and 1970s. In the Harlem of my youth, it was considered "fightin' words" to call some one "Black" or to imply that she had African features or were in any way connected to African. When I was growing up in Harlem James Brown's song "I'm Black and I'm Proud," which should have crescendoed in loud, joyous, sounds was initially only whispered in soft, shameful, hushed tones by fearful young people who gradually developed a growing pride and boldness.

Another factor in the ability to and support for the recovery from such horrific trauma such as the Holocaust may be an intact cultural history fostered by literacy and a tradition of written accounts of that history. African Americans were robbed of their history, their traditions, and their ability to record their experiences for posterity. Passing along information about our history and the atrocities imposed on us may have suffered because of the significantly lower levels of literacy than those found among Jews. Jewish people kept their history alive and were actively encouraged to be literate. Literacy among African Americans for the foreseeable duration of slavery was criminalized, and their formal education was made very difficult to obtain.

My first master's degree was in guidance and counseling from the City University of New York, where I learned much more than I did from my subsequent, much more expensive degrees. It was there that I learned how "to be" a psychotherapist. I became friends with one of my professors who was Jewish. To me, all of my other professors were just "White" and male, and he was no exception, although he did not consider himself White. He trained me and supervised my clinical work. My personal identity as a therapist was certainly influenced by him. This took place during the 1960s, and I was very active in the Civil Rights Movement, protesting and getting arrested for the cause. When I discussed with my White friend and professor my dilemma in and mixed feelings about our friendship, he seemed confused and both denied and enjoyed the idea that I considered him "White." To him, he was simply Jewish. To me, he was White.

It is difficult to determine how much of our shared personal identities as women, feminists, and as psychotherapists can account for our similarities and how much our different cultures may have influenced some discrepancies. I have never engaged in the Jewish practice of pilpul (as does Laura Brown) but I do ask questions and think critically. I have a strong commitment to social justice. Has that been influenced by *tikkun olam* indirectly via the many Jewish supervisors and clinicians that I have worked with and for? Several of the women in this volume consider themselves to be both feminists and psychoanalysts. Other feminists may question our decision as feminists to learn and practice psychoanalysis with its obvious sexist tenets, underpinnings, and training. The commonality of our histories of discrimination and oppression may provide clues to some answers to this query. The pain induced by such societal devaluation and inflicted cruelty may require special tools to excavate through the layers of shame, secrecy, trauma, pain, and defense mechanisms to try to uncover it so that it can heal. Such pain must need to bury itself from consciousness. A need to find "reasons" for the "irrational" or just to "try to understand" some things so incomprehensible as the Holocaust or slavery may somehow be an attempt to ease our own pain and disbelief of the horror and the inhumanity of our own life's herstory. Maybe if we can understand, we can heal it, be in control of it, "to speak and to name trauma is healing."

I would like to thank the editors for this insightful volume. I want to also thank the courageous women who dug deep into their often painful pasts to explore and share important issues and factors that can add to our knowledge as helpers and healers. One of my life's quests has been to determine how to develop "resilience" in people—particularly young people—so that we can cultivate and foster it. These very thoughtful, brilliant, and perceptive women have contributed a great deal to the kind of knowledge necessary to inform such an endeavor. By demystifying some of the mechanisms by which they and their families survived horrors to go on to succeed and prosper, they provide access to tools that others may be able to use to in order to succeed despite adversity. As a therapist, a woman, and a feminist, it has been an informative pleasure and a privilege to read and be asked to offer commentary.

Culture and the Self: On Paradoxes and Contradictions

ELAINE PINDERHUGHES

The narratives in this book express with abundant clarity some of the complexities, enigmas, contradictions, paradoxes, and felt sense of entrapment that are endemic in the cultural process and the search for a positive cultural identity. Each of the contributors addresses family of origin history, relationships with family members, and salient experiences from early life to the present that influenced what she experiences as her Jewish identity, her chosen profession as psychotherapist, and how she engages in professional practice. They are particularly informing in their analyses of how they use themselves in the therapy process and how that is connected to their identity as Jewish women. Each personal story provides us with a new prism with which to view the connection between social context, family history/dynamics, and individual identity in terms of cultural perspective and meaning. Together they demonstrate the complexity of Jewish identity and the often contradictory aspects of that experience. They also reveal how much one's personal experiences growing up and then later in life, which is uniquely interwoven with cultural identity and connection, overlaps with our training as psychotherapists and operates as determinants in our professional work.

The reader will learn through these narratives how our experiences of having power and lacking power in family of origin, community, and society (re: social status) and our need to gain a needed sense of power and agency can be pivotal in the evolution of that cultural sense of self that heavily influences our work.

There is an excellent articulation and exploration of the transgenerational transmission of loss, pain, trauma, and survivor guilt as consequences of Jewish cultural experience. As one author observes, there are the "'cutoff' affects belonging to my parents that took refuge in me." One poignant account after another reveals tales of passing as a non-Jew, of embracing another religion to avoid extermination and the consequences of those actions later in life, including Jewish identity formation itself.

The narratives also illustrate many aspects of cultural dynamics that include the relativity and changing nature of identity across the life span and across time for the culture itself. The narratives also reveal a cultural variability; for example, the variation among Jews in the range and degree of religious or spiritual practice to a complete rejection of any religious practice or belief at all. Many authors make a distinction between their identified cultural identity as Jews and their rejection of any religious teaching. While still others credit Jewish values for their own embracing of certain beliefs and behaviors such as ethical values, tenacity, independent thinking, social activism, preferences for certain foods and music, etc.

Another phenomenon illustrated in these stories is the personal struggle of many of the authors to integrate traumatic experiences, both inherited and personal, into a Jewish identity that is positive and clearly defined. There are many descriptions of efforts to reclaim Jewish identity that was relinquished in the search for a better life, in the struggle to avoid extermination, or in an effort to block out painful memories of trauma that had created a range of emotional cutoffs. There is even one example of managing ongoing, personal ambivalence regarding Jewish identity and fear of disclosure. There is also an example of what one author presents as sometimes a reluctance to openly reveal Jewish identity that turns into a dedicated attunement to conflicted identity in clients, a dedicated stance against misunderstanding and not hearing clients fully along with a love of Judaism and other cultures.

Among the many examples of changing a negative identity into a positive one are those describing working toward integrated intersectional identities, such as being Jewish, lesbian, and feminist or Jewish, bisexual, and female, thus embracing another complexity in the identity development of sexual minority Jewish women.

The authors explain how they used their understanding of their Jewishness to understand their attractions to certain treatment modalities, their way of thinking and working with clients, developing therapeutic alliances, and understanding both the client's transference and their own countertransference and as a barometer for the client's progress in treatment. Many of the contributors felt that their Jewish identity was central to their work as one stated, "All I am and all I do."

Among the important contributions of this book are a welcome sense of clarity regarding the application of psychodynamic concepts to cultural self-understanding and cross-cultural clinical work. Another is the way in which the narratives explicate possibilities for understanding the forces of history and transforming victim of history identity, both personal and collective, to agency as well as a transformation of humiliation to compassion for others that was observed directly in Glassgold's narrative. There is also an unusual clarity with which the dynamics of intersectionality as a dynamic in cultural processes is revealed. Overall, we have a collection of experiences that assist all of us in moving toward a perception of culture that is clear while complex and nuanced yet understandable in what is perhaps what Erikson called a human, wider identity.

Mazel Tov

JUDITH L. ALPERT

There is a flurry of interest in understanding how one's experiences, whether maturational, religious, cultural, or other, influence professional practice. Gabbard and Ogden (2009), for example, discuss their understanding of some of the maturational experiences that have contributed to their becoming psychoanalysts in their own terms. They point out that the development of the capacity to make use of what is exclusive and distinctive to each of them is most important in the process of their maturation as analysts. Bion (1987) said something close to this as well. He stated, "The analyst you become is you and you alone: you have to respect the uniqueness of your own personality-that is what you use, not all these interpretations" (p. 15).

Also on the bandwagon to understand how one's experience influences professional practice is my postdoctoral institute. The New York University Postdoctoral Program in Psychotherapy and Psychoanalysis recently held a symposium titled "How I Work as a Psychoanalyst: Personal Reflections on Formative Clinical Experiences" (Blechner, Hirsch, & Suter, 2010). In this symposium, two speakers (Mark Blechner and Irwin Hirsch) and one discussant (Barbara Suter) explored influences on their psychoanalytic work. While none of these folks (Gabbard, Ogden, Blechner, Hirsch, or Suter) focused specifically on religion, there was clearly an attempt to understand the myriad contributions to their work. Before I launch, a few introductory comments are in order.

First, the editors (Beverly Greene and Dorith Brodbar), along with the journal editor (Ellyn Kaschak), must be acknowledged for this creative volume. In general, there have been few narratives about the Jewish women's experience. Holocaust memoirs are clearly an exception. The point is that seldom do Jewish people write about themselves and their oppression. While anti-Semitism is alive and well, for example, it is seldom the object of our professional feminist discourse. Consider this: I teach psychology of women at New York University and have done so since 1973. For purposes of this course, I assign some readings that consist of women's narratives. Over the years, I have assigned different collected works. These readings include powerful and compelling stories of women who are Black, Hispanic,

Japanese American, Hmong American, Mexican women, and so on. These and other stories enrich our understanding of women's lives and counter master narratives. I am thankful for these collections of essays and recognize that many more are needed. However, what is missing in most of these compilations are the stories of Jewish women. Now do not get me wrong; there are other stories missing as well. However, here I am focusing on Jewish women's narratives. Now, finally, in this rich volume that reflects feminist scholarship at its best, Greene and Brodbar have given female Jewish psychotherapists a voice. Twenty-four distinguished psychotherapists have written narratives that enables us to consider the connections between family dynamics, Jewish identity, and the effects of Jewish identity on psychotherapy practice. Why is this important? In the absence of written narratives, one may fall back on stereotypes about what someone is like, where they have come from, what they are likely to do, and where they will end up. By means of this volume, Greene and Brodbar require that we throw away stereotypes of Jewish women therapists. For that I am thankful.

In preparation for this writing, I questioned 10 beginning master's level students in a school of health, nursing, education, and the arts professions. I spoke to them informally and individually. I wanted to hear their hunches about the backgrounds of Jewish women psychotherapists. This questioning, while not at all scientific, led to some interesting responses. In general, these beginning graduate students thought that Jewish women psychotherapists came from very privileged backgrounds. Clearly some do. But the full story is much more complicated as this anthology indicates. Where did their "hunch" come from? Perhaps it is related to some of the prevalent stereotypes for Jewish women. Two come to mind: "Jewish American Princess" and "shrewd businesswoman." This is clearly not the Jewish woman we meet in this anthology. This book makes it clear that the Jewish story is a complicated, rich, and diverse one. These women tell many different stories, some of which include rejection of Jewish identity, identification with Jewishness, liberalism, anti-Semitism, poverty, love of learning, oppression, transgenerational transmission of trauma and specifically transmission of the trauma of the Holocaust, protests against the Vietnam War, involvement with the civil rights and feminist movements, identifying with "the other," radicalism and liberalism, being working class and/or immigrant, social activism, and so on.

While there is clearly diversity among these narratives, there are some shared aims that seem to emanate from Jewish values. Take a detour with me for a moment. Consider an experience I had with Jake, my grandson. Along with his fellow classmates, nine-year-old Jake conducted a large portion of the Havdallah service, which is a ceremony associated with the end of the most important weekly holiday, the Shabbat. While conducting the service, Jake and I had eye contact. He would sing and read and meet my eyes. Then he would sing and read and meet my eyes again. When it was over, he approached me and he said that I looked like I was crying.

I thought about that. Had he sung and read in public school, I would have been proud but I would not have been as moved as I was in his synagogue, watching him carrying on the tradition of his grandparents and his great-grandparents. What became clear to me is that, while I do not regularly attend temple nor do I observe many of the practices endemic to Judaism, I have a strong identity as a Jew and my Jewish identity is important to me. This seems to be the position of many of the contributors here. While numerous contributors to this anthology were not observant Jews or even particularly knowledgeable about or educated in Judaism, I think they held Jewish values that influenced them in both their personal and their professional lives. Diversity in this anthology? Yes. But there is more. There is commonality. Each of the contributors could be called a *mensch*. The word *mensch* implies that a person has noble character and is moral and ethical. Being a mensch is not about being beautiful or popular or rich or successful. Mensch-like behavior involves such actions as visiting a sick person or bringing soup to someone who is hungry or returning a wallet that one found on the street. Being called a mensch is one of the greatest compliments. It involves doing good deeds, and such behavior derives from Jewish values. What strikes me is that Jewish values scamper throughout these stories. Of course, I recognize that what I am identifying as Jewish values may be important values to other groups and individuals as well. Three of the Jewish values that I recognize from a reading of this anthology and that I found in each narrative are (a) a strong sense of fairness, (b) a need to alleviate human suffering, and (c) a quest for knowledge and education.

Closing, I end where I began, in acknowledging the editors Drs Beverly Greene and Dorith Brodbar, the journal editor Dr. Ellyn Kaschak, and all of the contributors for an excellent and unique contribution to our literature. To all of you I say mazel tov, which is a Hebrew and Yiddish word used to congratulate one for a happy and significant event or occasion. The occasion here, of course, is the publication of the minyan.

REFERENCES

Bion, W. R. (1987). Clinical seminars. In *Clinical Seminars and Other Works*. London: Karnac.

Blechner, M., Hirsch, I., & Suter, B. (2010). How I work as a psychoanalyst: Personal reflections on formative clinical experiences. Presentation at the Symposium at the New York University Postdoctoral Program in Psychotherapy and Psychoanalysis, January 30, New York, NY.

Gabbard, G. O., & Ogden, T. H. (2009). On becoming a psychoanalyst. *International Journal of Psychoanalysis*, *90*, 311–327.

Epilogue

Intersectionality and the Complexity of Identities: How the Personal Shapes the Professional Psychotherapist

BEVERLY GREENE

I began this issue with the premise that family members are often the first people we know who are members of our ethnic group. It is family who are often the first bearers of the culture that we come to identify as a core part of who we are or who we are not and they teach us by both word, example, and in the dynamics of our relationships with them what we know about our culture (and others) in our early formative years. However, the personalities of those family members, their coping styles, and the history of psychodynamics in their own personal relationships, both personal and cultural past are mixed within what they present to us as our "culture." As we mature, extended family and community provide us with additional information about ourselves as well as about what our cultural identifications are or can be. Depending on the nature of our community, particularly if it is under siege, it can also provide a positive or negative mirror where we can see a range of images reflected back that is alleged to represent who or what we are and what we can become. As therapists we know from our work with clients that those images reflected back to many people were not always accurate representations of who they really were or could be at that time, whether those reflected images came from the social environment or loved and trusted figures in their lives or both.

While the external social environment is important, those early influences within our families are powerful. They often shape how we make sense of and respond to whatever the social and personal environment contain. I contend that our conflicts with, connections to, and internalized representations of ethnic, gender, as well as other identities are often connected to our internalized representations of, relationships with, and conflict with family members, particularly but not exclusive to those who raise us. With that idea in mind Jewish women who are psychotherapists and who are critical thinkers about cultural identity were sought and asked to consider how their family dynamics influenced how they see themselves as Jewish and what this meant to them. Furthermore, they were asked to consider how that identity or aspects of it expresses itself in their professional work with clients. For example, did it affect their initial attraction to this profession, and if so, why? Did it have a discernable effect on the kind of theoretical orientation or training they found compelling? In what ways did their identity influence their direct interactions with clients, such as the kinds of clients they worked with, the degree to which they explored this material in the client's therapies, their disclosure or lack thereof of information about their identity to clients, and if so, what information specifically and to whom? A group of diverse women who are distinguished scholar/practitioners for whom a focus on cultural, ethnic, gender, and sexual orientation identities are a focus of their professional work were then asked to read and offer us their "commentary" on the narratives. They were asked to explore what the narratives tell us about the complex issue of personal identities, the inter-sectional nature of those identities for Jewish women, and for others as well.

THE FIRST BLACK PEOPLE I KNEW WERE MY PARENTS

The first African Americans I knew were my parents and other family members. We were called Negroes then, sometimes "colored," later Black and now African American. When I was growing up, calling an African American "Black" or implying that they were descended from people of Africa would have been the highest form of insult to many members of the group who now use that term with great pride. Most African Americans had little direct knowledge about Africa, and the distortions about it purveyed by the dominant culture in the United States were easy to believe. That should not be taken to mean that African Americans accepted whatever they were told about themselves or lacked pride in our people. At that time to be considered Black or African was to be associated with all of the negative distortions of Africa and African peoples. Accurate information about Africa, its diversity of cultural practices, languages, and realistic depictions of its people and their contributions to civilization, and the exploitation of its rich natural resources and its people was unknown to most Americans. The Civil Rights movement of the 1950s and early 1960s and the Black Power/Black is Beautiful movements of the late 1960s and early 1970s changed previous negative attitudes to matters African that led to the proud acceptance of the label "Black" American and the proud claiming of African ancestry. However, during my early years, Negro was the most acceptable and for some of us the least offensive of the names used to refer to us.

All that I knew about what this meant, to be "Negro" was filtered through the eyes of family members even before I knew what that was or what it meant. How I came to label my experiences as having something to do with my being a Negro, Colored, or Black person, and later my subjective sense of *being* a Black person was largely dependent on how family members defined this thing called "Negro" or "Black." Of course this also came to be shaped by other significant people in the course of my development as I moved in larger and wider circles of peers and authority figures in our family and in the world. It was also informed by what I read. I was aware that I often valued and took on the perspective of those family members to whom I felt close personal bonds or identified with and less so with family members with whom I was conflicted, did not feel as close to, or regard as highly. This was particularly true when I was a child. When I was older I learned in my own therapy that those beliefs that were most difficult to challenge were the ones held by the people I felt closest to or valued most. One of the benefits of good therapy is that it can teach us that we can love and feel connected to people without having to uncritically accept their view of ourselves or the world. Fortunately, for me, my family represented a wide range of tastes, beliefs, values, and behaviors and ways of being in the world that, at least within our family, were never regarded as being culturally inauthentic or, for that matter, adverse to being an acceptable person. While that was not always true among my peers, it mattered somewhat less because I already felt a distinct and solid connection with Black folk and identity via my family's experiences in the Deep South, my own personal encounters with racism, and knowledge about our African and Native American ancestry. We had little written information about the Native Americans that are a part of our bloodline. We knew that our maternal grandmother, Flora's father Andrew and her grandfather Dan Melvin were either Lumbee or Cherokee, and our paternal grandmother, Prencie's mother Emma, had Native American lineage. That lineage was clearly present in the physical features of both of my grandmothers.

My maternal grandfather Dennie's mother, Mary Eliza Roberson, entered the United States from the British West Indies, intended for the auction block, just after the beginning of the Civil War. The state of war and the Carolina port of her entry complicated her legal status and left her in limbo until the war ended and slaves were declared free citizens. She settled first in North Carolina and then in Southern Georgia with my great grandfather Will. They had 7 children. The last of their children, my grand aunt Irene died in 2002 at the age of 102. Great-Grandma was a midwife and attended the births of hundreds of Black and White babies. She was still alive during the time I was growing up and I was fortunate to have spent time with her. The last time I saw her she was well over 100 years old and very active for someone of her advanced age. Indeed, when she died in 1966 she was, based on anecdotal stories and census records, between 109 and 113 years old. She was one of our family's tangible connections to the middle passage. Another direct link between our family history and to slavery was my maternal grandmother, Flora Roberson. She was the grandchild of a slave, Bella, and her master Mitchell Tyson. In my maternal bloodline going back to my great grandmother, Lucy Tyson, the women were skilled seamstresses known for their ability to design and construct garments from patterns they made themselves. The considerable constructional ability and talent that was clearly evident on both sides of my family was abysmally lost on me. Fortunately for me, literacy was also important. All but one of my mother's 11 siblings, of those who lived to adulthood, completed high school and performed well academically. Her elder brother and sister, Emmett and Lucy, finished high school, albeit in racially segregated schools of southern Georgia at the top of their class despite having to spend part of their mornings working to augment my grandmother's earnings. Their help was needed to support their 7 younger siblings in the aftermath of my grandfather's death in 1939. He was just 47 years old. Family members told us many stories about our history that left me with a deep sense of kinship and connection to many family members who have gone before me and anchors me in connection to something larger than myself. It also connects me to a struggle for rights and opportunities that began long before me. Knowing who they were and the lives they carved out of very few resources has no doubt given me a clear sense of my identity and fostered a connection to them despite the fact that many of them died long before I was born.

My paternal grandparents caused a stir in both of their families when they married. My grandmother, Prencie, was the daughter of Emma and Burke Howard. Emma was described as a mixed race woman of Black, Native American, and White admixture. Burke was described as "White" although we have been unable to discern whether he was actually White or so light skinned that he could easily pass for White and did so. My paternal grandmother considered herself Black, despite looking racially ambiguous to me, and was the darkest of her parents seven children who, we are told, were passing for White. My paternal great grandfather Cicero Greene and his siblings were dark skinned. Although my paternal great grandmother Emily was described as mixed race, their children were unmistakably black. In the eyes of Prencie's light-skinned siblings, marrying my grandfather Thomas meant that neither my grandmother nor her children would ever be able to pass for white. Neither side of their families favored the marriage because of the skin color differences between them and the feelings about skin color that were intense and not unusual in those days. According to family lore, my father and his five siblings could not be openly acknowledged by their maternal grandparents, aunts, and uncles as it would be disruptive for those who were passing. However, the Greenes were unusually literate and skilled and Prencie was illiterate. I am told that some of my grandfather's siblings thought he could do better than an illiterate girl 12 years his junior.

We were often told about our paternal grandfather, Tom Greene's, determination that his children be literate and that his daughters be educated enough to avoid having to work as domestics in White homes. Two of the three daughters did escape that fate. Black women employed in those situations were frequently the target of unwanted sexual advances by male employers who would threaten them with the loss of their jobs if they refused to comply with the employer's sexual demands. Tom kept a 6 foot chalkboard above the mantle and regularly drilled my father and his siblings in arithmetic and geometry lessons to be completed in addition to all of their chores. Thomas Greene appears in census records as a "sharecropper." He was, however, a skilled carpenter and builder. Dad is named for my grandfather's brother Sam, indicating the close bonds between them. Tom built the store that my grand uncle Sam ran until his last years. He was one of the few Black storekeepers in rural Mississippi where my father's family lived. He also built a house for his sister and her family as well as his own family dwelling and taught my father that skill. It was Dad's skill as a carpenter and builder that earned him a living and supported us for most of his working life. My grandfather drew blueprints for White contractors who then passed the drawings off as their own. He was paid for his work, but he was not identified as the person who created the blueprints because Black men were not permitted to do that kind of work, and Whites would not buy plans drawn up by a Black man. Being known as a "smart nigger," or one who possessed that knowledge would have put his safety in jeopardy. In contrast to my Jewish counterparts, being openly literate or "book smart" was dangerous for Black people, and they were often compelled to appear to be ignorant about matters that they knew a great deal about. The importance of keeping Black people illiterate can be traced back to laws during slavery that prohibited teaching slaves to read or write, in some states, under penalty of death. Maintaining illiteracy among Black people was and continues to be an important component of racial subordination. Black people, often with the help of some of the White members of slave-owning households, always persisted in becoming literate, however their intelligence had to be downplayed so as to not evoke the ire of racist Whites who were clearly threatened by literacy in Blacks. However, my ancestors, like other Black folks historically, placed a high value on being knowledgable and literate, even if you could not attain formal education. My paternal grandparents often raised the ire of neighboring Mississippi White farmers because they refused to keep their six children out of school to work in the neighbor's cotton fields during the times of the year that school was in session. One of my grandfather's younger sisters, Martha, graduated from Alcorn State College and attended Tuskeegee Institute during summers to complete a master's degree in education. She taught grammar school in Louisiana until her retirement. My father's eldest three sisters generally completed two years of what was then considered college. Rose, the eldest sibling, despite two years of college performed domestic work in the homes of Jewish professionals for most of her adult life. Whenever they discarded books, she brought them home to us. Hence we had James Baldwin, Henry Miller, Dorothy Parker, and other writers of the Algonquin Long Table as a matter of routine. It was my brown-skinned and blue-eyed Aunt Rose, who cleaned and cooked for well-to-do professionals for a living, who first exposed me to the special pleasures of the *New York Sunday Times* and its book review. Nothing about intellectual matters was with held from us. The love of literacy and learning was prominent among my elders and was passed along to my generation with an awareness of the sacrifices that many Black folks made over time to improve our access to opportunities. My direct experiences with family members and a litany of family lore left me with an awareness that Black folk represented a wide range of ways of being in the world with a wide range of different experiences but that we were all connected in some fundamental ways. My connection to family and our family's history was and is an intrinsic part of my connection to Black folk and my subjective sense of Black "identity."

My three younger siblings and I were raised by parents and elders who grew up in the midst of the fiercest forms of racism in the last century in rural Mississippi and southern Georgia. We were exhorted to be proud of our group as well as family history. Our struggles to negotiate racism as well as other dilemmas that are a part of the human condition were deemed a part of something larger than ourselves to which we were connected by the past and for which we had some responsibility to make the future a better place. Perhaps like the spirit of Tikkun Olam, we were exhorted to assume a sense of social responsibility for the world we live in. In this context we were admonished to learn from the struggles of the past so as not to have to repeat those mistakes in our own lives. The healthy psychological survival of our elders in the Deep South required that they understand how to negotiate the challenges of racism without losing their personal sense of dignity and humanity. We were taught to choose our battles carefully. It was an important survival skill.

Growing up in a multigenerational household, we were given great latitude to disagree with viewpoints of adults, debate the merits of our opinions and more importantly, to pursue our own dreams, and not theirs. Family members also communicated that we had a right to a place in the world, and respect as a human being despite what others might think and of course owed others respect in return. We were warned that many people did not think much of Black folks and that some even hated us, for no good reason. Such persons might challenge our rights to have the same opportunities that they were afforded and would attempt to undermine us both directly and indirectly. We were also taught that this behavior was not limited to White folks but that there were also Black folks who felt that Black people should accept being treated as inferior to Whites. If challenged about treating Black people as inferior, those doing so would likely deny it but that did not change the reality of what we learned was racism and what I later understood as internalized racism. In hindsight what was most significant about parental warnings was the notion that racist people could create problems for us but that neither *we*, nor our expectation of fair treatment was the problem. Racism was the problem and people who held those attitudes were the problem. Managing racist behavior in those who had the power to do so with impunity was defined as the problem. We were admonished that being part of the majority could make someone more powerful but did not mean that they were right or that their actions were just. In that context it meant that sometimes you would have to acquiesce to power but that this did not mean that those in power were "right" or that whatever they were asserting as a rationale to harm us was justified. They were simply more powerful. I had to learn early on in life how to manage the negative projections of others without internalizing them. As many of the contributors have observed, being an outsider gives one a very different view of the dominant group and also mirrors what is a part of the dialogue between client and therapist. The capacity to manage and understand what we evoke in others, what is true of us and what is not is an important skill for the therapist. Like many of the contributors and discussants to this volume, growing up as "other" helped me to develop capacities that have served me well as a therapist.

I grew up in a community in Northern New Jersey that during my formative years was both economically and ethnically diverse. While the demographics shifted as I approached high school to become gradually more African American, I grew up attending public schools with a diverse range of students as well as teachers. Hence I always had friends and teachers who were Jewish as were many of the merchants that served our neighborhood.

My public education was unusual in many respects. In my junior year of high school, Charles Herod taught us history. I do not say that he was our history teacher, rather, he taught us history. I do not recall how me or my classmates knew this but Mr. Herod, a Black man, had been an officer in the armed services. That alone was unusual for a Black man in that era. Perhaps because of his military background and a role he may have played in World War 2, he had an interest in those events and shared information with his classes that I later learned was not routine in high school history. He taught us that in addition to the concentration camps in Germany and the murders of Jews in the Holocaust, that anti Semitism was alive in the United States as well. He informed us of the role of the United States in turning Jewish refugees back to Germany during the war when it would most likely mean their deaths. Even more unusual, he told us about the United States holding Japanese Americans in internment camps on our soil and the practice of taking their belongings when they were detained. Not only did he teach us about the horrors of the war with respect to the treatment of Jews, from both Nazis and "allies" but he also shared a cache of audio taped interviews with Japanese detainees during their detention in US camps. I came away with the cogent lesson that anti Semitism was not restricted to Nazis or some evil empire far away from our shores.

A MINYAN OF WOMEN

I attended college in New York City at New York University against the background of the social unrest of the sixties and seventies where there were active conversations about identity, what constituted its authenticity and what that meant with a range of friends, classmates and teachers. It seemed a disproportionate number of my classmates were Jewish. In a brief ambivalent flirtation with Black Nationalism I found that its demand for prioritizing my racial identity at the exclusion of other identities that were important to me, its sexism and homophobia to be as repugnant as the racism of the dominant culture. As a result I did not see a place for someone with my multiple identities, all of which were important to me, within it. Feminist thought, while decidedly not as inclusive as it should have been in representing all women, at least held out hope for more inclusion and a way for me to make a contribution to that conversation about identity. Active dialogue about those issues continued during my graduate education and clinical training which also took place in New York City.

Perhaps the very first Jewish person that I had a direct relationship with was our family pediatrician. As a young child I knew, only because my parents said so, that he was Jewish and although it was unspoken it was somehow communicated that this was a good thing because Jewish people were "smart," and you wanted your doctor of all people to be "smart." Dr. Clement Schotland cared for my siblings and cousins from the time we were a few days old until we were nearly 18 years old. Twice a year he would examine us and chronicle the progress of our development, take note of and address anything unusual and express overall confidence in our development and our well being. He made personal visits to our homes when we were ill and came to be regarded as a member of our extended family. If we were ill and our parents called him he could be absolutely relied on to respond quickly with a phone call or house visit if need be. I recall that on one occasion when my younger sister and I were ill, our parents bundled us up and drove to his office. He gently told them that they should not bring us out into the cold to come to the office if we were sick, that *he* would come to us, as he did many times in the course of our childhood. Dr. Schotland was also the first person outside of my parents to heartily encourage my ambition to become a doctor and offered to assist me with letters of recommendation for colleges where he was an alumni when I applied for college admission, and he did so. I recall that when I was eight or nine years old he began asking me what I wanted to be when I grew up. At some point I responded that I wanted to study medicine and perhaps become a doctor. Typically that response coming from a latency aged "Negro" girl drew a range of reactions from people. Some just patronized me with admiration for such a worthy goal but assured me that I would change my mind when confronted with spending a long time in school in environments where Black people were not welcome and our intellect not valued. Others just dismissed it outright. Still others regaled me with tales of all the hardship that would assail me, despite their knowing little about medical or graduate education, only that preparation required a long time. There were always those folks who in hindsight were consistently doing things to encourage my ambition and progress in amazingly touching ways. Dr Schotland's response was enthusiastic and unlike many other people to whom I had expressed that desire, did not discourage me or remind me that this was difficult for "Negroes" or "girls" to do. He was emphatic that this was an important ambition because there were not nearly as many "Negro women" with doctorates as there should be. It was not just about there being too few Negroes to treat other Negroes but too few of us to make contributions that were important to the knowledge of others. *That* was different.

I was in college when he closed his practice and retired, hoping to spend more time with his grandchildren and leaving the care of the new babies in the family to another doctor. The new doctor was also Jewish, but was never quite regarded with the same level of affection or trust. When Dr. Schotland died unexpectedly in May 1970, we attended his funeral services and sadly said a last goodbye to someone whom we regarded as an old and trusted family friend. Any anti Semitic stereotypes I was exposed to about Jewish people were always filtered through my relationship with him and personal relationships with Jewish friends, teachers and merchants our family conducted business with. I understood that Jewish people had also been singled out for unfair and degrading treatment and that many of them had the capacity to understand some of what my experience as a Black person was like. I viewed anti Semitic sentiments as coming from a place that was the same as the source of racism about Black people. They came from people who were not to be trusted. Part of my racial socialization included being suspicious of what has been called White versions of the truth about Black people. It served to provide the basis for my questioning what the majority had to say about other people as well. Our family instructed us that we would hear things about Black people that were simply untrue and that we should not readily accept what we were told by others about "us" as they had a vested interest in disparaging us. Despite the fact that some of "us" might believe those racial and ethnic slurs we were warned that they were still untrue as there was good and bad in everyone. Despite growing up in the vicious climate of racism in Mississippi, my father often said to us that not all White people were the enemy and that not all Black people would be our "friends." "People" he said "are just more complicated than that". I also reasoned that if *they* or some conventional wisdom could lie about Black folks, *they* could be lying about other people as well and that Black people were not immune to believing things that were not true about themselves and about others. This was an important element in my awareness and acceptance of my minority sexual orientation despite not having that in common with family members that I knew of at that time. Overall I concluded that group membership or demographics was not enough to inform you about who could be trusted and who could not. Coming from the crucible of diversity of interests, temperaments, personalities, and even physical characteristics in a context of love and support from my family and the diverse environment I grew up in was not only empowering but freeing. It facilitated a way of being in the world that leaves me free to enjoy the special connections that I have with Black folks and our common cultural interests and still have a capacity to view human beings as having the possibility to be a wide range of things that their demographics do not always predict. That has also been important in my personal life as well as my clinical work in that I expect that any given client can be anything or believe anything and that I must get to know them to understand their experience of the world and to know who and what they are or are capable of.

CLINICAL IMPLICATIONS

My work as a psychologist over the last 25 years has included many clients from many different cultural backgrounds. I noticed that a great many beliefs, feelings, interpersonal dilemmas, characteristics, practices and dispositions were often attributed by many of those clients to being a part of the imperatives associated with national, cultural, religious, racial, ethnic, gender etc. authenticity. Often enough, the behaviors or beliefs in question were those that limited my client's capacities to see the world and other people more fully or to see many different parts of themselves as fully as possible. Many of those clients held beliefs, feelings and desires about themselves and others that they felt conflicted with having a sense of authenticity about some aspect of their cultural, gender, sexual orientation or religious identification. When we explored how they went about determining when something was a function of culture and when it was not, their concept often went back to family practices and both the importance and congruence or lack thereof between family and community injunctions about the meaning of membership in the group in question. They deemed this true about identities or beliefs about which they felt conflicted despite the fact that they held other beliefs and behaved in other ways that were also in violation of parental, family or cultural "rules". Often there were many visible examples of group members who did not define membership so narrowly however their existence or example was ignored or discredited. Clearly, in many clients this behavior can be a manifestation of their own defenses against what it would be like to see themselves in other ways, as a way of supporting a preexisting characterological position. For others it was sometimes a function of never really seeing or knowing anyone from their group who behaved differently.

These experiences awakened my sense, as a clinician, that for many people, behaviors and beliefs that are being referred to as "cultural" are often an amalgam of certain cultural standards and beliefs that exist on a spectrum, as they are mediated by familial figures, and characterological defenses. They are also related to the nature of one's relationships to significant persons in our lives during development and how those individuals represent what is defined as a part of our "culture" and what is not. I have also observed this phenomenon where practices associated with family dysfunction were presented to clients and then to me in therapy as though they were a part of the culture or religion. Many of those practices were often used by family members or peers to control clients in ways that did not allow them to develop constructive and more flexible strategies for problem solving.

CULTURAL PRACTICE VERSUS CULTURAL ADAPTATION

Many African Americans hold beliefs about practices that can be viewed as derivatives of African cultures, as well as those aspects of the dominant culture that have been incorporated by African Americans in their requirement to be bicultural. However many of those factors that are often deemed, "cultural" are not necessarily derivatives of African culture per se but are often adaptations to being a marginalized minority group in a hostile society. They are defensive attempts to survive racism that are perhaps useful short term that can become problematic when used chronically. They may have cultural relevance but they are not "cultural" per se in the way those terms are used by my clients and some clinicians. For example, the controversial practice of corporal punishment is not unusual among African American parents, however, it is not cultural per se. One of the tasks that African Americans face as parents is that of socializing their children to survive in a society that devalues and is often intolerant of them.

Many African Americans feel that the dominant society will be less tolerant of misbehavior in African American children than in White children and will punish the former more severely. In fact, depending on the historical period, a racial transgression like talking back to a White person, expressing anger, making direct eye contact etc. could easily result in your swift demise with no legal recourse. Many African American parents felt the need to teach their children to obey them and to behave in socially proscribed ways without question. They feared that if their children did not internalize the need to control themselves and to obey a parent in an absolute fashion, their very lives could be at stake. Corporal punishment was and is used by some parents to drive this point home and need not be abusive if done in measured ways with clear restraint on the part of the parent, and only for serious infractions. Unfortunately it can be abused when a parent disregards a child's safety by using excessive force, engaging in this form of punishment as a routine practice, doing so when angry or otherwise out of control etc. In some of my clients and the clients of therapists I have supervised, corporal punishment is taken to an abusive extreme but is explained as a culturally based approach to child rearing. No distinction is made between corporal punishment and abuse. My thoughts about these kinds of phenomenon over the years formed an important underpinning of the idea for this issue.

ORIGINS OF "THE MINYAN OF WOMEN": THE BACK STORY

This issue has its direct origins in a conversation over dinner in the spring of 2002 at the Knickerbocker Restaurant in New York City that included Dr.'s Louise Silverstein, Clare Holzman, Sara Zarem, Dorith Brodbar, and myself. For the purpose of this issue you could say they form the early core of what has come to be known among contributors to this issue as "the minyan of women." All of us are psychologists with an intense interest in cultural diversity and training clinicians to be culturally competent. To no one's surprise the conversation naturally went in that direction. We were discussing the ways that Jewish culture seems to be ingrained in the culture of New York City such that when people from other parts of the country refer to someone as behaving like a New Yorker, they are often using descriptors that are used to describe Jewish people. The descriptors are both good and bad. While I had my own ideas, because I am not Jewish and because I was curious about what that meant to *them* I asked them to tell me what it meant to be Jewish, how they would define it and what kinds of things are included in that definition. To my surprise each began their description by saying: "Well, I'm Jewish, but I'm not *really* Jewish." Of course I wanted to know what being *really* Jewish was and each had a different, vague idea but nothing really as solid as their responses to my original query would suggest. Whatever it was, they did'nt think *they* were *it*. Often, being *really* Jewish was organized around the degree to which they practiced Judaism. Each then told very distinct narratives about what being Jewish meant to them and those narratives were often organized around stories about people in their families.

As I asked more people the same question I kept getting a similar response. It seemed no one who *I* clearly saw as Jewish regarded themselves as *really* Jewish or Jewish enough, whatever that was. I wondered what a collection of those stories would look like and how it might inform practice and this rapidly took shape as this volume.

The purpose of the issue gradually unfolded and was clearly reflected in the subtitle, Family Dynamics, Jewish Identity and Psychotherapy Practice. In conversations with Dorith Brodbar about Jewish traditions, their meaning and connection to the issue, she proposed that the then small group of interested contributors formed a sort of Minyan . . . . of Women, hence the title. She also graciously agreed to serve as my coeditor. We wanted to develop these rich conversations into an issue in the hopes of extending a dialogue that was interesting to us, to others.

Our small group expanded to include Dr.'s Sophia Richman, Judith Glassgold, Ellen Cole, Laura Brown, Sari Dworkin, and Andrea Bergman. We presented symposia at the annual meetings of the American Psychological Association, the Association for Women in Psychology, the New Jersey State Psychological Association and recently the Eastern Psychological Association. We wanted feedback on our ideas and to determine if there was substantial enough interest in the topic to develop an issue. These presentations consisted of a panel of members of what is now referred to among us as "the minyan" and an invited scholar/practitioner, who often was not Jewish, to serve as our discussant and to provide us with "commentary." The symposia were well attended and responded to with great interest and enthusiasm. This further supported our assumption that there was a wider audience who would appreciate these ideas. A group of diverse and distinguished scholar/ clinicians were invited to serve as the issue's "discussants." They were asked to write a commentary on the narratives and to discuss how the narratives as a group inform us about Jewish identity, about the complex and intersectional nature of identity in general and what was elicited in them or reminiscent of their own sense of identity or struggles to understand some aspect of themselves.

THE NARRATIVES

One of the striking elements in the narratives was the diversity in the stories about what being Jewish meant to the contributor, *how* they were Jewish and how they were not. As an instructor and trainer of psychotherapists it can be difficult to convey the importance of understanding cultural imperatives and the way they affect our client's development and their lives without risking reinforcing stereotypes about those groups. The stories in this volume richly informed that which I have attempted to emphasize in cultural competency training. It is important to understand the nature of the client's group identification but it is as important to understand what that means to the client. In therapy, asking "how" a client is Jewish, Catholic, Black, White, Male, Female, gay or straight is perhaps more important than whether or not they are. That question can lead to a rich inquiry in which I always learn things about my client that I would never have anticipated.

As a Christian and a therapist with an interest in the development of cultural identity these stories became more and more interesting to me. I must also admit that I always thought of psychotherapy as having a particularly Jewish ethos. My own therapists were Jewish. I was never certain if my perception was based on the large and visible population of Jews in New York City where I live and where I was educated; if it was because so many of my mentors, friends and colleagues in the discipline were Jewish-it seemed a disproportionate number; if it was because I had a sense that a substantial amount of the psychotherapy literature, particularly but not exclusively in my psychodynamic training was written by Jewish psychologists and analysts, indeed, Freud and the early theoreticians were Jewish. I found it striking that Freud, in the viciously anti-Semitic climate of his time, worried that psychoanalysis would be viewed as a "Jewish science" and dismissed. It seemed to me that Freud had so little to say, considering how much he had to say in general, about the anti-Semitism of his time and that he and the other analysts were silenced, perhaps out of fear of being noticed. Being "noticed" as a Jew was not a positive event and even as I questioned contributors about their feelings about being "known" as a Jew many indicated that visibility is still associated with a certain level of trepidation about what might happen to you if you are noticed or if there is a perception that there are "too many" of you. Among my Black peers we refer to this as the "critical mass." Critical mass in this context refers to how many of you may be present and visible in a department, company, firm or neighborhood before you are perceived as "too many" and elicit feelings of anxiety, resentment or threat in members of the dominant culture that result in backlash. One of the ironies here is the focus on the effects of trauma and the resolution of trauma in the psychoanalytic literature. In that literature the ability to break silence about and speak, to name trauma is central to healing. Many of these narratives speak to the intergenerational transmission of trauma that is a legacy of Holocaust survivors replete with family secrets and tensions around whether Jews should be visible or invisible, whether you should speak out or be silent, what happens when you are silent and what happens when you speak out.

Dorith Brodbar discusses another form of silencing. She recounts the ways in which her mother's pain as a Holocaust survivor were silenced by minimizing them. Because she survived, her pain and her losses were deemed of less consequence and dismissed when she tried to talk about them. Because she was not taken to nor did she perish in the camps, because she survived her pain was trivialized giving her no healthy way to express her grief and trauma and heal from them. Brodbar points out that her mother was in some ways penalized for surviving and she describes the painful toll it has taken in her mother's life. This highlights the ways that we can forget that the dead may make the ultimate sacrifice but that their suffering ends with death. The living, those who are survivors, must live and cope with the pain of their experience every day. Whatever or however they make sense of that pain is often a focus of the therapeutic inquiry.

The psychoanalytic literature also explicates the many different forms of expression that trauma can take. In the stories in this volume they include somatization, perfectionism, denial and/or rejection of Jewish identity, claiming that identity in various forms, pursuing social activism etc. Another legacy of that period also includes living with so much realistic terror that it becomes a precursor for a kind of tension or hypervigilance about potential danger vs an inappropriate denial of the potential for danger that it leads to an inability to trust one's perception about when they are really at risk and when they are not. I often wonder what Freud and many of the other pioneering analysts might have had to say about those events and about Holocaust trauma if they were living in a time when their safety was not in immediate jeopardy. It is ironic that they were silenced, perhaps, by the very thing they may have been uniquely suited to explore.

Another one of the overlapping themes that emerged in the narratives in this issue is about the way that Judaism fosters a view of the world that compels one to learn. Unlike the unquestioning obedience to the deity and the acceptance of the literal word that represents the way that some Christian faiths are practiced, Judaism encourages a passionate dialogue about the creator's intent as expressed in the Torah. Group dialogue and discussion regarding the meaning of the word is encouraged and accomplished by reading, studying, thinking and learning the word but also constantly analyzing the word, generating alternative interpretations, exploring different perspectives, raising questions and more questions. Sound like psychotherapy?

Many of the contributors echoed the sentiment that this aspect of the practice and philosophy of Judaism is expressed culturally in the way that it encourages scholarly activity. It also encourages activity that is focused on healing the pain of others and making the world a better place expressed in the injunction "Tikkun-Olam," to heal or repair the world. Paula Caplan, Laura Brown, Shanee Stepakoff, Carol Heffer and others acknowledge the role of their Jewish identity in their commitment to social activism and a moral imperative to actively work to facilitate social justice. Heffer also points out that knowledge was an important survival tool for Jews because they were a routine target of hostility in many countries and were forced to leave their homes with little notice. Their level of literacy helped them survive wherever they went as their literacy and knowledge were always portable.

The narratives in this issue express both a diversity of life histories and experiences among Jewish women as well as many commonalities. While many Jewish women have White skin and benefit from the privileges accorded White skinned persons in the United States, they are also members of an oppressed group that has been the focus of hate, social discrimination and genocide in which not all Jewish women are White skinned. This can result in a heightened awareness of an identity that paradoxically may for some be concealed. Jewish women must negotiate the barriers of sexism, classism, heterosexism, and anti-Semitism that are similar to the challenges that are a function of social discrimination confronting women of color. This means that their experience of being Jewish is also colored by social class background, gender, geographic location, and other identities in ways that intersect with one another such that many different psychological and behavioral outcomes are possible. For many contributors being a woman heavily influenced their sense of Jewishness and how that was defined both within their families and in their communities. Because their ethnicity is usually very visible, women of color have fewer opportunities to avoid racist barriers by concealing their ethnoracial identity. Unlike most women of color, most Jewish women do not generally wear that identity on their skin where it is visible to everyone and as such they may find themselves in situations where they must consider whether or not to reveal that identity if it is to be known. Others, as Judy Glassgold observes, do not look like White women but do not look "Jewish" either and may be mistaken for a member of yet some other group. In this instance, they must make a conscious decision about whether or not to reveal that they are Jewish. Every choice, whether to reveal or conceal has psychological consequences. In some cases it may have psychosocial consequences as well.

Sari Dworkin and Beth Firestein observe that in a Christian society people are presumed to be Christian unless they say otherwise. Hence Jewish women, not unlike lesbians who are presumed to be heterosexual unless they say otherwise, must "come out" as Jews. Like lesbians and gay men they must make conscious decisions about when, where and how to "come out" as Jews in different situations across the lifespan. Unlike Lesbians, however, they do not have to come out to their family members as they usually share Jewish identity. What this means varies however from family to family. Hence a woman's Jewish self can be "mirrored" by parenting figures in positive and negative ways. How and what kind of mirroring takes place is implicated in the shaping of Jewish identity as well as personal identity and in some cases the two may be inextricable. Positive mirroring of course should predispose an individual to regard her Jewishness as a valued and positive part of the self. Negative mirroring may predispose one toward an ambivalent stance, denial or rejection of that aspect of the self. Mixed or idealized mirroring messages may predispose toward even more complex responses. Therefore, what is taught about what it means to be a Jew, how Jewish authenticity is defined, or how one's ethnic socialization is conducted is implicated in what evolves as Jewish identity. It is important for therapists to understand this.

How, when, and what kinds of messages about Jewishness family members or other important figures communicate to Jewish women about what it means to be a Jew and a woman, the extent to which one is in danger because they are Jewish, the degree to which one should be visible or less visible and what it means, the degree to which Jewish identity is imparted as a religious vs a cultural identity (and the meaning of this) all informs how Jewish identity itself comes to be experienced uniquely in individuals. How parenting figures and other family members experienced their own Jewishness is implicated here as well. While Jewish women and lesbians are obliged to "come out" and consciously disclose their respective often hidden identities, Jewish women do not have to come out to their families and unlike lesbians they receive "minority mentoring" from their families. There are other family members who are like them in this dimension of the self and those people are important sources of information and in-vivo tutoring as role models about how to manage the consequence of presenting oneself as a Jew. However, in public, like Lesbians, Jewish women are often required to disclose their identity as Jews, allow themselves or be mistaken for a member of the majority. Jewish families often have a shared history and understanding of anti-Semitism as well as the need and means to manage it. This means that there may be wide range of skills that family members have acquired to pass along, as well as in some families a denial of the need to manage anti-Semitism at all. Jewish women who are lesbians, who have disabilities or other identities may face a complex task in needing to be "mentored" in different places for different identities to learn how to manage the discrimination and danger that accompanies their multiple group membership. Jewish women with other salient social identities face a complicated path to a consolidated sense of identity that integrates different identities into a cohesive whole.

This issue explores the diverse manner in which family dynamics shaped Jewish identities for the chapter authors in ways that were unique and directly connected to their experiences within their families of origin and their development. Highlighted is the diversity of experience of ethnic identity within members of a group of women who are similar in many respects and who belong to an ethnic group that is often invisible. In the United States where White skin is privileged, Jews may be less readily identifiable to non Jews than people of color are to those outside of their group. Indeed, in the multicultural discourse, Jews are often considered White and their experiences are often conflated with those of members of White ethnic groups whose cultural history is nothing like that of Jews. The history of Jewish people reveals that when there was a desire to socially marginalize them, make them targets for violence, or attempt to exterminate them, it was not difficult for those who wanted them identified to do so. One of the themes in the narratives of this volume is organized around how family members were involved in the Holocaust, how they were affected by a climate of nothing less than unabated terror and how they responded. Common themes emerge, however we see that the responses are as diverse as the women in question.

Factors surrounding immigration status, the timing of departure from Germany, the proximity of family members to the Holocaust or pogroms, the number of generations one's family has been in the US differently influence the power of Holocaust narratives as well as their conspicuous absence. While it is important for therapists to understand the broad strokes of a culture and the general cultural imperatives claimed by group members, the heart of successful psychotherapy rests on coming to understand each client's unique *experience* of those things. The diversities of those experiences were explored by contributors to this volume and reinforce this point.

These narratives also highlight the ways in which the intermingling of family dynamics and subsequent Jewish identity in these women is manifested in their practice of psychotherapy. Each author has considered the extent to which these factors have a role in the way they practice psychotherapy, in their choice of theoretical orientation, the populations they are drawn to work with (or avoid) as well as the feelings elicited in the therapist when working with Jewish and non Jewish clients. They also explore the circumstances surrounding the disclosure of Jewish identity to clients, particularly the factors that influence disclosure or the decision not to disclose Jewish identity in ways that the therapist may or may not even be aware of.

Sara Zarem explores how she regards the spelling of her name as a reflection of her parent's ambivalence about their own Jewish identity (I am Sara, without the "h"). She discusses how that conflict and her mother's secrecy about her own parents is expressed in her therapy practice as a long-standing difficulty and reluctance to ask client's questions about secrets or other material that may be emotionally provocative, particularly if it may be painful. Overall, she views what she chooses to inquire about and what she chooses to avoid as having its roots in her relationship with her mother and her perception that she caused her mother pain when asking questions about family secrets.

Louise Silverstein grew up amidst a strongly identified Catholic family in the south and following her father's death when she was a small child, left the South and spent her remaining years among a strongly identified Jewish family in the Midwest. She discusses feeling like an outsider in each of those families and its influence on her affinity for family therapy as a theoretical orientation and her practice with families. Clare Holzman grew up post World War II in New York City in a predominantly Jewish community but in a family that shed all religious observance two generations before her. She was on her own to determine exactly what kind of Jew she was supposed to be. Sophia Richman spent her earliest years living in Poland with her mother during the Holocaust. With forged papers mother and daughter "passed" as Catholic. Her father, held in Janowska, a concentration camp, escaped, located them and hid in their attic for nearly two years. As a very young child, she would ask about the noises she heard coming from the cramped attic made as her father moved around the small space. "There is a hungry wolf in the attic" was the explanation, accompanied by a warning to stay away from the attic or "the hungry wolf will eat you." She explores the effects of those early years that her father spent in hiding in their house, at the height of the war, the secrecy, the ubiquitous danger, the fear and need for vigilance that she absorbed before she even knew language, and the trauma on both her parents, herself and their relationships with one another.

Andrea Bergman was born and raised in New York. Her family was not observant and she recalls that she rarely considered her Jewishness at all. That is until she started to travel and found that she had differing senses of awareness of her Jewishness depending on where she was. Julie Ancis echoes some of those themes. Living in the South as a Jew made going to Temple more important than it had been previously. Ellen Cole has lived and worked for the most part in Vermont, Arizona and now Alaska where she was and is often the only Jew. This contrasts her experiences growing up in Queens, NY where she was 17 years old before she knew anyone who was *not* Jewish.

Sari Dworkin, Beth Firestein, and Judy Glassgold are Jewish women who are also lesbian and bisexual and who discuss grappling with these issues from yet an "other" perspective. For those women in the volume who are also lesbian but chose not to focus on that in their narratives, one confided that she always felt more anti Semitism in the LGB community than homophobia in the Jewish community. All discuss the challenges of constructing identities whose boundaries seem deceptively simple to outsiders but to them is complex and shifts in salience in different contexts and different developmental periods of their lives.

Silverstein, Bergman, Zarem and others bring us back to my original question. What does it mean to be *really* Jewish? In what way are you Jewish and in what ways are you not Jewish enough to feel authentic. Perhaps the more important question is, who decides. Many of the essays are replete with themes around the tension of being an outsider, but not always wanting to lose some other aspect of identity to be "inside." I noted that many of these women struggled with the tension of feeling like outsiders as Jews, but also feeling at times estranged from other Jews, outside while on the inside.

SUMMARY

I hope this collection of powerful narratives addresses the mandate for therapists to be culturally literate, competent and to move beyond understanding just the broad cultural characteristics of groups and their members. More importantly, therapists must comprehend the client's subjective experience of the identity associated with group membership, the complicated interaction of diverse elements of that identity and identities and the broad diversity of subjective experience captured within any one group and its interaction with other identities much like the roux in gumbo. Each subtle variation in a combination of ingredients can produce a unique and unpredictable result.

I proceed with the assumption that healthy human identity is intersectional and complex, consisting of a stable but flexible matrix of multiple intersecting identities that may shift in salience depending on the complicated nature of both time, place, historical period and relationship context in interaction with developmental junctures and individual temperamental characteristics rather than a single unifying and static characteristic. I also maintain that insightful narratives such as these can powerfully illuminate and enrich our understanding of that complexity and multiplicity of identity. As psychologists, we often focus on the individual or an individual as a member of a group and do not give appropriate significance to social context. For Feminist psychologists understanding social context is essential to our understanding of behavior. Hence we must pay appropriate attention not simply to what a person brings to situations, but what the personal and historical context of that situation or dilemma is.

Individuals may bring many different dispositions to the world but what they do with the hand they are dealt can often rely on the opportunities available in society that affords them a chance to develop and express both their capacities as well as their distress in healthy ways. While they control some of what they bring to the table, they do not determine where the table is, what is on the table or if it is within their grasp. Hence, I want to underscore the importance of social opportunity in facilitating optimal development no matter what an individual's capacities or background may be as well as the role that social adversity plays in the development of both psychological resilience and vulnerability.

Index